D0381873

LIBRARY

Speech and Language Therapy Intervention
Frameworks and Processes

MW
HMW
0500955

4544561

Speech and Language Therapy Intervention

Frameworks and Processes

Karen Bunning PhD, Dip CST
University of East Anglia, Norwich

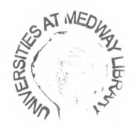

UNIVERSITIES AT MEDWAY LIBRARY

W

Whurr Publishers
London and Philadelphia

© 2004 Whurr Publishers Ltd
First published 2004
by Whurr Publishers Ltd
19b Compton Terrace
London N1 2UN
England

Reprinted 2005

All rights reserved. No part of this publication may be reproduced, stored in a retrieval system, or transmitted in any form or by any means, electronic, mechanical, photocopying, recording or otherwise, without the prior permission of Whurr Publishers Limited.

This publication is sold subject to the conditions that it shall not, by way of trade or otherwise, be lent, resold, hired out, or otherwise circulated without the publisher's prior consent in any form of binding or cover other than that in which it is published and without a similar condition including this condition being imposed upon any subsequent purchaser.

British Library Cataloguing in Publication Data

A catalogue record for this book is available from the British Library.

ISBN 1 86156 400 7

Typeset by Adrian McLaughlin, a@microguides.net

Contents

Preface

The closing decades of the last millennium saw the diversification of speech and language therapy practice into many different client groups. Specialist knowledge, skills and techniques have been developed to support innovations in practice; however, there is a tendency for knowledge to remain in isolated pockets and practice to be client group specific. The ever-growing bank of knowledge about communication disabilities and the demands on therapy services, present a dilemma for the profession, from pre-registration students and their educators to clinical managers and frontline clinical staff. For the educators the challenge is how to promote the integration of knowledge about communication disability and to establish crucial links across the range of clinical practice. For pre-registration students and frontline clinical staff it is about recognizing a core process for intervention such that knowledge and skills can be applied flexibly across client groups. The latter point is of course important to clinical managers in the recruitment of staff who are able to meet the needs of *all* people referred for speech and language therapy.

Polarization of specialist areas

The polarization that exists within the profession is exemplified by distinctions that are made between the different roles of therapists with contrasting client groups. The 'aphasia therapist' has little to do with the therapist who works with adults with learning disabilities. Conferences on speech and language therapy provide the potential for some urgently needed cross-fertilization between the specialisms, and yet it is usually the case that symposia are organized according to specialist areas. Students on clinical placement may find that the expectations of one clinical setting appear totally unrelated to the next. Distinctions between the different clinical areas of practice are frequently articulated, whilst commonality is ignored, making for a difficult learning process.

Integrated learning

Anecdote would seem to suggest that newly qualified therapists often feel most confident about the placement most recently experienced. Perhaps it is the *maturity* of the student, at a later stage in the training, which is critical to the development of clinical skills. Some students report the positive influence of an enjoyable clinical placement on their subsequent choice of employment. The question is, what was it that made the placement so 'enjoyable' and how does that experience relate to the learning process? Recruitment of speech and language therapists (SLTs) in certain client groups continues to be a problem, e.g. adults with learning disabilities. This may be due to insufficient attention paid to this particular area in the taught curriculum. Alternatively, despite the best efforts of educators, a lack of integration in the learning process may be the reason, so that knowledge and skills remain client group specific. Problems in recruitment to any one area of speech and language therapy will have implications for the service, for people who provide it and of course for those who use it.

Promoting commonality

This text seeks to promote commonality across the specialist areas and to reduce professional dissonance by looking across the different client groups. The use of a core conceptual framework for planning, describing and analysing separate aspects of intervention is advocated, which:

- establishes the use of a core vocabulary for describing aspects of the intervention cycle;
- asserts the value of problem-solving and clinical decision-making in the construction of interventions;
- identifies some core therapeutic techniques used by speech and language therapists across the client spectrum;
- examines the different levels at which intervention is pitched;
- locates the developing bank of theoretical knowledge in the foundations of clinical practice.

Structure of text

This book is divided into two sections: Section 1 focuses on the theoretical bases and frameworks of intervention; Section 2 looks at the processes of intervention and the different mechanisms for change.

The first chapter in Section 1 introduces a model for defining the cycle of intervention. Issues to do with cultural diversity, identity and psychological state are explored in Chapters 2 and 3. These are presented as critical areas for consideration in the range of intervention approaches. Chapter 4 presents a systems-based model for clinical decision-making and a conceptual framework for constructing intervention. Chapter 5 explores the process whereby therapeutic change is brought about.

Section 2 is ordered according to the centres of influence that are established in Chapter 1. The chapters move in an outward trajectory from the individual who has a communication disability, on to the level of communication partnership, then the social environment, and finally to the broader social and political arena of society. The final chapter concentrates on integrating the concepts explored in the text by presenting narrative accounts of intervention cycles that have been carried out.

Acknowledgements

The development of this text owes much to the inspirational work of Sally Byng, which provides the foundations upon which the conceptual framework of intervention is based. Her research on language interventions with people who have aphasia, her earlier contributions to the SLT curriculum in the Department of Language and Communication Science at City University London, and her ongoing work with Connect (the communication disability network), provide some much-needed direction to the study of intervention across the broad spectrum of client groups.

Special thanks go to Simon Horton for his generous contributions to the text. Sponsored by the PPP Foundation to explore and enhance clinical training across SLTs, occupational and physiotherapists, his work has provided useful insights into intervention practice. He also provided some of the transcribed examples of therapy sessions and case exemplars that are used in the text. Thanks must also go to the PPP Foundation for the use of transcribed video material of clinical sessions.

A number of people contributed clinical stories, professional insights and personal experiences to this text, for which gratitude is expressed to the following: Jill Bradshaw, Marie Gascoigne, Rachael Henton, Ros Herman, Mary Lee, Nita Madhani, Jane Marshall, Carole Pound, Joe Waring and Roberta Williams.

In order to protect client anonymity, the names and some details in therapy accounts and transcribed sessions have been altered.

Karen Bunning
November 2003

Transcription conventions

There are a number of transcribed samples of interaction in the text. Standard English orthography is used. In the case of phonological errors broad phonetic representations are given between / /, but International Phonetics Association (IPA) symbols are not used. Nearest approximations such as /?/ for glottal stop are used and are italicized. Transcription conventions have been derived from a number of different sources including: Atkinson and Heritage (1984); Goodwin (1981); Sinclair and Coulthard (1975).

Therapist is shown as T, and the client as C.

Each line is numbered (1, 2, 3, etc.). This is to help locate utterances or actions referred to in the body of the text. The numbers are generally of no other significance, i.e. they do not necessarily help to pinpoint an exact location in the transcription of the session as a whole.

(1.5)	Indicates time lapse in seconds and half seconds. This may be used to indicate a pause (within speaker turn) or a gap (between speaker turns). It may indicate time lag between utterances or other actions. Time lapse was measured from the video display counter.
(.)	Indicates a micropause.
<u>pump</u>kin	Indicates emphatic stress.
( )	Transcriber unable to hear what was said.
(word)	Indicates uncertain hearings.
((smiles))	Indicates transcriber's descriptions.
C: not [sure] T: [not]sure	[indicates the start of an overlap, and] indicates where the overlap ends.

=	Used to indicate continuity (no pause or gap between utterances). This is used in two main ways:

1) From one speaker to the next:

    C: I'm not sure=

    T: =not sure at all

2) To indicate a continuous major turn by one speaker, where there is a back channel response by the other (which does not overlap):

    C: I'm not sure=

    T: mhm

    C: =at all

so::   : is used to indicate lengthening of sounds; placed immediately after the relevant sound. The number of : used gives a rough indication of the length of prolongation.

quiet   * around a word indicates that it is spoken comparatively quietly.

...   Used to indicate that a part of the transcription has been omitted.

CAPITALS show written words or use of letter tiles.

Intonation

Symbols that indicate intonation are placed immediately following the word/s containing the relevant tonic syllable.

\\   A low falling tone, which may acknowledge a prior response, for example.

↓   A high falling tone, which may show strong agreement, surprise or sympathy.

↑   A rising tone, which may question a point or an answer.

/   A low rising tone, which may signal something more is required or to come, or is an invitation to continue, or it may indicate some doubt by the speaker about their own utterance.

^   A rising falling rising tone, which may imply doubt or reservation about a prior utterance.

SECTION 1
FRAMEWORKS OF INTERVENTION

Chapter 1
Cycle of intervention

Defining intervention is not easy. 'Intervention', 'treatment' and 'therapy' are terms that tend to be used interchangeably. There are many other words and phrases that are associated with it, including assessment and therapy programme, direct and indirect intervention, didactic or instructive strategies, and milieu approaches that concentrate on naturally occurring communication, amongst others. Most terms fail to capture the complex nature of intervention characterized by interacting factors, some of which are internal to the person who has a communication disability and some of which are external.

What is intervention?

Although definitions and operational terms for intervention vary, there is a shared intention to bring about change in an individual's existing situation by some means. Each is concerned with selecting and introducing the most appropriate method that will influence a positive outcome for the person concerned. Intervention is about the mobilization of specific resources to address the identified needs of individuals. Law, writing in Rinaldi (2000: 33) about pre-school children, states that 'Intervention refers to the allocation of additional services specifically directed at the needs.'

Movement and change

Movement and change are two important themes of intervention practice. Change infers the alteration or transformation of certain aspects in the existing situation, thereby making things better for the individual(s) concerned. Alternatively, it can mean that a predicted, undesirable outcome is prevented. Movement includes both a desired shift from an existing point as well as a delay or arrest in the natural course of a progressive condition. It is about the acquisition of new skills and the maintenance or modification of existing ones within a planned framework. Dockrell and Messer (1999: 237) describe it as 'any planned action designed to modify or prevent an unwanted outcome'.

Bray, Ross and Todd (1999: 12) define intervention as involving 'a decisive act to bring about change' which is underpinned by a strong theoretical base. The resulting course of action should reflect the presenting needs of the client and the professional knowledge of the therapist, and 'must be driven by a rationale or hypothesis'. It involves the deliberate selection and implementation of actions that are then evaluated.

Participants in the process

The person who has a communication disability, although at the centre of the intervention, is not the sole player. Jordan and Kaiser (1996: 55) propose a definition of therapy with an aphasic adult that includes not only the person who experiences communication difficulties, but also a range of key players as well. They stress the complex nature of therapy, which comprises:

> A range of aims and strategies initiated usually by a speech and language therapist... Therapy can be a complex, multi-faceted series of tasks and activities carried out between aphasic patient, therapist, relative and sometimes volunteer or friend.

Depending on the life-course stage of the individual, there will be different *other* people who have a relevant contribution to make to the intervention process: for the child it is likely to be the parents and professionals involved in developmental health or educational issues; for the adult, where significant others *are* involved, it is likely to be a partner, relative or parent and various professionals involved in aspects of health care and social support. The way an individual's intervention cycle progresses and the various weightings of activities towards assessment or therapy involves ongoing negotiation between therapist, individual and any significant others. Collaboratively, the key players work to define the most amenable next stage of the journey.

Universal vocabulary

Describing intervention is difficult without the use of a recognized and universally accepted vocabulary. Without such a vocabulary, there can be no common understanding of what intervention entails and what therapy really means. There are numerous intervention studies that have been published, covering a wide range of client groups, communication difficulties and therapy approaches; however, operational descriptions of therapy, particularly definitions of the practical strategies or techniques of therapy, frequently lack clarity (Byng, 1995; Enderby and Emerson, 1995; Law, 1997). Horton and Byng (2000), commenting on the inadequacy of the *language of therapy*, assert that a shared core vocabulary would promote both consistency in therapy practice and therapist self-awareness of what they call 'enactment processes', e.g. interactions between the therapist and the person with a communication disability.

In order to establish consistency in the use of terms within this text, a differentiation of the terms 'intervention' and 'therapy' is provided initially. *Intervention* is an over-arching term that is taken to mean the cycle of activities carried out by the therapist and client and/or significant others. *Therapy* is one aspect of this cycle, *assessment* another.

Purpose of intervention

The main purpose of intervention is to bring about tangible benefits to the person's existing situation. Yoder (2001), writing about augmentative and alternative communication approaches, attempts to capture the aspirations of intervention: 'the hope of a language system that allows one to communicate competently with family, friends, teachers and employers' (p. 4).

In relation to the same clinical area, Martinsen and von Tetzchner (1996: 39) define the purpose as providing children with 'the best opportunities for developing language and communication'.

This phrase is applicable across the range of communication disabilities. Intervention is about constructing optimal conditions for individuals to develop and use their available communication skills so that they are able to access and participate in social opportunities of personal value.

Intended outcomes

According to Dockrell and Messer (1999), there are two dimensions to the underlying purpose of intervention:

- Preventing or modifying unwanted outcomes, e.g. early language stimulation to promote the communication development of the child with severe learning disabilities, or direct speech work to prevent or reduce deterioration of intelligibility in adults with acquired deafness.
- Promoting the maintenance and acquisition of skills and knowledge, e.g. teaching total communication strategies to a child with learning disabilities or an adult with an acquired language impairment.

Additionally, there are other elements that are integral to the intervention process (Byng, Pound and Parr in Papathanasiou, 2000; Pound et al., 2000) including:

- Psychological adjustment and accommodation of the individual and significant others to the prevailing situation and to changes as they occur, e.g. the parent of the newly diagnosed child with severe learning disabilities; the person with aphasia who is no longer able to work and is now dependent on state benefits; the person whose progressive neuromuscular disease means a decline in skills over a period of time; the person who is learning to communicate with oesophageal speech post-laryngectomy.

- Development of personal autonomy and self-actualization in relation to those changes as evidenced by use of communication skills and other behavioural indicators, e.g. the dysfluent child who learns to defend his speech against the taunts of a peer; the child with profound and multiple learning disabilities who rejects a stimulus for the first time, demonstrating a change from earlier compliance; the adult with aphasia who negotiates personal goals of therapy with the therapist.
- Reduction in barriers with a consequential increase in participation at different levels of community and society, e.g. the new user of an alternative communication system, such as a voice output communication aid (VOCA), who commences going to his local pub once more; or training of communication partners so that conversations are more accessible to the individual.
- Development and maintenance of health and wellbeing, e.g. the dysphonic adult whose therapy includes a voice hygiene regime that helps level of hydration, the parent who takes part in a support group to relieve the stresses of caring for a child with a disability.

Reflecting real needs

Intervention is designed to reflect the real needs of the person, taking into consideration other concomitant factors such as age, the nature and severity of the communication difficulty, and any causal or maintaining factors (Dodd, 1995). Bray, Ross and Todd (1999: 75–78) provide a useful description of each of these factors. It is the evaluation of these factors both separately and collectively that prompts a tailoring of intervention purpose. Consequently, variations in speech and language therapy (SLT) across the client groups may be seen:

- Improving access, efficiency, quality and capacity of communication (for example children with cerebral palsy using augmentative and alternative communication (AAC): von Tetzchner and Martinsen, 2000; living with and beyond aphasia: Pound et al., 2000; using total communication with adults with learning disabilities: Bradshaw, 1998; van der Gaag and Dormandy, 1993; and children with learning disabilities: Abudarham and Hurd, 2002; Mitchell and Brown, 1991).
- Maintaining the utility and function of communication for as long as possible (for example in people with progressive neurological conditions: Armstrong, Jans and MacDonald, 2000; Johnson and Pring, 1990; in elderly people with dementia: Bryan et al., 2002; Bryan and Maxim, 1996; Orange et al., 1995).
- Promoting progress in underlying or overt aspects of the communication system to an acceptable or targeted standard (for example language processing in people with aphasia: Maneta, Marshall and Lindsay, 2001; Marshall, Chiat and Pring, 1997; Robson et al., 1998; phonological processing in children: Bowen and Cupples, 1999; Dodd

and Bradford, 2000; Frazier-Norbury and Chiat, 2000; therapy with people who have voice disorders: Dunnet et al., 1997; fluency work in pre-school children who stutter: Onslow, O'Brian and Harrison, 1997).

Expectations of service users

The expectations of service users are an important consideration. Porter and McKenzie (2000), writing about interventions with children, point out that parents may have certain beliefs about the long-term outcomes of therapy that are unlikely to be realized, e.g. 'early intervention means that my child will not experience difficulties later on'. The same might be true of almost any other client group. Where there are firmly held but unrealistic beliefs about the outcomes of therapy, engagement in the actual process of change may be constrained. For example, a belief that speech is the only positive outcome for the person with aphasia may hamper attempts to establish the use of total communication strategies.

Effects of intervention

The effects of intervention are defined as 'changes in behaviours associated with communication difficulties and is equivalent to outcomes, a term more commonly adopted in the UK' (Law, 1997: 1).

In determining which aspects of the service user's communication to evaluate, the therapist makes reference to the mechanism for change that has been targeted for modification, e.g. is it the specific speech and language processes of the individual? Is it the interaction style that significant others use with the client? Is it particular aspects of the communication environment? Each stakeholder in the intervention process, whether the individual, the parent, partner or therapist, has a different perspective to contribute to the evaluation.

The therapist carries out assessment activities in order to evaluate change in the individual's communication skills or the main target of the therapy. The idea is to make before and after judgements about the effects of the intervention. This includes not only the direct assessment of the client's speech and language abilities, but also communication taking place between client and significant others, use of environmental strategies, etc.

The client may have a view on what the intervention has achieved for his or her communication skills and associated lifestyle. To this end self-evaluation methods may be used such as questionnaire, rating scales and in-depth interviewing.

The significant others, including parent, teacher, partner, carer or support staff, may have an opinion as to the effectiveness of the intervention. Similar evaluation methods to the client's may be used as well as basic observation schedules.

The relative success of an intervention will vary across the different stakeholders involved in its enactment. Each occupies a different position from which to make value judgements about the intervention. It follows, therefore, that differences in interpretation may occur between the separate perspectives – the service user may assess therapeutic success differently to the therapist.

Lack of change

Where there is a lack of evidence to support positive and measurable change and a perceived failure to achieve the identified goals of intervention, critical inspection of the content and implementation of the intervention is needed. A lack of change may be due to:

- Misconceived decisions in the construction of intervention that have not adequately or appropriately reflected the individual's profile in context. Communication skills are seen as part of the whole person's functioning in daily life. For instance, a decision about the timing of the intervention demands an appreciation of the person's personal and environmental circumstances as well as the clinical presentation of communication skills, e.g. working with a person on their language skills at a time that coincides with intensive medical treatment may be undesirable.
- Poorly articulated goals and objectives of intervention, such that the fidelity of therapy enactment is called into question. Implementation is inconsistent with the defined plan. This may be because the aims and the proposed route of change have not been conveyed clearly to the client and significant others. This is particularly important when significant others are involved in the delivery of therapy. In order to promote reliable and consistent implementation, the therapist's understanding of the therapy needs to be mirrored by the people who are responsible for carrying it out. There is room for error because it is not clear what exactly needs to be done, e.g. articulation drill work is carried out inconsistently by the parent.
- Inadequacies or inconsistencies in the targeted mechanism for change such that the supported practice element of therapy is not carried out according to the recommendations. This may be due to a number of reasons, including competing priorities experienced by the key players, issues to do with uptake of responsibilities, or individual value systems that are at odds with the plan of action.
- A lack of ownership of therapy goals may lead to the disengagement of the client and/or significant others. A goal that is imposed on an individual by the therapist rather than defined through partnership negotiation may negatively affect individual energies, interest and application.

Role of generalization

Naturally, change is desired beyond the parameters of the clinical session. Generalization refers to the transference of therapeutic effects across settings, communication partners, events and conditions, and over time. It is a frequently ignored aspect of intervention studies (Leonard, 1981).

Generalization of therapeutic gains is not something that happens as a natural consequence of therapy. The automatic transference of new skills acquired in one situation, e.g. the clinical setting, into another, e.g. the home, classroom, workplace or other context, cannot be assumed (Calculator and Bedrosian, 1988). It requires deliberate planning as part of the mechanism for change. Bricker in Warren and Reichle (1992) comments that it is insufficient to teach children communicative behaviours that are dependent on specific cues. Change that restricts itself to the controlled condition within the clinical setting will not necessarily have an efficacious effect on the person's functioning at other times. The therapy plan that does not include a forecast of how generalization will occur is incomplete.

A number of methods may be employed to promote generalization of outcomes that may be used separately or, more usually, in combination. These include:

- Bringing about change to the mechanistic processes of communication so that new paths are laid down and self-monitoring is established, e.g. a change in the way an individual processes or produces speech and language generalizes across settings and communication partners because change is applied to internal mechanisms.
- Involving significant others in the therapy process so that the responsibility for change can be shared between the client and the main communication partners, e.g. joint development of new ways of communicating and interacting in different settings and communication situations because change is applied to the partnership.
- Affecting the infrastructure of the communication environment by manipulating points of access and opportunities for participation, e.g. reduction in barriers to communication access and participation and provision of suitable communication support because change involves adapting the environment.
- Affecting identity and self-advocacy through activities to enhance self-image and raise awareness of rights so that the individual is able to push change forward beyond the parameters of the familiar communication environment to society.

Intervention cycle

The cycle of intervention usually involves a number of components. A traditional view of intervention would usually start with assessment and diagnosis whereby some measure of the person's communication skills is taken, then move on to analysis and interpretation of assessment data, before planning and implementing therapy. This describes a sequential process where certain activities precede others.

Organic intervention

Horton and Byng (2000) propose an alternative view of intervention. They describe it as being an 'organic' process where there is a constant interaction between factors (Basso and Marangolo, 2000; Byng, 1995). Speech and language therapy intervention moves, from the first contact between client and therapist, through the progressive disclosure and exposure of the individual's skills and difficulties. Gerard and Carson (1990: 74) propose that assessment and diagnosis be seen as '(an) integrated part of managing a complex system'.

Assessment and diagnosis are part of a continuous and dynamic process whereby the individual's profile is added to, refined and modified at different levels of functioning. The transactions that take place between the individual and relevant setting events help to build up the bank of information about the individual. Diagnosis is part of this complex system and occurs as a systematic appraisal of the critical factors exposed at any particular point of the intervention cycle. It is not a remote procedure that only occurs at the completion of the first formal assessment; rather it is a continuous review of a changing profile. A person's profile varies and mutates according to changes in internal condition and external context.

Dynamic cycle

Although it is possible to identify the starting point within the cycle, e.g. the referral, there is no fixed chronology to the remainder of the components. They are viewed as component activities that occur at various points in the intervention cycle according to the presenting needs of the individual and the clinical decision-making of the therapist. At the centre of the cycle of intervention is the individual profile, which comprises not only data relating to the person's speech, language and communication skills, but also information concerning identity, psychological state, cultural background, and contextual and health-related issues. Figure 1.1 provides an illustrative summary of the intervention cycle.

Entering/referral

The initial point of access to speech and language therapy (SLT) is represented by **A**. This is the most usual way for an individual to contact a service in the first instance and usually involves a recommendation from one agency to another. Referrals to SLT come from a variety of sources, including another professional (such as health visitor, medical personnel, teacher, day centre officer in a social services setting or residential support worker) a concerned parent or partner, or the individual as a self-referral. The referral provides the service with brief details about the focal person together with the reason behind the recommendation. The

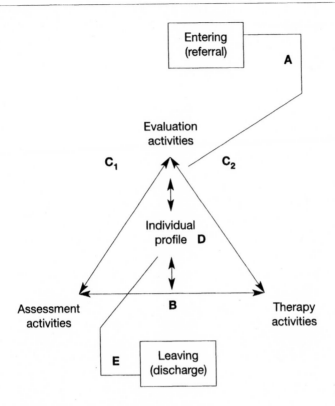

Figure 1.1 Dynamic cycle of intervention

content of the referral provides initial information for **D**, individual profile.

Assessment and therapy activities continuum

The continuum **(B)** refers to a variety of tasks and opportunities that are variously weighted to assessment or therapy. Activities range from procedures (structured and unstructured) that are designed specifically to explore, reveal and test the communicative abilities of the person, to tasks and opportunities where specific therapeutic techniques are employed to extend the available communication skills of the individual. The interface with evaluation activities is marked C_1 and C_2.

- *Assessment activities*: The aim is to explore the individual's communication skills, the positive factors that may be built on, the points at which breakdown occurs and the setting factors that influence performance. It is a process of revealing the skills and deficits that are characteristic of the person's presentation and that say something about his or her identity. An assortment of methods is used in the pursuit of information gathering and hypothesis testing:

- *Information gathering* by interview or case history from or about a communication impaired person – from the focal client and/or significant others. With the aphasic adult, Pound et al. (2000) recommend prefacing these more formal methods with an informal conversation approach. The therapist can use this opportunity to 'tune-in' to the person's communication style and to experiment with the most relevant forms of facilitation that may be usefully employed in later information gathering activities. This approach is applicable across the range of client groups and provides a comfortable lead-in for both client and significant other. Information gathering covers a range of topics including social/family/educational/ health background of the individual, current communication strengths and difficulties, discussion of leisure/work/social interests and needs, and identification of physical/communication/structural/ social barriers causing access problems.
- *Structured and unstructured assessment activities* include nondirective play with children and open conversation with adults, carrying out a formal assessment to test out certain communication aspects, using observation and recording as a method of enquiry.
- *Individual profiling* whereby salient factors to do with the person's communication and daily living skills are summarized in an orderly way. This is a process of mapping the positive factors and the difficulties that the client faces in living with the communication impairment. This is a critical aspect of the intervention cycle that involves client and therapist jointly prioritizing units of information. The summarizing and interpreting phase relates to the differential diagnosis whereby the bank of information is evaluated and a judgement is made about the nature and extent of the communication difficulty. Hypotheses are formulated for testing.

- *Therapy activities*: Two main aspects of therapy activities are identified:

  - *Planning therapy*, which requires an interpretation of the data collected so far, in the context of individual and environmental characteristics. The therapist considers the client's situation and the potential to acquire new behaviours or to modify the use of existing skills in some way. Therapy planning involves decisions regarding the content of therapy (the goals of therapy and what will be done), the process of therapy (the supporting actions and how it will be done) and the context of therapy (the conditions of therapy and other setting variables). Materials and activities are selected, facilitation strategies are invoked, and conditions of therapy are devised for testing out the hypotheses.
  - *Implementation* of the therapy plan is not necessarily the sole responsibility of the therapist. Others who are relevant to the communication skills, life-course stage and lifestyle of the individual may be involved in the delivery of therapy (Dockrell and Messer, 1999).

Evaluation activities

Evaluation of assessment activities (C_1) reveals new information and confirms clinical hypotheses for inclusion in the individual profile (**D**). Evaluation of therapy activities (C_2) involves appraising the individual's responses, thereby introducing new information to **D**, the individual profile, or confirming existing information. A synthesis of all available information is carried out, including data reported from other agencies and members of the multi-disciplinary team. The effects of intervention are measured. This can be carried out during and after assessment or therapy activities. Evaluation of assessment and therapy activities involves appraising the individual's responses at a number of different levels:

- *checking online* during an assessment procedure as in a dynamic assessment that explores the learning potential of the person, or during therapeutic interactions so that the contributions of both therapist and client can be monitored and modulated as required;
- *checking post-activity* so that the individual's range and quality of responses to an assessment procedure or therapy activity/interaction opportunity can be calculated, and in the case of the therapy activity, modified as required;
- *checking post-session* so that the individual's range and quality of responses to assessment and/or therapy activities can be calculated and used to inform the content of the next session;
- *checking post-episode of intervention* so that the effects on the client's communication skills and identity can be calculated. Ideally, change beyond the clinical session should be explored, e.g. across communication partners, events, conditions and settings.

Individual profile

The individual profile (**D**) is what is known about an individual at any one point in time, e.g. communication skills, cognition, identity, health and psychological state. It is informed by **A** (referral) in the first instance and built on by what is revealed by C_1 and C_2 (evaluation of assessment) and **B** (therapy activities). In turn, the individual profile influences **B**, the selection and implementation of assessment and therapy activities and **E**, the decision to close an episode of intervention.

Leaving/discharge

Leaving/discharge (**E**) describes the closure of a person's episode of intervention. Pound et al. (2000) state their discomfort at the use of the term 'discharge', because it confers power on the professional and diminishes the central role of the client, whereas 'leaving' portrays the individual as active agent rather than passive respondent.

The reason for leaving is informed by D, the individual profile. The therapist assesses the appropriateness of closure and negotiates the procedure with the individual and significant others (Williamson, 2001). Consideration is given to the attainment of therapy goals, the assessed effectiveness of intervention, the wishes of the individual, other aspects of the individual's lifestyle that may be relevant to the individual's progress in therapy and any conflicting priorities, the degree of compliance with therapy recommendations, and the expressed commitment of the service user.

Cycle of intervention: Donald, an older man with aphasia

Donald was a 74-year-old retired bank manager. He was married and lived at home with his wife. Donald was referred to speech and language therapy by the neurologist following a CVA and multi-infarct episodes and a recent development of severe epilepsy. He had a working diagnosis of multi-infarct dementia.

In the initial stages, sessions were weighted towards carrying out a range of structured and unstructured assessments in order to arrive at a differential diagnosis of the dementia and dysphasia. Instrumentation used included the Psycholinguistic Assessments of Language Processing in Aphasia (PALPA: Kay, Lesser and Coltheart, 1992), Test of Reception of Grammar (TROG: Bishop, 1982), British Picture Vocabulary Scale (BPVS: Dunn, Whetton and Pintillie, 1982) and the Middlesex Elderly Assessment of Mental State (MEAMS: Golding, 1989). Informal assessment procedures involved conversation and interview of the client and his wife. The data arising from assessment activities suggested that Donald had a severe receptive dysphasia involving auditory processing deficits and 'word deafness'. Expressive language was impaired by severe word-finding difficulties. His visual processing was better than his auditory processing.

Donald experienced frequent seizures and transient ischaemic attacks (TIAs) that resulted in a fluctuating presentation. His dysphasia was degenerative and therefore the over-arching aim of intervention was to support Donald's communication skills for as long as possible by:

- maximizing functional communication within the home environment;
- utilizing communication channels available to the client, e.g. visual processes rather than auditory ones;
- promoting communication between Donald and his wife and significant others;
- providing a means of emergency communication, e.g. for general public or hospital/emergency services.

Therapy activities focused on the development of a meaningful vocabulary of Makaton signs supported with symbols that Donald and his wife could use together. A communication book was devised to cater for those times that Donald felt unwell, was lost or required help from the general public or emergency services. Donald was usually seen with his wife in weekly hour-long sessions, which concentrated on the functional use of signing and symbols. They were encouraged to interact using question/answer and instruction/response sequences. Occasional individual sessions were carried out with Donald in order to monitor any change to communication skills, particularly following a new infarct. Donald also attended a communication group for people with dementia on a weekly basis.

Because of the degenerative nature of Donald's condition, evaluation of intervention focused on functional use of communication skills in relation to the defined goals. As such the reports of Donald himself, his wife and hospital nursing staff during times of admission were relevant. During the episode of intervention, changes were recorded in the following areas:

- The acquisition and use of an extensive range of Makaton signs and symbols in a variety of meaningful utterances meant that Donald was able to communicate functionally and interactively with his wife and significant others.
- Donald's wife was able to communicate more effectively with him.
- Donald became more confident in his use of communication skills and contributed to group activities although he remained reliant on the therapist to interpret his meanings for much of the time.
- During hospital admission times, Donald was able to use his communication book with symbols to communicate with the nursing staff.

The cycle of SLT intervention was brought to a close when Donald's overall health condition declined with a corresponding decrease in functional use of skills. Strategic maintenance of communication gave way to priorities of personal care and medical treatment.

Conceptual framework

It is clear that the broad scope of intervention demands a variety of skills and domains of knowledge (Byng, 1995). Using ethnographic methods, van der Gaag and Davies (1994) examined the working practice of four SLTs specializing in the field of learning disabilities. Broad recognition was given to many different domains of knowledge and skill, such as the use of demonstration and modelling techniques; strategies for managing challenging behaviour; social skills training; use of the community setting to achieve objectives; and maintenance of the client's interest and motivation. However, the practice of these techniques and approaches has not been defined explicitly, therefore variations in their interpretation and use by the SLTs reporting are likely.

Clinical decisions

Timely and relevant clinical decisions ensure the relevance of assessment and therapy activities to the changing needs of the person. Williamson (2002: 8) outlines the judgement and decision-making competencies expected of the qualified SLT practitioner at different career stages. It is about 'determining the best course of action at any one time given the particular set of circumstances'. Williamson states that describing therapy in 'absolute terms' can never be achieved, because of the unique demands of individual cases and the distinctive features of the broader service context, including caseload pressures, available resources and service ethos. Professional considerations and reasoned judgements will include the 'need to interpret test results along with a wealth of information from a variety of sources' (Gerard and Carson, 1990: 61).

The therapist's theoretical interpretation of the underlying deficit is a probable source of influence over the resulting therapy. For instance, the Hanen programme (Manolson, 1983) and the Swedish Early Intervention programme (Johansson, 1994) are based on responsive interactions within a social constructivist model of communication. Nevertheless, identification of the theoretical base of therapy is not sufficient to account for differences in the therapeutic process.

Externalizing the process

A number of speech and language therapy researchers have been concerned with externalizing the process of intervention (Bunning, 1996; Byng, 1995; Byng and Black, 1995; Enderby and Emerson, 1995; Horton and Byng, 2000). There is a shared incentive to articulate what it is that we do. How can any one type of therapy be replicated if it is based on a knowledge base and skill set that varies from therapist to therapist?

A systematic approach to decision-making for working with children was developed by Gerard and Carson (1990). It incorporates both the content and process of intervention: 'What objects, events, people and interaction patterns should be altered and how will they be altered' (p. 73).

Dockrell and Messer (1999) also identify the same components as distinct entities in their intervention framework: (i) the target of therapy (or what is changed) and (ii) the process of therapy (or how change is brought about).

Distinct levels

Two levels are identified for looking at intervention – construction and enactment (enactment is a term first proposed by Horton and Byng, 2000):

- At the *construction level*, a universal framework for planning and reviewing intervention is provided. It gives a structure that includes critical planning stages and key decision points. At this level, a completed cycle of intervention may be described and evaluated. This forms the focus of Chapter 4: Construction of intervention.

- At the *enactment level*, a local framework for looking at the detail of implementation is provided. It gives a structure for examining the therapist's use of technical skills with the client. At this level, the interface between therapist and client may be described and analysed. This provides the focus for Chapter 5: Enactment of intervention.

Goals of intervention

The cycle of intervention involves a process of constant sifting and revealing of 'truths' about the individual that affect the course of action. In keeping with the integrated view of intervention, where assessment, diagnosis and therapy are integral to the process, goals emerge and change. They are defined as a result of the negotiations between client and therapist. Throughout the intervention cycle, as new information is added to old information, decisions are made with or on behalf of the individual. This is a fairly fluid process, where:

- At the beginning of the cycle, little is known about the individual although there may be some information about aetiology, basic background information and reason for referral.
- On the assessment–therapy continuum, there is the gradual and ongoing exposure of positive factors and deficits associated with the individual's presentation. It is revealed where aspects of skill support communicative success and where breakdown is an outcome of the communication difficulty. Differential diagnosis is viewed as an essential part of that process, where communication 'truths' are revealed systematically.
- Interactions between the individual and significant others are observed and interpreted, leading to timely and meaningful judgements about the person's communication skills so that clinical hypotheses may be formulated. This informs the next stage of intervention.

Interdependence of goals

One or more aspects of human functioning are targeted for change or moderation and this is then linked to a particular centre of influence. Goals of intervention are interdependent and supported by decisions that weigh up a range of assessment data, personal characteristics, contextual issues and prognostic information based on what is known about a given condition. Importantly, a goal refers to a *process* and not an arbitrary set of standards representing an outcome.

Approaches to intervention have become more holistic in recent times, embracing a number of different aspects of communicative functioning. Adapted from Byng, Pound and Parr (in Papathanasiou 2000) to be applicable to any client group, the following areas are identified as the main goals of intervention:

Developing and enhancing communication – the development, extension and maintenance of existing communication skills, taking in to consideration the broad spectrum of modalities that are relevant to communicative exchange and social participation. The goal of developing and enhancing communication is not confined to the person who has a communication disability. Communication is viewed as a mutual process of social co-ordination that is essentially interactive (Grove et al., 1999). As such, communication is located at the levels of individual, communication partnership, environmental setting and society. It seeks to build on positive aspects of the person with a communication difficulty and to address areas of difficulty or to overcome complicating factors and barriers.

Developing and supporting autonomy – the encouragement of individuals to express internal judgements, and to assert their ideas and needs. The autonomy goal is viewed as realizing the empowerment potential of the person so that he or she is able to make choices, contribute to decision-making in various aspects of daily life, assert and protect their rights, and exert control over their lives.

Promoting health – the development and maintenance of a healthy state of being. The promoting-health goal combines physical and psychological health. Physical health refers to the physical condition of the person and psychological health refers to emotional stability and adequacy of resources to deal with difficulties. The prevention of ill health is also included in this definition. It is about accommodating change in lifestyle due to the onset, development or progression of disabilities so that ill health is not an automatic consequence.

Developing and adapting identity – expressing, asserting, maintaining and adjusting sense of self in relation to presenting difficulties. This is about the interaction of the person's individuality with their unique experiences of communication disability. The developing child who experiences difficulties with speech and language needs to express the distinctiveness of his/her character. The adult with aphasia needs to preserve a sense of self whilst, at the same time, adapting to the change in personal circumstances.

Identifying barriers and promoting participation – recognizing the obstacles to participation and using strategies to minimize the effects of barriers. This is about exploring and dealing with the effects of a communication disability beyond the impairment itself. It looks to effect change in the centres of influence that surround the individual who has a communication disability so that it is easier to use available skills.

Goals of intervention: Leah, a young woman with learning disabilities

Leah was a young woman of 26 years of age. She had severe learning disabilities associated with Turner's syndrome. Leah lived at home with her parents and attended a social education centre during the week. Leah's mother and her keyworker at the day centre, citing her lack of social inter-action and her disruptive behaviour as the reasons, made a joint referral to speech and language therapy. They both wished to see an increase in Leah's signing and social skills.

Assessment involved interviewing significant others and systematic observation using momentary time sampling (Martin and Bateson, 1986; Brulle and Repp, 1984). The latter involved looking at Leah's interactive behaviour in a range of natural contexts, interacting purposefully with other people and objects, and non-purposeful behaviour when she was doing nothing in particular or else emitting behaviour considered to be injurious to herself or disruptive to others.

Leah's profile consisted of some positive factors to build on:

- one or two Makaton signs and body, facial and vocal gesture;
- attention for solitary activity;
- visual and tactile exploration of environment (messier the better!);
- expression of affect: smiles, laughs, screams;
- intense eye gaze directed to other person on occasions;
- staff team willing to participate in intervention.

And difficulties to address:

- high level of stereotypic and self-injurious behaviour (pulling out own hair by the roots) with accompanying risk of scalp infection;
- some aggressive behaviours: throws objects and strikes others;
- dependence on non-conventional communication behaviours, which was not reflected in the communication environment;
- limited interactions with staff who expressed some reluctance to inter-act with Leah, citing her aggressive behaviours and limited com-munication as challenging;
- limited interactions with peers.

Leah's intervention goals focused on:

- developing and promoting Leah's identity through establishing oppor-tunities for positive and mutual social interaction with staff and peers;
- manipulating the barriers to social interaction that were identified in staff communications with Leah (there was a high dependence on con-ventional linguistic forms that inhibited Leah's participation in social interaction);
- promoting a state of health and wellbeing in Leah by effecting a reduc-tion in her self-injurious behaviour, i.e. pulling her hair out by the roots;
- developing Leah's autonomy by setting up opportunities for her to express personal likes and dislikes.

The goals were enacted through a twice-weekly therapy group that ran over a four-week period. The groups were fashioned as a series of interactive workshops where the therapist worked in partnership with members of staff, modelling new ways of interacting with Leah and providing feedback on the interactions taking place. Therapy activities focused on a sensory-based approach (Individualised Sensory Environment: Bunning, in Fawcus, 1997) whereby sensory opportunities for interaction were provided. This involved a deliberate approach to interaction that included:

- sensitive responding to Leah's non-conventional communication behaviours;
- use of minimal verbal code to support Leah's processing of sensory information;
- use of tactile stimulation and, to a lesser extent, vestibular stimulation.

Repeated assessment measures revealed a reduction in Leah's non-purposeful, disruptive behaviour and gains in her purposeful interaction. Leah and her communication partners had developed new ways of interacting using the potency of the sensory stimuli.

The emergence of some basic signs and functional gestures was noted. Staff experience of 'purposeful' interaction with Leah challenged any previously held negative attitudes. As her likes and dislikes of sensory stimuli were revealed, so Leah's identity as someone who becomes animated when 'messy' sensory activities are on offer, and her emphatic choice of certain items over others, became established. With the growth of positive social interaction between Leah and the staff and peers, her self-injurious behaviour decreased and, consequently, her hair started to grow back.

Mechanism for change

In partnership, the therapist and client work to identify the most appropriate route for the intervention process. This is referred to here as the *mechanism for change* (Byng and Black, 1995). Based on what is known about the client's communication skills and personal situation, the mechanism for change, or how the therapy will work, is defined. This is sometimes inferred by the directness of approach. A direct approach has a primary focus on the interaction between client and therapist. An indirect approach would usually involve significant others as intermediaries in the therapy process. A combined approach features aspects of both. It is acknowledged that goals are interdependent and that the process of change is not confined to the target of therapy. There may be collateral growth or modification in other areas related to the focus of intervention.

Centres of influence

Based on Bronfenbrenner's (1979) ecological system of human development, change is sub-divided into centres of influence illustrated in Figure 1.2. It starts with the individual at the centre, moves out to the immediate

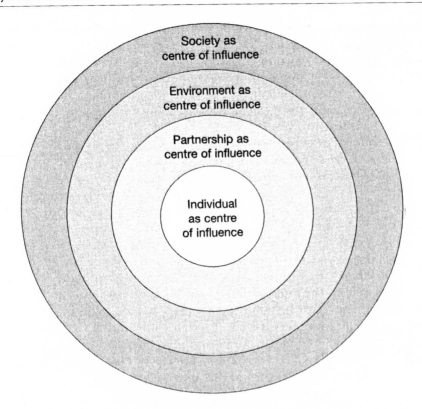

Figure 1.2 Centres of influence

context of communication partnerships, then to the communication environments that are part of the person's life and finally to society. A centre of influence is defined as the primary site of the intervention (assessment–therapy) activities. More than one centre of influence may be targeted at any one point in time. Change is not restricted to any one centre of influence and may traverse different centres that will variously affect the functioning of the individual who has a communication disability.

Individual as centre of influence: The approach focuses on internal processes of the individual that affect the way information is received, organized and interpreted. Individual competencies and functional use of skills are of primary interest. Examples of an individual approach may include language therapy, articulation work and motor speech training.

Partnership as centre of influence: Communication is viewed as a mutually co-ordinated process, whereby the ideas of each partner are exchanged and interpreted. The therapeutic process is a negotiated course of learning and change where both client and significant other(s) are contributors and assume shared responsibility. Usually the therapist works with the client and partner(s) together. There is exploration of the unique communication partnership so that new ways of interacting are tried and developed. Examples of the partnership approach can be seen in a range of approaches, including intensive interaction (Nind and Hewett, 2001), conversation analysis (Lesser and Perkins, 1999), phonological therapy – 'parents and children together' (PACT: Bowen and Cupples, 1999), individualized sensory environment (Bunning, in Fawcus, 1997) and the Lydcombe programme for stuttering (Onslow, O'Brian and Harrison, 1997).

Environment as centre of influence: The focus is on environmental manipulation or alteration of the context in which communication takes place. The environment includes the activities and opportunities that are available for communication purposes as well as the skills used by other people. The ecological approach may involve manipulating a contextual barrier so that communication access and participation are promoted. An example of such an approach might be developing accessible ways of presenting information to people with learning disabilities who have low levels of literacy, by introducing visual imagery to represent the same meanings as text. The intervention effectively deals with the difficulty and promotes client access by removing a literacy barrier. Skills development amongst significant others is also included with the aim of affecting the way people communicate with and respond to the person who has a communication disability. The mechanism for change lies in modifying the communication skills of others so that more relevant and balanced communication partnerships are established. Examples of this are conversation training offered to volunteers who support people with aphasia (Pound et al., 2000), and managing the communication environment of people with learning disabilities who exhibit challenging behaviour (Bradshaw in Abudarham and Hurd: 2002).

Society as centre of influence: This is about promoting the self-worth of individuals such that they are able to effect positive changes in lifestyle (Mosely, 1994). Commonly referred to as advocacy, this involves interaction between the individual and the relevant social, educational and political environments. Opportunities are both created and supported, so that questions are asked, authority is challenged and needs are communicated. Advocacy work can be seen on a continuum where the scope of influence increases gradually. It starts at the level of self-advocacy and interpersonal exchange and moves on to assertion of views in the societal and political arena. The recent trend of involving service consumers as participants in research and as service consultants is a form of advocacy in action.

Although the options for centre of influence have been identified here, they are set within a negotiable framework. Intervention with a client may include a combination of mechanisms whereby individual competencies and context are viewed together as artefacts of change. Defining the dynamics of the therapeutic process is critical to its success. Without conscious and planned consideration of the agents of change, the therapy process is incomplete and any subsequent outcomes will remain a mystery.

Moving across centres of influence: Marius, a pre-school child with language delay

Marius was a three-and-a half-year-old boy who lived at home with his parents. His father was a cab driver and the mother was a full-time parent. The health visitor had made the referral to SLT because of a shared concern, with the parents, regarding Marius's very slow language development. The mother was reported to find Marius 'difficult to handle at home' because of his lack of speech. This difficulty was compounded by the father's long working hours, and the mother felt the pressure of being the main carer for her child.

Conversation with the mother revealed a very tired parent who was finding it difficult to manage her son's disruptive behaviour at home. Marius had regular temper tantrums that appeared to be related to a frustrating inability to express himself. The mother articulated feelings of remoteness from her child and admitted that she had found it difficult to bond with Marius. She had suffered some medical complications at the time of the birth, which had meant that Marius had been separated from her for two days afterwards.

Marius was observed in a non-directive play session with his mother and with the SLT. The following characteristics were noted:

- Marius engaged in car play, making accompanying engine noises;
- Marius sought the attention of his mother by grabbing at her clothing followed by syllable strings that were usually unintelligible;
- Marius's play was quite destructive at times; for example he would unscrew all the heads of the dolls and throw them into a corner of the room;
- the mother was extremely tentative in approaching her child and seemed unsure how to relate to him;
- Marius had demonstrated an interest in picture books with the therapist and pointed at items of interest.

The goals of intervention were focused on: enhancing Marius's communication skills; identifying and adjusting the barriers at the level of the communication partnership; supporting the development of a positive identity for both Marius and his mother in recognition of the challenges in their relationship; and boosting the mother's confidence as a parent and a primary communication partner to her child.

The main centre of influence to be targeted was the communication partnership of Marius and his mother. The aim was to facilitate a positive relationship between Marius and his mother through non-directive play. Early on in the intervention cycle a nursery place was secured for Marius, which helped to relieve some of the pressure on the mother. This introduced another centre of influence for consideration, i.e. the communication environment of the nursery. The therapist made regular contact with the nursery and advised the staff on developing relevant communication partnerships with Marius. Although it was only a morning placement, the mother was greatly encouraged by the respite this afforded her relationship with Marius. In a sense, it took some of the stress out of their relationship. Individual therapy sessions were offered to Marius and his mother, aimed at promoting:

• shared attention for activities, in particular looking at picture books;
• non-directive play where the mum was encouraged to follow Marius's lead;
• a responsive communication partnership whereby the mum responded to Marius's communicative attempts regardless of whether she understood what he was attempting to say, i.e. allowing him to direct the adult's attention.

During the sessions the therapist and mum worked together with Marius, with the SLT providing loose models for the mother to observe and try out. Therapy continued on a weekly basis over an eight-week period followed by monthly review in the nursery context with the mother. Both mother and child made a number of gains:

• looking at picture books together had developed into a routine activity that both derived some pleasure from. Marius had started to label pictures that he pointed out to his mother who in turn reinforced this. For this type of activity, Marius would frequently sit on his mother's lap;
• the mother appeared more relaxed with her child and he with her. Although the difficult times still persisted, the mother stated that these times were becoming less so;
• the destructive element in Marius's play was not as noticeable. His play had extended beyond simple car play and the nursery reported his regular use of the soft play area and the home corner.

Philosophical backdrop

The underlying philosophy – the principles and values of the service – is a major source of influence on intervention practice. How disability is defined and interpreted and where it is located is crucial to the conceptual framework of intervention. Both will affect the content of intervention and the process whereby change is brought about. The way we respond to people with communication disabilities and the values that underpin SLT services are relevant to the individual's progress (Byng, Cairns and Duchan, 2002).

Concept of disability

The philosophical direction of a service goes hand in hand with the way disability is conceptualized.

In 1980, the World Health Organization (WHO) published its first version of the International Classification of Impairment, Disability and Handicap (ICIDH), summarized in Table 1.1. Although it aimed to capture the variety of experiences of people who live with health conditions, it was focused almost exclusively on a biomedical model for cure and treatment.

Table 1.1 Terms and definitions used in ICIDH (WHO, 1980)

Term	Definition
Impairment	Any loss or abnormality of psychological, physiological or anatomical structure or function
Disability	Any restriction or lack (resulting from an impairment) of ability to perform an activity in the manner or within the range considered normal for a human being
Handicap	A disadvantage for a given individual, resulting from an impairment or disability, that limits or prevents the fulfilment of a role (depending on age, gender, social and cultural factors) for that individual

Criticisms of ICIDH

Oliver (1990) criticized this framework for allying itself to the 'medical classifications of disease–disability–handicap'. Because disability is located with the person, it is the person who is seen as requiring intervention to reduce any limitations brought about by the impairment. Oliver (1990: 6–7) goes on to state that 'these schemes, whilst acknowledging that there are social dimensions to disability, do not see disability as arising from social causes'.

Alternative definitions

In the revised edition, ICIDH-2 (WHO, 1997) introduced the idea that disablement and functioning are outcomes of interactions between health conditions and contextual factors. Two sorts of contextual factors were identified: social and physical environmental factors (social attitudes, architectural characteristics, legal and social structures, as well as climate, terrain and so forth); and personal factors that include gender, age, other health conditions, coping styles, social background, education, profession, past and current experience, overall behaviour pattern, character style and other factors that influence how disablement is experienced by the individual.

After extensive field-testing, the International Classification of Functioning, Disability and Health (ICF) was published (WHO, 2001), providing a revised framework for the description of health and

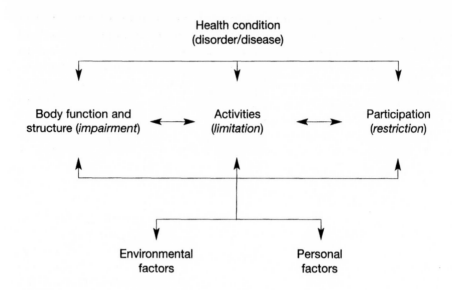

Figure 1.3 Interaction of ICF concepts (WHO: 2001)

health-related states. *Impairment* as a construct is replaced by body structures and functions. The new framework is depicted in Figure 1:3 and
describes an interactive model of human functioning, not merely disability.
Features of the ICF include:

- a *social model orientation* where the impact of contextual factors is
  recognized as a root cause in disablement and functioning of disability, together with the health condition. The interaction is complex,
  bi-directional and dynamic. The model does not posit a causal linkage
  between the three dimensions of disablement; rather, at each level, disablement occurs within and by means of contextual factors.
- the employment of *neutral terminology* supporting the social model
  orientation, where 'activity' is preferred over 'disability' and 'participation' replaces 'handicap'.
- the use of *flexible operational definitions* where disablements include
  losses or abnormalities of bodily function and structure (impairments),
  limitations of activities (disabilities) and restrictions in participation
  (formerly called handicaps).

Location of disability

Differences in the location of disability are seen in the medical and social
models. The medical model interprets disability as a personal problem,
directly caused by disease, trauma or other health condition that requires
individual treatment by professionals. It locates the problem within the
impaired individual. There is a focus on individual deficits, inabilities and

symptoms with a corresponding drive towards cure or adjustment and behaviour change by the individual. Oliver (1998) identifies two important functions: first, the initiation of rehabilitation programmes designed to return individuals to 'normality' and second, assistance in the psychological accommodation of a 'disabled' identity. Impairment is the fundamental construct, seen as causing disability and handicap, and *in need of cure and treatment*.

Within the medical model, disability is portrayed as a static or fixed property. There is an implicit assumption that the individual is adaptable, whereas physical and social environments are not, i.e. individual must adjust to the status quo. However, normality and disability are social and relative constructs that are difficult to measure. As Oliver (1998) suggests, individual preference or environmental circumstances may be the main reason for an individual's condition rather than some organic or intellectual pathology.

The social model is based on the principles of inclusion and empowerment. There is greater acknowledgement of diversity and the complexity of individuals' lives, needs and choices (Clark, 2001). It locates the problem within society where oppression is linked to disability. Disability is dissociated from the body and there is no causal link with impairment. Instead, there is a focus on disabling the barriers in the environment that contribute to participation limitations. A positive 'enabled' identity is portrayed that promotes autonomy and control with an interest in social action, exertion of rights and choices.

Disabling barriers

The identification of material, cultural and attitudinal barriers is crucial to a social perspective of disability (Oliver, 1990):

- Environmental barriers include poor accommodation of individual support, and access needs restricts participation, e.g. a lack of Braille, lack of sign language interpreters, no ramps for wheelchair users.
- Attitudinal barriers mean that the attitudes and behaviours of others can lead to opportunity restrictions and constraints on independence, e.g. a parental belief that the child will never achieve because of a learning disability, or use of language that is considered to patronize or stigmatize the person.
- The way things are done can impose structural barriers by ostracizing individuals and limiting their participation, e.g. the meeting that is conducted in a way that precludes the contributions of the person with a disability, as in the failure to signal speaker turns, which confuses the person who relies on lip reading to access a conversation.

Culture of empowerment

So what does the model of disability say about the context of intervention? There are certain features that influence the culture of the SLT service. Their interpretation variously contributes to the empowerment of service users and the assertion of individual rights. This empowerment process includes language, partnership, diversity and the provision of appropriate settings for intervention.

The *language* that is used to describe a service or the people who use the service denotes the tenet of that service. The principle of putting the person first *before* the disability humanizes and personalizes. Sutcliffe and Simons (1993: 23) quote a self-advocate as saying: 'If you put "*people* with learning difficulties" then they know that people want to learn and to be taught how to do things.'

The *partnership* of professional and service user in the design and delivery of services operates in such a way that the views of the 'experts', i.e. those people living with disability, are represented and services designed accordingly. This includes a negotiated procedure whereby clinical decisions are made and goals are identified.

Diversity is recognized at a number of different levels: the individual's communication needs and the intervention activities to support them, and sensitivity to the many different cultural and ethnic needs of individuals.

Settings for intervention where potential barriers to participation have been identified and appropriate adaptations put in place. The 'enabling environment' is crucial to the process of empowerment. It has been defined as the setting that provides complete access and the opportunity to use available knowledge, skills and abilities (Corker in Swain et al., 1993). Furthermore, the knowledge and skills of staff and clients is said to outweigh in significance the physical attributes of the setting. Communication ramps are provided to promote skill use by the person with a disability. This includes all forms of alternative and augmentative communication. Examples of communication ramps are simple language use, use of gesture, sign, objects of reference, pointing, pictures and symbols, communicating at a slower pace, guessing what a person's behaviour means and checking out an interpretation, etc. One feature of the London Centre of Connect – the communication disability network, is the provision of wall-mounted note pads with attached pens. These are located throughout the building to facilitate total communication.

Cycle of intervention

The cycle of intervention is an intricate journey that is the result of an interaction between numerous factors associated with the client. Because of this, each person's experience of intervention is unique. The word 'intervention' is used as an over-arching term to describe any or all of the potential activities that may occur in the delivery of SLT. There is no chronological order to the components of the intervention cycle, i.e. assessment does not necessarily precede therapy; rather, it is an organic entity that moves and shapes itself according to the collective contributions of the therapist, client and/or significant other(s).

Chapter 2
Cultural diversity

An intervention cycle that is relevant and responsive requires consideration of the full spectrum of individual need. This means attending to individual characteristics that make up and influence participation in the immediate family context, the local community and the broader society. Recognition of the setting variables helps the therapist to build a comprehensive and context-based picture of the individual: one that is connected to the person's lifestyle and situation, and which ensures the relevance of interventions. Neill (2000: 162–163) recommends that culture be 'viewed as a vital factor in gaining any appreciable understanding of people in a given place'.

Cultural definition

Culture refers to the lived experience. There are certain distinctive features that are shared by some individuals, which alternatively support inclusion within a cultural group or demarcate exclusion:

- people who live in a particular *geographical location*, such as an inner city housing estate, or else who favour a transitional experience, e.g. the community of travellers;
- people from different *ethnic backgrounds* who may share religious convictions, value systems, family practices and social activities;
- individuals with a *particular attribute* that demarcates them as different from mainstream society but also allies them with others with similar attributes, e.g. the deaf community and the disability movement.

Cultural definition not only distinguishes one particular way of life from another; it also helps to inform others of the thinking and behaviours that are integral to that way of life (French Gilson and Depoy, 2000). Culture is a word used to represent the experiences, beliefs, values, social networks, activities and customary practices that are embraced by a group of people. It influences the way an individual responds to a set of circumstances and interprets personal experiences. It also affects the way individuals relate to each other (Neill, 2000). 'Our sense of citizenship and community is defined by boundaries which demarcate zones of inclusion and exclusion' (Marks, 1999: 153).

Understanding of culture and ethnicity

Effective service delivery in the public domain demands an understanding of ethnicity and sensitivity to cultures that are different from the familiar or dominant one. It implies acute awareness of culture as an integral part of a person's presentation and the tailoring of services so that relevance to service user may be achieved. Neill (2000) refers to the 'crucial role' that cultural sensitivity plays in international health programmes. It is about being aware of and valuing difference in such a way that services are amenable to the prevailing culture of individual service recipients.

A lack of understanding of cultural differences and ethnicity may lead to manifest indifference. Coll and Child in Bhui (2002) go further and state that an inability to perceive and accept racial difference can lead to inferior treatment of some people, which is akin to racism. The result is that the things that are important to an individual or a group of people remain hidden and are therefore not respected or attended to by others. This can lead to problems in communication between people, poor uptake of services and eventual alienation from provision in mainstream society.

Consequences of a constrained interpretation

The way a culture is construed by others may affect their responses. Neill (2000: 163) points out that culture can be defined in 'an excessively elementary and inert way', situated in traditions of the past. Assumptions are made about the way a person is likely to respond to a set of circumstances *because* of their cultural background. A set of beliefs about a particular group of people can become predictive and lead to them being denied the same opportunities as others. Ahmad, Atkin and Chamba in Ahmad (2000) provide an example with the debate on consanguinity and health amongst the South Asian population. They state that evidence of a link between family formation based on consanguineous marriage and childhood disability is inconclusive; yet popular belief that first-cousin marriages contribute to the prevalence of conditions such as thalassaemia and deafness prevails in society.

When such a narrow definition of culture is employed in the development of interventions there may be what Neill (2000) refers to as a 'straight jacketing' effect. A constrained interpretation of a people's cultural needs means that 'real' needs may elude those in a position to meet them. The options and choices given to people from the dominant culture in society may not be offered to those from a smaller constituency, because of a stereotyped view of their requirements. Ahmad, Atkin and Chamba in Ahmad (2000: 31) draw on the experiences of Asian women receiving obstetric care, and comment that: 'Health professionals' stereotype of Asian women and terminations lead to discretionary withholding of certain tests.'

Inequalities

A fixed and narrow view of a people's culture may lead to discriminatory practice so that they are denied the same opportunities as others. Systematic inequalities in health care provision to minority ethnic communities have been well documented (Ahmad, Atkin and Chamba in Ahmad, 2000). Recipients of health care appear to be variously disadvantaged by virtue of their ethnicity. Bhui (2002) comments on the additional suffering and struggle experienced by ethnic people with mental health problems. Prejudicial attitudes, narrow interpretations of need, limited understanding of culture and ineffective communication skills are cited as some of the core issues within service provision. Ahmad, Atkin and Chamba in Ahmad (2000: 30) were concerned with birth outcomes amongst the Pakistani population and talk about the need to recognize the potential effects of 'racism in everyday life and service delivery'.

They elucidate by giving the example of the later registration of Asian women at all stages of obstetric care compared with their white counterparts. A lack of relevant and accessible information is cited as a contributory factor.

Fazil et al. (2002) looked at the issue of service access regarding the care of a disabled child. The majority of the Bangladeshi and Pakistani families in their survey experienced difficulties at some time in establishing contact with appropriate services. Sources of difficulty are attributed to language barriers and the 'failure of service providers to work equally effectively in languages other than English' (p. 239). This imposes limitations on the information available to potential service users from different ethnic and cultural backgrounds. Referral rates and uptake of services may be negatively affected.

Risk factors

Differences in health and wellbeing exist between ethnic groups (Acheson, 1998). Some behavioural risk factors have been attributed to ethnic differences (Dundas et al., 2001). Stewart et al. (1999) looked at the incidence of stroke across ethnic groups in the UK. They found that black Caribbean and black African people are not only much more likely to have a stroke, but also that the age at onset is ten years earlier than for their white counterparts. Such evidence requires the development of services that will attend to the needs of any vulnerable section of the population. The development of initiatives in response to local need might include a range of health promotion activities and targeted screening. Whatever the initiative, it will always be dependent on the perceived amenability of the service to the ethnic or cultural group.

Inappropriate and unresponsive services

Interpretations of health needs based on a constricted view of culture can lead to inappropriate service responses. Fazil et al. (2002) comment that the lack of uptake of respite services by ethnic minority families of disabled children is more likely due to a lack of confidence in the services' ability to meet their needs rather than the commonly assumed 'cultural preference'. It is clear that each interpretation will lead to contrasting courses of action.

An interpretation that attributes lack of service uptake to 'cultural preference' prevents service introspection, e.g. Is the service relevant to people from this culture? What measures are in place that facilitate access and engagement with the service? In short, the onus is on the *user's difference* and a service response is not expected.

Conversely, concluding that poor uptake of service is due to a lack of confidence in its relevance is more likely to prompt a response from the service.

The power of separate interpretations to influence different courses of action is clear. Ideas about a culture may be alternatively prohibitive or facilitative. This is an important principle for therapists to remember when working with people from diverse cultures and ethnic groups.

A paradox exists in the provision of health, social welfare and educational services (Fazil et al., 2002). The families who are vulnerable to material deprivation, and people from minority ethnic groups such as Bangladeshi and Pakistani families, are those who are least likely to have their needs met: 'Different dimensions of structural and individual discrimination, based in disability, "race" and gender, interact to create inequality and unjust suffering' (Fazil et al., 2002: 250).

Cultural dominance

The phenomenon of 'ethnocentrism' is prevalent in health, social and educational organizations (Ahmad, Darr and Jones in Ahmad, 2000). This is where the main culture in society is maintained in an elevated position such that contrasting cultures are subordinated. It is a term that is often used to describe the domination and powerful influence of Western European culture in public services. Coll and Child in Bhui (2002: 142) state that 'white supremacy' is evident in many societies. Ethnocentrism in the public service domain can be seen in failures to acknowledge difference associated with ethnicity and culture. This is demonstrated by inflexible service provision that does not look to the demography of its users, but instead shapes itself on professional ideology and the dominant culture in society.

Walmsley and Downer in Ramcharan et al. (1997) provide the example of the forcible Anglicization of people with learning disabilities in the institutional care settings of the past (before the advent of the new styled community services: DoH, 1980). Although service users came from a range of cultures and ethnic groups, little or no regard was given to differences and preferences associated with their backgrounds. Meals, activities, personal care, dress, and educational and religious opportunities were fashioned on the dominant white-English culture. In this context, 'ethnocentrism' is seen as an oppressive force that restricts and even denies expression of cultural diversity. In a contrasting move away from Anglicization, the inaugural conference of 'Black People First', a self-advocacy organization representing black people with learning disabilities, asserted their racial identity by producing a charter that listed a number of minimum care standards, including sensitivity to language and culture, and responsiveness to dietary preferences (Black People First, 1993).

Misunderstandings

Misunderstandings may arise where people from two or more cultures come together. Differences in behaviour, communication style, relationships and activities may appear strange and incomprehensible to people who are not of the same culture. Interpretations of behaviour are made on the basis of the familiar or dominant culture and are therefore likely to be inaccurate. This lack of understanding or appreciable awareness of a culture outside our own can lead to mistrust, separation and even hostility between cultures. Communication breakdown is a common side effect of such cultural ignorance (Bhakta, Katbamna and Parker in Ahmad, 2000).

Variations may exist in the way individuals from different cultures express their own views of their particular circumstances and in relation to ill health and disability. The person's position in the family and any culturally implicit expectations on that person are relevant factors. Health concerns may be diminished alongside family responsibilities that are informed by the culture. Lantsbury (2001) cites the case of Mr A, an Asian Muslim who, following a head injury, described his concentration problems as 'having a headache'. This was stated against a background of expectations that 'it is solely his responsibility to provide for his family, which he can no longer do ... as it is unacceptable for his wife to work' (p. 7).

Individual communication styles may alternatively cause offence and bewilderment to participants. Lantsbury (2001) provides a concrete example of different cultural interpretations of the word 'no': 'In some cultures it is rude to say "no" or to admit that you have not understood something that has been explained to you, such as what to do next, or when the next appointment is' (p. 7).

Importance of cultural awareness

Neill (2000: 166) draws on examples from international health programmes that demonstrate 'apparent ignorance of the recipient culture'.

Citing Brady (1995) he comments on how the lack of Aboriginal health workers in state hospitals and community clinics in Australia in the past 'led to charges of racism and insensitive treatment'. Although the problems have been somewhat remedied since the 1970s, poor accessibility remains an issue. Wright and Sherrard (1994b) surveyed therapists working with children and adolescents who stutter. They reported reduced attendance amongst stuttering clients from Asian backgrounds and with a perceived lower success rate. Even the shared ethnicity and culture of the therapist appeared not to make a difference. The authors do not attribute this to any one factor and suggest that a number of variables are likely to be responsible, such as 'basic cultural differences in concepts of stuttering and therapy between therapist and client, inadequate interpreter services, and lack of training and experience on the part of the therapist' (p. 336).

Cross-cultural communication

In contrast, there are examples where successful health programmes have been established on the basis of cross-cultural communication. Neill (2000) quotes an article by Bastien (1987) that illustrates how contemporary medicine was successfully combined with traditional practices. Bolivian practitioners engaged in negotiated planning and decision-making with Andean peasants. Joint workshops were developed so that each party in the partnership could learn about the practices and rationales of the other, in order that interventions should be relevant and amenable to the recipients. Neill (2000: 168) observes that 'Perhaps the greatest success Bolivian doctors achieved was devising, with the help of social scientists, health education methods that allowed Andean peasants to understand health concepts and make related decisions within their own cultural concepts of disease and health.'

Clearly, the message is about the importance of collaboration between cultures. This implies a mutual process of information sharing and learning, so that the service is acceptable to the recipient culture.

Responses from SLT services

Various initiatives have been put in place to promote service amenability to people from different ethnic and cultural groups. Lees (2002) points out that cultural sensitivity is not about image-building but a learning process whereby knowledge and experience are acquired. Listening and observing are critical aspects of that process.

Wright and Sherrard (1994a) report the findings of a nationwide survey of SLT services provided to Asian children and adolescents who stutter. They describe a number of initiatives identified by respondents, designed to bridge lingual and cultural gaps, including:

- discussion of cultural issues as part of the negotiation between therapist and client and/or significant other(s) so that therapy plans are relevant;

- translation of appointment cards and other written information into Asian languages, e.g. Urdu, Punjabi, etc.
- additional home visits promoting 'a better understanding of their way of life and more co-operative relationships' (p. 317);
- allocating more time for assessment and therapy activities to support working through two languages and addressing any associated issues;
- arranging appointment times with recourse to family lifestyle, e.g. one therapist considered family mosque attendance after school when booking appointments for the child and parents;
- introducing social routines that are amenable to the person's ethnic and cultural background, e.g. one therapist was reported as learning routine phrases in Urdu for greeting and meeting Asian families, for establishing basic case history information and building up a rapport.

Rahman-Jennings and Hulme (2001) describe how service users from the Bangladeshi community of Camden and Islington, London, were involved in the design of an early years SLT service. The first author was employed as a Bengali-speaking co-worker. Prompted by a desire to improve the Bangladeshi community's access to the SLT service, semi-structured interviews were conducted with thirteen families to ascertain their perceptions and understanding of SLT. Poor attendance of services was attributed to a number of reasons, including language barriers, a lack of confidence, inadequate information about the reason for an initial appointment and the service location, lack of family concern or alternative beliefs about the nature of the problem and what will support its resolution, and the pressure of other family commitments. Based on the views of those interviewed, the SLT service put in place a number of initiatives designed to reduce any language and cultural barriers that contribute to poor uptake of service:

- Information and appointment letters translated into Bengali.
- In-house training for existing advocates and interpreters who are employed on an ad hoc basis.
- Involvement of the Bengali-speaking co-worker in organizing initial appointments and following up missed ones, fulfilling an interpretation role in assessment activities and checking the understanding of families regarding the purpose and outcomes of therapy.
- Specific adaptations to packages of care (Hulme, Rahman-Jennings and Thomas, 2001).

Lees (2002: 12) provides some examples from SLTs working in Sure Start schemes in the north of England, including:

- employing male workers to facilitate contact with 'hard to reach' fathers, whilst also bearing in mind that 'the subculture of childcare may still be very female oriented';
- providing SLT as part of a whole-team approach so that domination by any one profession is avoided and priorities are calculated and responded to with reference to the individual's cultural background;

• establishing a presence in the local community and the places fre-
quented by those likely to access SLT services, such as community
centres, libraries and religious venues.

Not an 'empty vessel'

Health and educational services in inner city areas bring therapists into
contact with people from a range of ethnic and cultural backgrounds.
Service users are not 'empty vessels' waiting to be filled by the professional dictates of a service (Mull, 1995, cited by Neill, 2000). Personal
experiences, values and beliefs, and familiar practices and patterns of
behaviour, are established variables that the user brings to the professional consultation. Awareness of ethnicity and cultural background is
germane to a comprehensive understanding of the person's needs, particularly where negotiated decision-making and partnership practice are
at the centre of the intervention process.

Listening to service users is central to contemporary approaches to
service delivery (DoH, 1998). Their views are critical to the design of
locally responsive services. Ali et al. (2001: 949) explain this as a natural
consequence of the 'increasing emphasis on human (adult and children's) rights' as evidenced in recent legislation (Human Rights Act,
1998). Hulme, Rahman-Jennings and Thomas (2001) designed an SLT
intervention package that was responsive to the solicited views of the
local Bengali community (see Rahman-Jennings and Hulme, 2001). Prior
to the user involvement study the same service was offered to all families
regardless of ethnicity and culture. One outcome of listening to the service users was the introduction of a Bengali-speaking co-worker who
assumed responsibilities at critical stages in the intervention cycle, e.g.
initial appointment, assessment and parent/child interaction therapy.

Disability, race and culture

The experience of disability is culturally variable. The system of values
that are embraced by a culture will affect the individual life-course experience and the responses of others. Consideration must also be given
to the pervasive influence of the dominant culture in society and how it
interacts with the immediate ethnic and cultural context.

Oppression

The barriers faced by people with disabilities have already been explored
in the previous chapter; however, differential treatment may be meted out
because of 'one or more aspects of their perceived identity' (Ali et al.,
2001: 950). Prejudicial and discriminatory treatment is experienced
across many different cultures. People from black and minority ethnic

communities are disproportionately represented in a number of areas and experience:

- Higher rates of unemployment than their white counterparts (Commission for Racial Equality: CRE, 1997a).
- Over-representation in the criminal justice system (CRE, 1997b).
- A stronger likelihood of being excluded from school.
- Poorer socio-economic status due to lower pay levels and poorer access to state benefits compared to white people (Nadirshaw in Bhugra and Cochrane, 2000).

Double jeopardy?

People from minority ethnic groups are at risk of being marginalized in health and social care provision (Daker-White et al., 2002). Both disablism, i.e. differential treatment of people with a disability because of a perceived difference, and racism, i.e. differential treatment because of the person's perceived ethnic and cultural identity, may be experienced (Ali et al., 2001). Individuals with disabilities who originate from ethnic minority groups face multiple sources of oppression (O'Connor, Fisher and Robinson, 2000). Vernon (1999: 387) refers to this as a 'minority within a minority'. Oliver (1996) criticizes what he calls 'additive approaches' used to describe the experiences of disabled people who also share characteristics with other oppressed groups in society, such as gender, sexuality, race, etc. Terms such as 'double discrimination' are felt to be inadequate because they separate out the individual's experiences according to the type of oppression. Oliver (1996) makes the point that it is impossible to compartmentalize experiences.

Stuart (1992: 179) favours the term 'simultaneous oppression' for its interconnectedness. It supports the idea of an individual's collective life experience even though there may be multiple sources of oppression (Hill, 1994). Vernon (1995; 1999: 387–388) argues that this implies that 'disability and race are experienced invariably at the same time'. Recognition is given to the fact that 'one or the other may predominate in different circumstances'.

Multiple oppression

Vernon (1999: 395) rejects the term 'simultaneous oppression' because it denies the significance of context on the type of oppression experienced. Vernon provides a concrete example of this:

> When a black person is in the company of non-disabled black people, s/he may experience disablism but not racism. Similarly, when s/he is in the company of white disabled people, s/he may experience racism but not disablism. In the labour market, s/he may be refused a job in consequence of disability or race related discrimination, or both.

The term 'multiple oppression' encompasses the idea that a person may experience different sources of oppression. It considers that an individual's experience of disability may be modified or exacerbated by the values society places on other contextual factors, e.g. class, culture, race, etc. Vernon (1999: 395) goes on to say that attributes which denote a privileged status, such as higher social class status or male gender, may modify the intensity of oppression experienced.

More than one culture

Individuals who share attributes with different groups may find themselves with a foothold in more than one camp. They may have interests in common as well as conflicting lines of thought. For instance, Ahmad, Darr and Jones in Ahmad (2000) comment that ethnic diversity is virtually unacknowledged in the deaf community. The deaf identity is constructed on the basis of shared experiences of language (BSL) and oppression from a predominantly 'hearing' society. People from ethnic minorities experience other influences in relation to their cultural background, e.g. religion, social and cultural activities.

Ahmad, Darr and Jones in Ahmad (2000) conducted interviews with parents of hearing-impaired children recruited from minority ethnic communities. Some parents expressed tensions between the 'hearing' ethnic group and the 'deaf' culture. The language used by deaf people was not always shared by the home culture, leading to problems in communicating about religion, cultural history and social activities. This prompted one Pakistani mother to write to deaf organizations for materials to support religious education.

Connecting with peers

The need to identify with peers is strong. Social contact, emotional support and joint problem-solving are just some of the drivers (Vernon, 2002; Rai-Atkins, 2002). Bignall, Butt and Pagarani (2002) provide a direct quote from a young Asian deaf woman: 'My mother and father, they don't know sign language, they can't teach me about my own religion and my own culture.'

They describe the usefulness of peer support groups for people with disabilities from black and minority ethnic groups. Amongst the benefits reported by the young people interviewed (from Asian, Caribbean and African backgrounds), were having the opportunity to explore identity issues related to both culture *and* disability and meeting people who really understood because of a shared life experience. The importance of cultural identity is borne out in one woman's comment that 'I feel better mixing with my own'.

Vulnerabilities

Public services are usually constructed with reference to the dominant culture, although used by people from multi-cultural communities. The fact that people with learning disabilities originate from all races and cultures was ignored by service providers for many years (Baxter et al., 1990). Institutional treatment in the UK meant the centralization of all people according to the predominant white English and Christian culture. Repercussions for black service users include causing psychological stress, identity confusion and a lack of self-confidence (Ferns in Brown and Smith, 1992).

Institutional racism occurs when the practice of an organization either fosters negative attitudes towards one section of the community or else fails to address or eradicate any issues that arise. One example is the stereotyping of people from minority communities, leading to poor or negative experiences. This in turn may translate in to disempowerment, a lack of confidence in services and poor uptake of treatments offered.

For people from minority ethnic and cultural backgrounds, there is a basic problem in using public services that are framed on a single dominant culture. To start with, the relationship between the two is an uneven one: the public service – being larger and highly bureaucratic but with usually one main over-arching purpose, e.g. health or education – overshadows the smaller group of people with their cultural framework. Not surprisingly, points of tension and difficulty may occur.

Language and ethnicity

Language is the medium whereby connections are made, relationships built and information exchanged. A lack of shared code is an automatic barrier to building up the partnership between client and practitioner. Daker-White et al. (2002) urge professionals to reflect on the difficulties of assessing cognitive function in people where English is not the first language. The assessor needs to have cultural awareness and particular language skills appropriate to the individual client. Without these two prerequisites, a secure diagnosis cannot be made. Fazil et al. (2002) report that where families identified ethnicity of the practitioner as a critical factor in service provision, the main reason put forward was 'language' barriers. Furthermore, there is evidence to suggest that people are more likely to want and respond to intervention when they are relevant to the culture and language of the target group (Molkhia and Oakeshott, 2000).

It is self-limiting to isolate language as an obstacle to interventions with people from diverse ethnic and cultural backgrounds. True understanding is not simply dependent on shared linguistic code, but entails an appreciation of culture and its effect on meaning (Bhui, 2002). Rao (2001: 544) urges that language and culture be seen in close association with each other: 'While language has been traditionally viewed as a vehicle to communicate meaning, its functions and purposes extend beyond the domain of mere semantics and communication.'

She explores the use of colloquial language in 'appropriately supporting the inclusion of people with disabilities within a particular cultural context'. Bengali mothers are reported to use the term 'inconvenience' to explain a child's difficulties. Rao (2001) identifies two main inferences of this word:

1) To help others to understand the difficulty or challenges that a child experiences in a particular situation.
2) To prompt others to respond in accommodating fashion to the needs of the child in a natural and unobtrusive way.

The facilitative nature of the term 'inconvenience' could be said to be in 'stark contrast' with the clinical labels and medical terminology that are more commonly used.

Channels of communication

Communication between service providers and people from minority ethnic and cultural backgrounds may be problematic or weak. Fazil et al. (2002) report that the parents of disabled children in their survey experienced infrequent contact with the schools. Differences in parental expectations regarding their child's academic achievements and the views of the educational establishment were apparent. This is explained by the lack of regular and effective communication between service provider and user.

The Bangladeshi parents in a small-scale study conducted by Warner (1999) felt that their working relationships with teachers at their child's special school were basically positive because the school understood the difficulties they faced. Potential language barriers were ameliorated by the presence of a Sylheti-speaking school assistant in the nursery; however, none of the parents in the survey wished to be involved in school-based activities. Warner (1999) identifies several possible reasons for this lack of engagement, including health issues, competing family demands and home circumstances, although none of these are verified. It is possible that there were unexplored issues to do with cultural divisions and understanding of roles.

Accessibility

> ... hardships caused by barriers to communication ... the inability of services to respond to the needs of nonspeakers of English. (Chamba and Ahmad in Ahmad, 2000: 83)

The individual's facility with English may be a factor in gaining access to the services that are needed (Fazil et al., 2002; Sproston, Pitson and Walker, 2001). Proficiency in the use of the English language in speaking, reading and writing varies considerably across different ethnic groups (Office for National Statistics: ONS, 1996). This is supported by Chamba and Ahmad in Ahmad (2000), who report variations in the use and command of English amongst South Asian carers of disabled children. A lack of adequate information about services affects the quality of care given. They recommend that special attention should be paid to the linguistic accessibility of service organizations for people whose first language is not English.

Difficulties and hardships may arise as a consequence of linguistic difference. Individuals whose native language does not coincide with the language used by public services may experience problems in understanding the available options, and identifying and making actual contact with services that are needed (Chamba and Ahmad in Ahmad, 2000). The repercussions of unmet need may be far-reaching; quality of home life and familial relationships may be placed under duress.

Lack of knowledge

It is widely recognized that knowledge and understanding help people in coming to terms with a disabling condition (Jordan and Kaiser, 1996; Parr et al., 1997). Jones, Atkin and Ahmad (2001) reported the difficulties experienced by parents of Asian deaf youngsters in obtaining information about their child's condition and the sources of available support. Ali et al. (2001) warn of the limitations imposed by language barriers regarding educational and intervention choices. It is important to provide information for parents in their native language wherever possible (Warner, 1999). With reference to Chamba, Ahmad and Jones (1998) and Smith (1994), Ali et al. (2001: 965) comment that 'Access to and knowledge of services is low amongst ethnic minority disabled people and their carers in comparison to white families, with detrimental consequences for the child's development.'

Fazil et al. (2002) observe that the families in their survey experienced uncertainty and confusion regarding the role of service providers. Cases of families knowing nothing more than the name of a domiciliary worker are cited. Details regarding the designation and host institution of the professional worker eluded some service recipients. This lack of concrete information makes for a confusing and insecure picture of service provision. The credibility, integrity and authority of the provider are challenged and user confidence is negatively affected.

Inappropriate services

An inappropriate service is one that fails to take into consideration the cultural and social needs of an individual. Critical needs may remain hidden because of language or cultural barriers. Even when they are revealed, a lack of cultural awareness may lead to problems of interpretation. Both scenarios may lead to the wrong services being provided. Read (2000: 66) comments that 'Culturally responsive and appropriate services are often simply unavailable to Black families.'

Professionals within the health, educational and social welfare sectors have a responsibility towards the identities of service users. For SLTs it is not just a case of dealing with an individual's communication difficulty in isolation; it is about recognizing the effects of other personal and contextual factors, of which race and culture are a part.

Interpretation of disability

The need to understand the nature of a loved one's disability is not confined to any one culture. Proffered explanations of the circumstances and effects of a person's communication difficulty are processed variously according to the value system held by the individual. An interpretation is made with reference to the broader cultural context (Katbamna, Bhakta and Parker in Ahmad, 2000).

Diverse values

Attitudes to disability are affected by the underlying value system that has prominence within a culture. Just as variations in beliefs and activities occur across cultures, so do the underlying values that relate to those practices. For example, the degree of abnormality and dependence acquires different meanings in different cultures. Porter and McKenzie (2000) observe that the way achievements are valued may be dependent on the dimensions of the endeavour, whether individual or co-operative. In some cultures a greater emphasis is placed on collaboration than on singularity.

Diverse perspectives

Differences may exist in the way certain cultures ascribe values to life-course events and achievements. In the same way, disability acquires different meanings depending on the cultural context in which the term is used. Miles (2000: 616) comments that 'Religious and philosophical models continue to serve some purpose in explaining disability in much of the world.'

The literature frequently asserts the difference in the way black and Asian communities view disability as opposed to the white community. For instance, alternative beliefs and inherited practices may explain some of the differences in parenting practice. Read (2000: 82) discusses the cultural variability in mothering: 'The history of particular groups and the social structures within which they live make sense of their approaches to mothering and why it is different from dominant definitions.'

Katbamna, Bhakta and Parker in Ahmad (2000) investigated caregiver perceptions of disability amongst South Asian communities. Many female carers who were interviewed reported that 'blame' had been apportioned to them for the disability of a child. Warner (1999) observes how Bangladeshi parental views of a child's disability are influenced by their origins. She cites the example of a mother of an autistic child who talked about seeking help from a religious person (*pir*). Ali et al. (2001) point out the complexity of understanding attitudes to disability within a cultural context. Reports of negative attitudes shown towards disability, especially within the Asian community, need to be assessed against the limitations of stereotyping. Other relevant factors may be neglected – including home living conditions, employment and family dynamics. Begum (1992: 2) recommends that 'caution needs to be exercised when trying to interpret the evidence'.

Cultural dislocation

Routine cultural practices are not immune to the advent of disability within the family unit. Lantsbury (2001) comments on the cultural dislocation that may occur when one family member has a brain injury. Impairment of memory may make the observation of certain religious or cultural behaviours difficult. The position of individual members within the family unit may be threatened or disrupted by one person's disability.

Dislocation within the family unit

Oyedele was a 22-year-old man who experienced severe cognitive and communication difficulties as a result of a head injury. Oyedele was the oldest child of three. His parents had moved to England from Nigeria five years previously. Prior to his road traffic accident, Oyedele was studying for his A levels with a view to going to university to study medicine. His parents acknowledged that his position as eldest male child imposed a number of expectations on him.

One year after the accident that caused his head injury, Oyedele and his parents were still seeking a cure for the situation so that Oyedele could occupy his rightful place as eldest son. Oyedele was still striving to prove his former abilities to his parents. His conversations with the SLT focused on medically related topics and his position in the family. The parents were anxious to know the time-scale for improvement in their son's condition.

The tension between the effects of Oyedele's disability and the cultural values held by the family was evident. It represented a major disruption to 'the way things are supposed to be'. The demands of the present situation – accommodating Oyedele's special needs, and the cultural expectations on the first-born male child in the family – were in direct opposition. Learning to live with disability represented a massive challenge to both Oyedele and his family. It ultimately meant foregoing some cultural ideals and altering the expectations on Oyedele as the oldest male child in the family.

Service versus culture

Tensions may exist between the beliefs and life-course principles of the home culture and the commonly held views that prevail in society (Porter and McKenzie, 2000). A common tension that occurs in services for people with learning disabilities is the goal of independence. Cultural and professional views on a young adult 'leaving home' may be in direct opposition to each other. For some Asian cultures, the act of a daughter leaving the family home in pursuit of self-determination and independence is unacceptable. Only by the act of marriage, where parental responsibilities for a daughter shift to the new husband and his family, can such a move be accommodated.

Self-determination in opposition to family values

Shakira was an Asian Muslim woman with moderate learning disabilities. She was 33 years old and lived with her parents in the family home. A period of respite care, where she experienced new opportunities regarding social and leisure activities, led her to request a more permanent move to a local residential facility. Effectively she refused to return to her parents, stating her desire to have a boyfriend, to continue her newly experienced social life, and to experiment with make-up and new styles of dressing. Her social worker was caught between a need to listen to her client, i.e. Shakira, whilst also respecting the dictates of her home culture. Communications between Shakira and her family broke down. Her parents were furious with the social worker, who they saw as interfering with Shakira's family life and cultural beliefs. Her brother was very angry at the position his sister had taken and talked of disowning her. Shakira radically changed her appearance and diet and refused all contact with her family, viewing them very much as the enemy to her aspirations. The situation was fraught with pressures and sadness on both sides. The social workers were anxious to facilitate a negotiated agreement between their client and her family. This led to a compromise where the parents agreed to respect Shakira's decision to live away from the family home and she agreed to a resumption of family contact.

Valuing diversity in SLT practice

Valuing multi-culturalism needs to be addressed at every level within society. French Gilson and Depoy (2000: 210) identify four principles that provide the foundations of multi-cultural thinking:

1) Culture exists and is an integral part of the 'human experience'.
2) It 'is founded on the notion of pluralism'.
3) Multi-culturalism attributes value to diversity.
4) At the centre of the debate on multi-culturalism is the issue of inequality related to the balance of power between individuals and cultures.

If the place of culture is accepted as central to communication and interaction, it follows that ways of addressing and improving cultural sensitivity in therapy services are necessary. Fazil et al. (2002) propose that 'education' is a pivotal part of any change process. A broader definition of education incorporates:

- the gathering and sharing of information and experiences across cultural divisions such that service providers are in a position to listen to and learn about the significance of ethnicity and culture in a person's life, and service users are clear about the role and designation of the therapist;
- the opportunity for questions, answers and mutually worked-out solutions that draw on ethnic and cultural experiences;
- a dynamic consultation process that develops according to the presenting needs of the individual.

Cultural responsiveness

Cultural responsiveness is about observing the presenting needs of individual service users with respect for diversity and *without* the constraints of stereotyped images. Porter and McKenzie (2000) add that it is important for the professional to be aware of his/her own cultural biases and the potential to influence situations. This is consistent with Fazil et al. (2002: 252) who recommend that 'service providers should not make assumptions about the services which a particular family might want or value'.

The meaning of cultural awareness

Lees (2002: 11) questions what cultural awareness means to a profession such as SLT, which is dominated by white, middle class personnel. In the context of the Sure Start initiatives, she comments that it is a 'stumbling block' in reaching, not only families from ethnic minority groups, but also 'white working class families'.

The therapist needs to be aware of the cultural milieu of communication. Differences in communication and interaction styles may exist at the various levels of representation affecting the unspoken rules of social interaction (the way in which verbal and non-verbal skills are used). For example, communication in Western culture tends be 'low-context': there is an emphasis on open, direct communication with explicit meanings attached. On the other hand, communication in Eastern culture tends to be 'high-context', where the style is more indirect and self-concealing. Much of the meaning is implicit and attached to relationships and situations rather than the actual words that are being said (Hargie, 1997).

The linguistic content of therapy sessions and the associated materials need to be amenable to the individual's culture. A lack of consideration of the ethnic and cultural background of the person may lead to disastrous consequences for the intervention. It may result in a lack of engagement and uptake by the client and significant others, simply because the content and supporting material of therapy are not relevant to lifestyle. It is like using the language of chemical engineering with a prima ballerina!

Developing meaningful and functional vocabulary

Parimal was a 14-year-old boy with Down's syndrome attending mainstream school provision. He was from an Asian background. The therapist and teacher were working together to expand his functional vocabulary. Cookery lessons were initially targeted as the teacher explained that although he was always co-operative, he often appeared passive and quiet. She had not really managed to *engage* Parimal in these sessions. The therapist discovered that the food used in these sessions had been selected on the basis of his learning disabilities, e.g. basic culinary fare such as 'baked beans on toast'-type meals. With the teacher, she arranged for the next session to reflect his Asian culture by using the ingredients for a potato curry. Parimal's response to the session was totally different: mere co-operation changed to enthusiasm! He was openly interested in the array of Indian spices, opening up the packets and smelling and tasting them. Although he still needed some help to employ his vocabulary functionally, he was an active and confident contributor to the session.

The meaning of behaviour

Sensitivity and respect for people from minority ethnic cultures requires the therapist to have an open mind that is alert to cultural issues as they arise. Trained advocates are sometimes used to draw attention to cultural issues that may help the therapist to interpret client behaviour and responses to a set of circumstances. Lantsbury (2001: 7) provides a useful account that highlights some of the issues:

> In our day centre we had a young Egyptian attendee who kept pointing to a painting on the wall and getting agitated. An Arabic-speaking volunteer told us what she was saying and explained that in her culture it was unacceptable to have a picture of a woman on display. Without this explanation, her agitation could have been interpreted as a result of her brain injury.

Cultural influence on play

Kai-yin was a three-year-old girl from a Chinese background. She was an only child and her parents had recently settled in an inner city area of England. Kai-yin was referred to SLT by the health visitor because of her general slow development. The main language of home was Cantonese, although the father spoke relatively good English. Initial sessions with Kai-yin and her mother were carried out with a co-worker of similar lingual and cultural background. It was observed that Kai-yin's symbolic play reflected her cultural background. In large doll play, she disregarded the plate and spoon, and first put her hand in the bowl and then to the doll's mouth. She later attempted to place the doll's hand in the bowl and repeat the sequence. The father and co-worker confirmed that this was their usual way of eating.

Although a small example of culturally related behaviour, it nevertheless illustrates the importance of cultural sensitivity and informed interpretation of the person's behaviour. The same child also demonstrated a preference for sitting cross-legged on the floor, which once again the father confirmed was the habitual seated position in the family home. Subsequent therapy sessions observed Kai-yin's familiar position, which helped to establish optimal conditions for Kai-yin to respond and for encouraging carryover in the family home. In a sense, the SLT sessions reflected key aspects of the child's family background and culture thereby making them more amenable to those concerned.

Support network

Any interventions that require family collaboration should go beyond the nuclear family to members of the extended family where relevant. The support network of an individual is built up on the tenets that are implicit in the immediate family culture. It may be usual for a family to confine resolution activities and any difficulties experienced to the immediate context, i.e. moving outside those accepted perimeters is not the 'done thing'. Katbamna, Bhakta and Parker in Ahmad (2000) observe that accessing and receiving help from outside the home culture may not be customary practice. Alternatively, a lack of confidence in the wider community brought about by previous experiences may affect access and uptake of services. Of course it may also be the case that seeking help outside the family unit may be routine procedure and the role of extended family members is highly relevant.

Pathways of opportunity

Neill (2000: 170) states that 'Culture is more of a pathway of opportunity for the acceptance and success of health programs rather than a barrier.'

The design and infrastructure of local services must have recourse to the community that they serve. The importance of tailoring interventions, in particular any health promotion activities, to reflect both individual and community needs has been stressed (Dundas et al., 2001). Targeting change on the observable behaviours that are assessed to contribute to a particular condition or circumstance is too simplistic and unlikely to be effective (see Neill, 2000). As Dundas et al. (2001) point out, the underlying motivation and attitude to change that already exist are of paramount importance to the achievement of positive outcomes. In this sense, the SLT needs to learn from the clients and significant others about their needs and cultural practices and to make sure that any intervention is in keeping with them. Porter and McKenzie (2000: 131), citing Seligman and Darling (1997), stress that 'Before we can begin to meet the needs of families from cultures other than our own, we need to understand how they perceive their needs within their personal and cultural context.'

Confidence in service

Inspiring confidence in service provision means being alert to any other variables that may affect the individual or family's response to existing circumstances. The experience of communication disability may be compounded by difficulties in accessing appropriate services because of linguistic or cultural barriers. Where a struggle is experienced in finding a service that is relevant to a problem situation, frustration and even anger may follow. Alternatively, individuals may resign themselves to the belief that 'this is how things are'.

Working with multilingualism

Proficiency in the use of spoken English varies amongst people from diverse cultures, although spoken English is likely to be the primary means of communication with professionals. In their survey of parents of disabled children (n = 570), Chamba and Ahmad in Ahmad (2000) found that over a third experienced some difficulties with spoken English. Competence varied by ethnicity, with more black African/Caribbean parents having complete understanding of spoken English compared with the Asian groups in the sample. Religious denomination was also a determining factor, with Muslims rating their use of English lower than the Hindu group. Looking at the use of primary care services by Chinese people living in England, Sproston, Pitson and Walker (2001) found that the strongest predictor for going to see a general practitioner was the ability to speak English.

Although sharing of a common linguistic code seems to be important to users of health and educational services, meeting the needs of people from ethnic and cultural minority groups goes beyond the provision of a series of translations from one language to the other. As Chamba and Ahmad in Ahmad (2000: 92) put it: 'Effective communication requires not only a knowledge of language but also the cultural and service context in which communication takes place.'

Working through an intermediary

Interpreting is not just a straightforward translation or mapping from one language to another. Winter (1999: 89) refers to such practices as 'certain shortcuts' and advises against the use of translated assessment materials and employing bilingual personnel to administer them. The demands of working with individuals from multilingual backgrounds are much greater and involve knowledge and understanding of the individual's immediate circumstances against the backdrop of the person's culture and ethnicity. For service users it involves entrusting information to a third party for accurate translation to the service provider. The primary client, whether child or adult, and regardless of presenting communication difficulty, entrusts their experiences of communication disability to the integrity of the interpreter. Significant others, whether the parent of a disabled child or the partner of a language-impaired adult, expect the needs of a loved one to be represented faithfully. This requires some understanding of the individual's condition on the part of the interpreter.

A further challenge, to service users and therapist is participating in an interaction of altered dynamic: one that involves an intermediary. Communication shifts from a two-way to a three-way exchange. This demands skilful use of non-verbal and verbal skills by the therapist. Focus is maintained on the primary client's agenda whilst also taking in the contributions of the interpreter.

Lay interpreters

Sometimes the services of a 'lay interpreter' will be employed, with various degrees of success. The parents of disabled children in Chamba and Ahmad's survey in Ahmad (2000) reported how a family member or friend would often fulfil the role of interpreter. However, maintaining the prominence of the service user's agenda may be problematic if the intermediary is related in some way and therefore has a vested interest in a particular outcome. Jones, Atkin and Ahmad (2001) found that the Asian young deaf people in their study expressed concern about the presence of a parent as a broker of services because of communication difficulties:

> The reliance on gatekeepers complicated communication and young people felt they could not fully express themselves. Several of the older respondents, for instance, believed it was difficult to convey complex thoughts to a practitioner when going through a third party. Consequently, they felt communication was superficial and rarely met their needs (p. 58).

This raises some important issues about the distribution of power: the service is for the young deaf person and not the person negotiating the agreement. Differences in personal agenda may be problematic. The parent is required to fulfil two separate roles that are not necessarily in accord: parent *and* service broker.

Skilful interpreting

The interpreter undertakes an intermediary role between two parties, representing the views and ideas of one to the other. This demands the conscious subordination of any personal agenda and an absolute focus on the agenda of the primary players in the intervention process, i.e. the therapist and the service user(s). Chamba and Ahmad in Ahmad (2000) recommend that professional interpreters should have a comprehensive knowledge of:

- The service, its overarching purpose and context.
- The role of the therapist and any goals that are implicit in the role.
- The cultural context and ethnic background of the service user.
- The individual's communication difficulty or the reason for referral as well as any associated difficulties experienced.

Co-workers

Bilingual co-workers have a key role to play within an SLT service. Co-workers are usually recruited from the local community and trained and employed within an SLT department. Bray, Ross and Todd (1999: 152) summarize the advantages brought by a member of staff who possesses 'in-depth knowledge of the community languages, they may also be able to provide a wealth of knowledge about cultural issues and the local community'.

Access to skilled, culturally sensitive co-workers is vital to the SLT service that serves multi-cultural and diverse ethnic communities. They are usually trained by the SLT service to carry out a range of duties that render the intervention cycle accessible and relevant to the needs of the service user, including: taking a case history in the client/carer's home language, carrying out assessment and therapy activities as appropriate to the SLT's recommendations and with recourse to the home culture, interpreting information between the service user and professional, and offering written translations as appropriate (*Communicating Quality 2*: RCSLT, 1996: 294).

A responsive and relevant service?

A responsive and relevant service is one that is shaped according to the diverse needs of the population it serves. This means avoiding the assumption that Western ideas about disability and functioning have the same meaning for all cultures (Hussain, Atkin and Ahmad, 2002). Equity of access and optimal uptake of service is an important consideration when thinking about cultural and lingual diversity. Specific attention needs to be given to certain critical aspects of provision, including:

- *Service information*: providing information leaflets and posters on a range of relevant topics, including what the service provides, how to make contact, explanatory leaflets, advice on management of communication disabilities, translated into a range of languages that are relevant to the needs of the local community. The distribution of information may need to target locations that individuals from different cultures are most likely to frequent, e.g. local community centres and parents' groups.
- *Referral and leaving intervention procedures*: providing procedures for opening and closing an episode of intervention that are reflected in the published information and support linguistic and cultural differences amongst service users.

- *Assessment and therapy activities*: selecting, devising and using activities that are compatible with the ethnic and cultural background of the individual. Cultural sensitivity demands consideration of the effects of ethnicity and culture on intervention practice, including:

  - involvement of the family and consideration of the presenting difficulty from the perspective of the home culture and ethnic background;
  - the activities that are employed, the therapeutic techniques that are invoked and the setting that is used;
  - the goals of therapy, articulated according to cultural values that are prominent in the individual's life;
  - choice of suitable and relevant materials and resources that mean something to the individuals concerned;
  - selection and use of appropriate techniques that are amenable to the cultural background of the individual.

The therapist needs to gather the best possible information about the individual and to gain a holistic and meaningful view of the person. The involvement of co-workers will provide some useful insights into cultural background and will help to bridge the gaps that may exist between service provider and user; however, nothing can replace raised awareness of possible cultural issues in the mind of the therapist. This means actively seeking cultural insights from the individual concerned, the parents or significant others, so that a meaningful interpretation of the client's communication skills and difficulties can be made, and a quick interpretation based on the dominant culture in society is avoided.

Chapter 3
Identity and psychological state

The importance of a holistic approach to intervention with people who experience difficulties with communication has long been recognized. This means not treating the communication difficulty as a clinical entity distinct from the person and their immediate circumstances. The term 'holistic' describes an approach to intervention that is sensitive to the multiple sources of influence on the person's functioning. It involves the conscious and planned consideration of the individual and/or significant other(s) and their life experiences, because 'Communication and related disorders can lead to a loss of independence, a change in life style, confusion, frustration, failure at school, adverse reactions from others and difficulty with relationships' (Bray, Ross and Todd, 1999: 5).

Influential factors

The planning, implementation and evaluation of intervention requires careful consideration of the inner emotional state of the individual and significant other(s). The therapist is alert, not only to any change in circumstances experienced by individuals, but also to their reactions to those altered circumstances. The way someone responds is dictated by the individual's sense of self and past experiences, together with numerous setting factors. This is evident within each aspect of the intervention cycle.

Circumstances of referral

The focal reason for the referral, i.e. the person's communication difficulty, should not be viewed in isolation. The process of seeking help can in itself be a source of stress to the person and his/her family. A loss of valuable time to access professional services may have a profound effect on anxiety levels, e.g. the parent who waits for three months to receive an initial appointment for a child's speech and language therapy; or the adult who, after discharge from hospital following recovery from a stroke, awaits the reactivation of their speech and language therapy from a local service. There may be a range of factors that colour the circumstances of the referral and affect the psychological state of the individual and significant others:

The age, lifestyle and occupation of the individual provide information about the life-course stage of the individual. Collectively, these aspects reveal something of the personal circumstances at the time of the referral. They might denote impending change in life course, as in the case of the pre-school child who is nearing school entry age. Alternatively, a referral to SLT may represent a disruption at a time of comparative stability in the person's life course. The therapist needs to be alert to the possible meaning of a referral in the context of the life-course stage of both individual and significant other(s).

The onset of the person's communication difficulty may affect their psychological state. The nature of the onset, whether developmental or acquired in a sudden and acute way, gradual or progressive, will affect individuals variously. A gradual onset may mean that concerns are slow to surface and may even be dismissed or minimized over a period of time. A sudden and acute onset may stultify or even shock the persons concerned, leaving no time for adjustment to the new set of conditions that have been imposed, as in the case of the person who has a stroke.

Conditions associated with the onset of the communication difficulty such as ill health, poor social and economic situation, and constraints on social participation, are relevant to the circumstances of the referral. External events or other factors within the person's immediate context may affect the individual's emotional wellbeing. Personal energies may be consumed by or diverted to the source of other problems, which may or may not be directly relevant to the referral reason, e.g. a rent increase that provokes anxiety in the parent of a child, the general poor health of the person referred with aphasia, the demands of a stressful job that depresses the person with a voice disorder, etc.

The efficiency and accessibility of the referral procedure are critical to the individual who seeks help. The amount of time that has elapsed between emergent concerns and the formal referral to SLT may be a source of stress to both individual and significant others. Once a problem has surfaced and is recognized, a response is required. A perceived lack of response, or delay, in the referral procedure can leave the individual 'in the dark', having to deal with their concerns alone. This may be compounded by any difficulties in accessing a service in the first place. The existing support network of the individual, including family, friends and colleagues, may help to alleviate personal anxieties and is therefore an embedded factor for consideration.

Factors in assessment and therapy activities

Jordan and Kaiser (1996) point out that the intervention itself may give rise to tensions between the set of demands and the individual's usual lifestyle. Intervention by its very nature infers that something new or different is being introduced to an existing situation.

Revealing competence and need

For some people, the very process of revealing communicative competence and exposing corresponding needs may be stressful. Nicoll (2001) tells the story of Ron, who had aphasia as a result of a stroke. He attended a rehabilitation centre where he was offered an individual programme and activities organized for a whole day. Ron resented his dependence on others forced by his use of a wheelchair at this time. He expressed his dismay and frustration at therapy demands presented to him in speech and language therapy sessions, whilst also recognizing his need: 'I couldn't believe I couldn't do this. After a while, I thought, wait a minute, this has happened, so you just have to do it. I didn't particularly like it but thought it would do me good' (p. 14).

Subsequently, Ron moved on to participate in an expressive arts project working with two speech and language therapists, an artist and an illustrator. New constructions of aphasia were achieved by personal expression through art. Through his illustrations Ron found expression for his experiences of having a stroke and the resultant loss of skills.

Influential factors

The possible factors that may affect the psychological state of those concerned are wide ranging:

- *Understanding of the communication difficulty* is important to the individual's acceptance and participation in the therapy process. An incomplete or inaccurate understanding of the facts may give rise to a range of feelings, including anxiety, false hope and frustration. A diagnosis or prognosis that is felt to be 'hopeless' may affect the energy an individual is able to contribute to activities.
- *Understanding the rationale for assessment and therapy activities* is relevant to the way an individual is able to approach the demands presented to him or her. It is linked to what is understood about the underlying difficulty. Where the aims or reasons for a therapy session or particular activity remain elusive to the individual concerned, then active engagement and participation is less likely.
- *The perceived broader implications for the individual's lifestyle,* including occupation, education, domestic arrangements, social participation and leisure pursuits, refer to the possible effects of intervention on the continuation of the person's life course and that of significant others. The time required for attending appointments and carrying out therapy activities may present some difficulty. Personal circumstances, such as the child's parents both working full-time, may be problematic.
- *The impact on family members and significant others* needs consideration. Individual capacities to deal with new or altered circumstances may vary. Conflict may arise between key family members; for example,

the mother who is keen to introduce Makaton signs to support her learning-disabled child's slow language development may be in opposition to the father's view that this will deter verbal development and make the child seem 'more abnormal'.

- *The availability, accessibility and support of other agencies* may be relevant to the needs of some people, e.g. education, day services, counselling, home help, relatives support group, etc. An existing support need may render the demands of therapy as unimportant; for instance, the partner of the person with advanced-stage Alzheimer's disease may find it difficult to modify conversation skills when stress levels in relation to care remain high due to a lack of support from other agencies.

- *The allocation of roles within intervention activities* may mean a change in status for the individual and/or significant others that is difficult for a variety of reasons, e.g. the teacher who is now the learner, the parents who receive advice on their role with their child, the manager who must now relinquish former controls and participate in negotiated decision-making with the SLT, the grandparent who receives therapy from the therapist who is young enough to be a grandchild, etc.

- *Conflicts with the individual's personal value system* may happen. A therapeutic goal may clash with the personal ideals held by the individual, e.g. a goal to work on drawing as a means of communication is felt to be of little value compared with speech. The personal style of the SLT and the resultant quality of rapport established between client and therapist may affect the individual's ability to contribute to assessment and therapy activities. A positive rapport between client and therapist is evidence of mutual appraisal and regard, and acknowledgement of the other person's right to contribute.

Factors in evaluation activities

Enderby and John (1997) developed therapy outcome measures (TOM) that were based on the International Classification of Impairment, Disability and Handicap (ICIDH: World Health Organization, 1980). In acknowledgement of the integral part played by psychological state, they added a separate domain termed 'well-being/distress'. Seltzer et al. (2001: 265) recognize the importance of this dimension: 'It has long been recognised that exposure to stressors at various points along the life course has long-term consequences for well-being.'

This is echoed by Jordan and Kaiser (1996: 63) who emphasize the importance of capturing 'not only results using standardized tests or test–retest of performance on specific items related to therapy but also the aphasic person's opinion on whether therapy has been of benefit to his or her every day life'.

Regardless of client group, the individual's own appraisal of the situation, as the beneficiary of the intervention, is as important as any objective measures that may be employed. This may be carried out with the primary recipient of the intervention, e.g. adults with a communication difficulty, or in some cases the secondary recipient, e.g. significant others including parent, keyworker or teacher, where individual appraisal is done by proxy.

Differences of opinion

As the individual's performance is continuously appraised and evaluated during the intervention cycle from initial contact, through a range of assessment and therapy activities, to discharge, there are client/significant other-centred factors to consider, including:

- Any personal goals held by the individual that are at odds with the evaluated outcomes, e.g. 'I want him to be as good at talking as his peers'.
- Differences in self-perception and objective measures, e.g. 'Your assessment might say that my communication is more fluent but it doesn't feel like that to me!'
- Any expectations that remain unfulfilled by the intervention and are therefore a source of disappointment or dissatisfaction to the person, e.g. the parent who is disappointed by the lack of a diagnostic label to explain in orderly fashion the 'confusing array of symptoms' displayed by their child (Porter and McKenzie, 2000: 101).

Circumstances of 'leaving intervention'

The ability to deal with the closure of an episode of intervention and the demands of 'moving on' may be affected by:

- The preparation of the individual and/or significant others, readiness for SLT closure and confidence in the outcome.
- The individual's ability to look beyond the active course of SLT.
- The ongoing support network of the individual and significant others, including any input from other agencies.
- Other circumstances and any collateral activities that may impinge on the individual's ability to move forward, e.g. another major life event that disrupts the closure of intervention such as illness or loss of job.

The influence of identity is seen in the circumstances of the referral, the setting factors of assessment, therapy and evaluation activities, and the circumstances of discharge. It shapes an individual's response to each set of circumstances as they arise. The ability to deal with a new or altered condition varies according to differences in individual capacities.

Identity

Identity is the set of descriptors, characteristics and constants that one sees as belonging to him/herself, and that render one recognizable and unique to others (French Gilson and Depoy, 2000: 210).

Identity can refer to an individual persona or a collective identity. It is a term used to refer to the individual's sense of self. Identity is made up of a complex system of constructs that is formulated by the interaction of personal experience and social narrative. Social identity theory (Tajfel, 1981) describes personal identity as encompassing the perceived unique individual attributes of personality, personal values, preferences and aversions, competencies and difficulties. Jordan and Kaiser (1996: 21–22) talk about self-image as being 'shaped by the interaction of personality factors with aspects of life that a person considers important, such as employment, family and leisure activities'.

Developing sense of self

Peters in Barton (1996: 228) identifies three major places where personal identity, as a 'self-centred activity', takes place: the church, school and family environment. Each is characterized by rituals and symbols derived from cultural and societal values and practices. They influence the formation of identity over the course of time, from the earliest stages of childhood. It starts off with a growing awareness of self and recognition of own name, family, gender and age (Griffiths, 1994). Ideas and attitudes develop and change according to the experiences of the person. The accumulation of self-knowledge and the act of 'speaking about ourselves' contribute to identity formation (Priestley in Corker and French, 1999).

Transitions take place at critical times within an individual's life. Starting nursery and then school mark major changes in the lives of young children. It is often the first real separation from the parents. Subsequent moves over the life course involve the broadening of the individual's social horizon as biological maturation interacts with altered roles, new demands and responsibilities associated with each change. Hanley-Maxwell, Whitney-Thomas and Mayfield Pogoloff (1995) comment that the transition from school to adult life is one of the most important transitions in society.

Narratives in society

Experiences through the life course shape our responses to present and future situations. Each personal experience is coloured by the narratives that are current in society. Thomas in Corker and French (1999: 55) summarizes this interactive process: 'Numerous other social narratives – all produced in particular social times and social spaces – interact to constitute the ontological narratives of those who live these times and spaces (narratives about gender, age, class, 'race', social status, place and so on).'

There are external discourses embedded within society. Somers (1994) refers to these as public narratives. Societal images of disability and associated values will affect the way both an individual and others perceive him- or herself. The discourses that individuals encounter in different life situations influence their self-concept and their understanding of disability as a social construct (Priestley in Corker and French, 1999).

Social construction of disability

It has been suggested that the medical model has had a profound and negative effect on the self-image of people with disabilities (Campbell and Oliver, 1996). Critics of this model state that it locates the problem with the person, instead of looking at the effects of social organization. For example, it is not the simple fact that the person with aphasia has limited ability to express their needs; it is the failure of society to accommodate difference (Dowling and Dolan, 2001).

The social construction of disability represents a move away from the idea that a person with disabilities *disables* those around them. Instead, the construction of disability is located within the strata of society (Dowling and Dolan, 2001). The importance that society attaches to membership of the mainstream social group is evidenced in three areas:

1) the study of eugenics – the strengthening of a biological group and the prevention of 'wrongful births' through prenatal screening, e.g. for Down's syndrome, euthanasia for people with a terminal illness;
2) the high value placed on physical fitness, image and cognitive function, gives rise to debates on human tragedies where someone who is disabled may be considered to be 'better off dead';
3) the low value that is accorded to disabled people, e.g. the seriousness of crimes against disabled people is often diminished so that the victim of rape is referred to as 'sexually abused'.

Media representation

Media portrayal of world events and legislative themes has an all-pervasive influence. One debate that has been going on for some time concerns people who have a mental health problem. The report of a few extreme cases, where fatalities to members of the public have occurred, has given rise to a powerful narrative that embraces the notions that: (i) mental illness means *violence*; (ii) community care means *killers on the loose*; (iii) mental illness means *crazy all the time* (Source: Mental Health Foundation video – Myths in Madness, 2000). Britain in 2002 saw a government-led debate about the introduction of new measures for the protection of the public. The fact that people with mental health problems are far more likely to self-harm than harm others is *not* the high-profile narrative.

Role of public narratives

Public narratives may alternately promote or constrain the development of identity. Images and icons used in charity advertising in the past have conveyed an image worthy of public pity and sorrow. Marks (1999: 167) argues that the demeaning portrayal of people with disabilities by charities contributes to their exclusion. A narrative that focuses on difference and abnormality reinforces the view that such individuals are outside the mainstream of society. The not uncommon view of disabled people as 'unfortunate, different, oppressed and sick' poses a direct challenge to some commonly held societal values, such as the importance of work in Western culture. This can lead to prejudice, which expresses itself in discrimination and oppression.

During the Victorian era, the popular public narrative regarding people with learning disabilities and mental health problems dealt with 'difference and abnormality' by segregating them from society. People were housed in large, long-stay institutions. These were indestructible environments with high fences and bars on the windows. Uniform provision meant a lack of privacy and opportunities to express self. Difference and abnormality translated into a subhuman class of people. In contrast, a narrative that is primarily centred on human beings and the civil liberties that are shared by all supports the *right* to a place in society. The dispersal of residents from large hospitals to community-based services in the 1980s sought to re-establish people with learning disabilities in society.

Power of language

If what Peters in Barton (1999) says is true about 'the power of language to convey values and beliefs' (p. 110) and 'language is linked to power and ideology' (p. 113), then its contribution to the divisions in society cannot be underestimated. Priestley in Corker and French (1999: 93) observes that during the course of any one day, a disabled child will come across different 'ways of speaking about disability' that will have an impact on personal experience and sense of self.

There are other disability narratives in the public arena that have been around a long time. The philanthropic model promotes the notion of personal tragedy. It endorses the types of narratives where disabled people are plucky, admirable, courageous, victims or heroes. The medical model incorporates stories where abnormality, rehabilitation and adjustment may feature. It gives rise to narratives where there is a desire to 'normalize' or to conceal any imperfection. More recently, there has been a conscious effort to focus on human rights rather than deficiencies, with alliances growing up between disability organizations and UK charities, e.g. Mencap and Scope (Marks, 1999).

Formation of attitudes

The interaction of life experience and public narratives gives rise to personal beliefs and value systems out of which attitudes are formed (French, 1996). Attitudes provoke intentions and behaviours. The observable behaviour of the person accessing the SLT service should be seen in this light: as a possible indication of internal thoughts and beliefs about the current situation or the reason for the referral. French identifies the three commonly cited components of attitude:

- cognitive, which refers to individual beliefs about an object or person;
- affective, which refers to the evaluation of an object or person according to prevailing ethical codes, social and cultural norms that make up an individual's value system;
- behavioural, which refers to the overt expression of inner judgement.

Beliefs may also be held at the level of institution and therefore inform particular professional behaviours. For instance, there are certain practices within care services that appear to promote dissociation from the people in receipt of care. Menzies Lyth (in Trist and Murray 1990) described various distancing devices used by nursing staff with patients in their care, including the use of reductionist language, e.g. 'the liver in bed 12', and the domination of standardized procedures that constrain individuality and spontaneity of practice. These practices might be explained by a desire to avoid becoming emotionally involved with the patient.

Conflicting narratives

Juxtaposing narratives may be part of the experience of disabled people and their significant others. Swain and Cameron in Corker and French (1999) draw parallels between the 'declaration of identity' by disabled people and the 'coming out' process experienced by many gay men and lesbian women: 'It is a declaration of belonging to a devalued group in society. Coming out has meaning against alternative processes of internalisation of dominant ideologies' (pp. 68–69).

The attitudes, beliefs and responses of significant others are a powerful source of influence over the way an individual responds. There is no guarantee of agreement between the accounts of family members and that of the individual. Conflicts may therefore occur. Depending on the maturation of the individual and the nature of their disability, there may be risks associated with aspects of lifestyle and the uptake of opportunities. Primary carers seeking to open up lifestyle opportunities to a child frequently have to weigh the benefits to the individual's independence against any possible risks (Seltzer et al., 2001). Similarly, the partner of an adult with an acquired disability may find it difficult to be a passive observer when a loved one asserts his/her independence. Despite existing potential or competencies, the individual's right to use them may not be recognized by other people, which in turn leads to disempowerment.

Importance of inclusion

Marks (1999) states that the shaping of our psyche is contingent on the range and quality of life experiences in the social environment. She refers to the *colonizing practice* that is commonly applied to people with disabilities and their exclusion from full citizenship. Borland and Ramcharan in Ramcharan et al. (1997: 88) identify two major types of identity: the 'excluded identity' and the 'included identity'. The concept of the 'excluded identity' is said to be a product of two inter-related themes: inclusion in society and the development of a self-concept. Although writing about people with learning disabilities, they assert the applicability of this maxim to all human beings. Self-awareness and identity is affected by social opportunity restrictions. Citing the studies of feral children who grow up outside human society, Borland and Ramcharan (1997) discuss the relevance of social group interaction and life experiences to the development of self-concept. When an individual or group of people are segregated from society for a long period of time, it may lead to 'irremediable breakdowns in capacity for reintegration and resocialisation' (p. 89).

Narrative identity

Thomas in Corker and French (1999) presents the personal narratives of disabled women. What comes across in each story, regardless of the nature of the person's disability, is the tension between personal experiences (ontological narrative) and the public narrative, i.e. the narratives that are commonly 'attached to cultural and institutional formations larger than the single individual' (Somers, 1994: 618). In each woman's story there is a strong sense of the ontological narrative being challenged by the public narratives of society. Discussing the narrative of 'Joan', who has ME, Thomas (1999) observes the interplay of two different types of public narrative:

(i) The shattering effect of the more negative perspective –

... public narratives about 'the impaired body and person': not normal, of lesser value, impaired people as other (p. 51).

(ii) The supportive perspective to counter the negative –

... those (narratives) told to her by other people with ME – and she found a way to re-tell her story to and of herself (p. 51).

Shared identity

Social identity refers to the characteristics shared by the members of a social group, e.g. people with learning disabilities, children with fluency problems, adults who have had a laryngectomy (Swain and Cameron in Corker and French, 1999). Membership of a group may be a double-edged sword. It may help people to identify the sources of oppression in society, to share experiences and embark on mutual problem-solving, and to mobilize social pressure for change. Conversely, it may also label the person in such a way that they are stigmatized by others in society, e.g. people with schizophrenia as a group are frequently vilified in the media.

Turning points

The advent of disability in a person's life may have far-reaching consequences. The continuation of a life-course pattern may be disrupted to varying extents, such that personal goals and aspirations may appear unattainable, and individual status and abilities seem unrecognizable or even worthless. These effects are not restricted to the person who experiences the change, but also include significant others:

> In life course theory, a turning point is conceptualised as a point when a person's life takes a sharply different direction. Having a child diagnosed with a disability is an example of such a turning point because parents' lives may be forever altered. (Seltzer et al., 2001: 266)

A lack of control

Eileen was a woman of 70. When she was 64 she was found to have base-of-the-tongue carcinoma for which she received extensive radiotherapy. As a result of this intervention, six years later she was no longer able to swallow safely apart from very thick purée. She was referred to SLT for advice regarding her dysphagia. Eileen was very upset at the side effects of her radiotherapy and said that nobody understood what it felt like to kill yourself slowly because you simply wanted a drink of water. For her, not having something as basic as a cup of tea was a major disruption to her life. She was, after all, a cup-of-tea person! There were clearly issues around Eileen's identity and her perceived lack of control in her life due to the emergence of problems six years *after* she thought she was past the worse.

Transitions

Griffiths (1994) observes that the transition of individuals with learning disabilities from adolescence to adulthood is a protracted and complex transition that does not encompass all aspects of life at once. Change is not a single event, but rather a series of small changes in status and recognition of progress towards adult status, which brings both new opportunities and varied responsibilities.

No matter whether the disability is acquired at a stage in an individual's life, e.g. as a consequence of stroke, or it is introduced incrementally into the family unit as in the case of the child diagnosed with a developmental problem, the life course of the individual and/or significant others will be affected. In each case, there is a turning point that will influence future directions of the life course, even though subtle differences may exist because of the *timing* of the change.

Challenges to self-concept

An individual's self-concept may be challenged by the onset and consequences of disease or trauma. Altered physical appearance, the impairment of skills, and difficulties in everyday functioning may affect the person's sense of self. The person, who was familiar before the onset of the life-changing event, may not be recognizable any more. Jordan and Kaiser (1996: 22) comment that 'A significant change in any one aspect of life is likely to lead to some modification of that self-image. Becoming disabled may affect every aspect of life.'

The effects of altered appearance

Deirdre was a 45-year-old woman who underwent a partial mandiblectomy and partial glossectomy as a result of facial cancer. She survived the surgery and presented as quite euphoric afterwards. A period of radiotherapy followed during which she approached her treatment sessions with noted stoicism. Her speech intelligibility was badly affected due to the disfigurement of her facial muscles and structures. She was subsequently referred to SLT. In an initial session she expressed her anger at those who had 'done it' to her. She referred to herself as having 'a face like a monkey' and questioned whether it had all been worth it. Her survival from cancer had in no way prepared her for her change in appearance and altered way of communicating. How Deirdre felt about herself and her experiences of the previous eight months were entwined with her communication difficulties.

Altered life course

Hogan in Corker and French (1999) highlights the altered direction of the person's life course and the change in customary social position. He comments on the relevance of both individual and social perspectives in shaping the identity of a person who experiences acquired disability: 'Acquired disability signals a massive change in a person's social position and constitutes a personal crisis for the individual. Identity as a social phenomenon becomes apparent as individuals are perceived by themselves and others as different' (p. 80).

The loss of language and communication skills may have a devastating effect on some people. Changes to lifestyle may result, such as altered status at home and work (Sarno, 1993). There may be a perceived reversal of roles between partners when one person becomes disabled, e.g. the management of household accounts switches from one to the other, or the major financial contribution shifts from husband to wife, any of which may challenge the established balance in a relationship. It may interfere with formerly held values in relation to self, i.e. the various ways that an individual measures personal worth. Parr et al. (1997: 112) state that 'The experience of aphasia suddenly interrupts the biography of the person who develops it. It is associated with many aspects of life: work; education; relationships; domestic organisation and even personal attributes such as wit and ease of conversation.'

Changed roles

Prior to his stroke, George managed a small firm of civil engineers. He was used to issuing instructions to his employees and managing multiple contracts of work simultaneously. At home, he was a dominant personality. His wife reported that he frequently had the casting vote in any disciplinary action to be taken with their two teenage children. After his stroke, George had a right-sided weakness and severe expressive aphasia. Suddenly, he was no longer manager at work or home. His wife assumed a co-ordinating role in terms of his support needs, as well as managing the discipline of their two children. His personal status had been severely disrupted on two major fronts: work and home. Furthermore, in the initial stages of his recovery, his wife observed the 'different' attitudes and behaviour of neighbours and friends, with pity and sorrow being the overriding emotions. George was reported as becoming withdrawn and morose during this period.

Family vulnerabilities

Encountering disability can affect the significant people in the family context:

> The normal life cycle can be disrupted for the first time when the family becomes aware of their child's disability. This can precipitate a crisis affecting the whole family, perhaps immobilising it for a time as members devote their energies to dealing with the powerful emotions that they are experiencing. (Porter and McKenzie, 2000: 48)

Certain vulnerabilities are exposed in families of a child who has a disability, particularly at times of transition. Porter and McKenzie (2000) identify a number of reasons for this. The parental experience of the child's initial diagnosis may resonate at transitional stages when anxieties about the next stage may surface. A lack of predictability in the disabled child's life course means that preparing for change is made difficult. Conversely, attempting to plan for transitional stages too early may also add to the stress experienced by the parent.

Comparisons may be made between the familiar service that is left behind and the new, less familiar service that is introduced. The experience of uncertainty about the services on offer, the emotional maturation of the child and the changing of needs over time is common (Hanley-Maxwell, Whitney-Thomas and Mayfield Pogoloff, 1995).

Family relationships

The advent of disability may bring about a shift in family relationships and the designation of roles. The people who are in close and regular contact with the individual are vulnerable to the effects of change, whether it is parent–child, husband–wife, partners or siblings. Porter and McKenzie (2000) observe that as a child's disability comes to the notice of the family unit, tensions may be widespread. The change in circumstances may threaten existing patterns of daily life.

Transactional effects of the individual's experiences on the responses of family members have been reported. Olney and Kim (2001) comment that an individual's uncertainty and doubt may be reflected in the responses of others. The challenge of living with disability may cause significant others to assert the importance of a realistic approach to personal goals and expectations. The desire for a loved one to succeed runs alongside a wish to protect them from struggle and disappointment.

Sources of stress

Porter and McKenzie (2000) identify a number of stressors in the families of children with disabilities. The particular needs of the child may compete with the demands of other family members, the roles that individuals used to play before the turning point, and external pressures in the community and society. The time involved in devoting parental energies to a disabled child's care may leave less time for other family relationships, e.g. between parents, between siblings and between parent and child. The perceived value that is attached to the time and attention given to the person with a disability may engender feelings of resentment amongst siblings and other family members. Hayes in Ashman and Elkins (1998) observes that dealing with the reactions of other family members is sometimes more difficult for the parents than managing their own responses. Family constructs may alter and roles may be reconfigured, although this is by no means inevitable (Porter and McKenzie, 2000).

Isolation and discrimination

Providing support for a child or adult with a disability can be an isolating and lonely experience. Parents who are the primary carers of disabled children are vulnerable to various mental health crises (Dowling and Dolan, 2001). Care demands may compromise lifestyle. It may be harder for the primary carer to organize alternative care for the child, both practically and emotionally.

The sometimes devaluing experience of having a disability is not always confined to the individual. Significant others or those in regular, close contact with the disabled person may also experience discrimination in society. As Goffman (1963: 43) points out, 'The loyal spouse of the mental patient, the daughter of the ex-con, the parent of the cripple ... share some of the discredit of the stigmatised person.'

Making sense of disability

Those affected by a 'turning point' in an individual's life will have a unique perspective on the situation. It is the discrete identity of the person and their incumbent strategies for dealing with transformed circumstances that colour a response to change. Olney and Kim (2001) explored the ways in which people with disparate diagnostic labels make sense of their disability. Three processes were considered to be critical to the integration of all aspects of self:

- self-definition;
- appraisal of individual abilities and limitations;
- management of the perceptions of others (pp. 568–569).

Complex process

Making sense of disability is an extremely complex process. Parr et al. (1997) observe that people with aphasia use different identities and accounts of aphasia according to the situation in which they find themselves. Certain features may affect an individual's internal accommodation of difference and/or change in life course.

Type of disability and its visibility

The extent to which a disability is perceived as visible and the type of disability may be factors in self-recognition and the perceptions of others. There are both advantages and disadvantages to be gained from having a hidden disability (Olney and Kim, 2001). There may be the chance for greater control of identity when a person's disability is not obvious to others. They are less vulnerable to the negative attributions of others simply because the disability is concealed from public view; however, this can also represent a barrier to the person who seeks assistance from others. Shakespeare, Gillespie-Sells and Davies (1996) comment that the person whose disability is not obvious is less likely to *come out* as disabled because it is easier to pass as *normal*. The lack of obvious disability may lead to questions and doubts expressed by both the individual and others concerning the legitimacy of the individual's need.

Conversely, the visibility of a disability may provoke immediate judgements based solely on the individual's appearance, e.g. the implication is that the person who is profoundly physically disabled must also be of limited intellect. Holloway (2001) comments that the positive experiences reported by disabled university students were largely attributed to their learning needs being recognized by staff and through the provision of appropriate equipment. Therefore it would seem that some sort of balance between recognition of need and assertion of personal rights is desirable.

Perspectives on disability and view of what is 'normal'

Disability affects the level of competence regarded as necessary for achieving former or age-equivalent status. Society has a set of normal standards for competence in the adult world. It is assumed that adults can manage their own personal care, handle money and tell the time, get about independently, read and write, develop social relationships with those that matter, to name but a few!

The parent whose child is failing to keep up with peers experiences frequent reminders of the child's delayed development and any abnormalities in social behaviour. Childhood peers in school or in the local neighbourhood provide natural comparators. The accepted view of 'normality' may be at variance with the reality of the child's development. The individual may be precluded from the same achievements as others because of limited access to learning experiences, and his or her right to use competencies not being recognized by others. Olney and Kim point out that 'Assumptions and attitudes of others can have a strong influence on self-perception, causing individuals to feel guilt, anxiety, self-doubt and ambivalence, particularly in regards to receiving assistance' (Olney and Kim, 2001: 564).

Environmental factors

Baker and Donnelly (2001) observe that children with disabilities are more likely to have social experiences of a poorer quality than their peers. They suggest that inclusive education in itself is not sufficient to guarantee positive social experiences. Diverse environmental factors contribute to the degree of success or failure in a child's social encounters, including the attitudes of others and the teaching–learning infrastructure of the educational establishment.

The person with an acquired disability may feel the pressure to resume the activities and occupations that were part of their lifestyle before the onset of their difficulties. A return to *normality* may be the principal measure of successful rehabilitation. Individuals and significant others are driven by the desire to resume a previous life course from the point at which it was disrupted.

Dealing with difference

Barnes in Hales (1996) recounts his personal experiences of living with a visual impairment. He recalls that he 'only acquired a sense of difference when I went to school' (p. 38). The theme of segregation recurs throughout his narrative as he is transferred from special boarding school to the 'partially sighted unit' where 'the sense of being somehow abnormal was only marginally less oppressive' because he was now living at home. Barnes identifies at least three strategies he used to overcome his visual impairment:

1) Minimization, whereby he developed the use of particular techniques in pursuit of the appearance of normality.
2) Overcompensation, whereby he developed 'socially valued attributes to deflect from subjective limitations' such as putting in more hours than the average worker (p. 40).
3) Openness, whereby he was honest about his visual difficulties and revealed them in the public arena such as soliciting the help of staff in the university library.

He recommends the last strategy as the only really effective way of dealing with the experience of disability and states that, although not simply achieved, 'This is something that can only be learned from people with similar experiences' (p. 43).

Adjustment

Adjustment would seem to be an active process that runs through the cycle of intervention. What does the term 'adjustment' mean? Research into the self-perception of people with disabilities has largely concentrated on the experiences of those with physical disabilities (Olney and Kim, 2001). Livneh (1991) developed a unified theory of adaptation comprising five distinct stages. It describes a process of changing self-awareness and internal conflict resolution that starts with the initial impact, defence mobilization followed by initial realization, then retaliation and finally reintegration.

Reorganization of personal constructs

Naugle, in Martinelli and Dell Orto (1991: 142), defines adjustment as 'a reordering of priorities and a reintegration of the self with a renewed sense of self worth'.

This seems to infer a reorganization of personal constructs in the light of the experience of disability. Charmaz (1995) makes a clear distinction between *living with disability* as opposed to living for it. It is about incorporating the effects of disability into the sense of self. This implies that lifestyle experiences are not separate from disability experiences – disability is a part of who the person is.

Adaptation on a continuum

Various models have been put forward to explain the process that parents go through in accommodating their child's disability. Hornby in Mitchell and Brown (1991) proposed the stage model of adaptation to loss. Parents are thought to pass through a continuum of reactions as their feelings towards the child develop. Although the experience is qualitatively different for every parent, certain phases have been identified in the literature (Cunningham and Davis, 1985; Hornby in Mitchell and Brown, 1991; Gompertz in Fawcus, 1997).

Not a normalizing process!

Adjustment does not refer to a 'normalizing' process whereby the individual learns to conform to familial and societal constructs. That is not to say that society and culture do not influence the ways we respond to change and difference – they do. The immediate value system of the family and the broader constructs of society provide the conditions for adjustment. Olney and Kim (2001) point out that the literature on disability and adjustment tends to confine itself to the limitations brought about by an individual's disability, rather than the attitudes of self and others towards disability. The latter is surely important to the construction of self-perception and the discernment of others.

A continuous process

Adjustment is not a fixed entity, i.e. you've either adjusted to this turning point in your life or you haven't! It is a continuous process of accommodation and resolution in relation to an inconstant environment. As new situations are experienced and different social contacts are made, so the individual and significant others shape their responses.

Reconnecting life

Nigel was a 42-year-old man. He worked as a sales representative for a firm marketing sports equipment. Nigel was single and enjoyed socializing and flirting with women. He was a good-looking man who was popular with women. Following a diagnosis of carcinoma of the larynx, he had a full laryngectomy. Nigel felt that when he lost his natural voice, he also lost his sense of self because now he had to do 'different things' to communicate. Nigel had surgical voice restoration and subsequently achieved good speech, but the disruption to his identity remained. One year later, he still refused contact with the professionals involved in his care, the exception being the SLT. There had been a complete absence of predisposing factors in his history and Nigel was in a state of disbelief at what had happened to him. He was also angry and felt 'hard done by', questioning the competence of those who had managed his case. An early misdiagnosis by the GP had meant a delay in Nigel's treatment and consequently much of his anger and resentment was directed at the medical profession.

Nigel attended SLT on a once-weekly basis that moved to twice weekly at certain critical points in his rehabilitation. In the initial stages, he rejected outright the idea of receiving counselling. Accordingly, SLT focused on the concrete and mechanical use of his 'restored' voice mechanism. Although the therapist recognized his need for expert input from the counselling service, she also acknowledged that he was not ready for this. Although therapy sessions concentrated on direct voice work, by the very nature of the work the sessions also involved 'talk', which was important

to the development of much-needed trust between Nigel and those in a
position to help him. Early on he stated that he preferred to text the therapist regarding his appointment times because, as he stated, 'text is more
normal – everybody does it'.

Issues to do with the loss of Nigel's natural voice gradually crept into
the sessions: he revealed that when his voice had been removed, he felt
as if the surgeons had physically ripped out his identity as well – the person he used to recognize as himself. It bothered him that no woman
would find him attractive any more. Later he started to pose questions
such as 'What am I going to do with the rest of my life?' At this stage, the
therapist successfully negotiated with Nigel to let in another professional,
a counsellor. His counsellor was also a qualified Macmillan nurse and
Nigel embarked on a journey of reconnecting his life with her support.

This case emphasizes the importance of a holistic approach to therapy.
Where loss or change is part of the individual's experience, the identity of
the person is as much in the foreground as the communication skills.
Continuation of life course is made possible by consideration of all the
factors that impinge on the person's current condition, e.g. in the case of
Nigel, the lack of predisposing factors for the cancer, the misdiagnosis at
the level of general practice, the perceived change in self-image before
and after surgery, the sense of loss experienced by Nigel, running alongside a sense of disbelief, all contribute to a profile of complex and
intertwined issues.

Transitions in dealing with loss

Walker (1995), writing about the transitions that feature in the recovery of
the sexual abuse survivor, identifies a resolution process that leads to the
expression of grief and mourning before healing, forgiving and moving on.
In the earlier stages, it involves reflecting on and understanding what has
happened, trusting oneself, and relating the experience to the broader context of one's life in an effort to make sense of it, before the outlet of anguish.

These stages could be equated with the experiences of the adult who
becomes aphasic as the result of stroke or the person who has had a laryngectomy and must rely on alternative means of voice production. In both
cases, the individual develops some understanding of the cause and
nature of their changed circumstances. Information is provided at critical
stages in the intervention to support a growing understanding of what
has happened (in the case of the person who has had a stroke) or what
will happen (in the case of the impending surgical removal of the person's larynx). Trusting oneself implies a belief in one's own ability to
respond to the new set of circumstances. It is about getting in touch with
one's own sense of self in order to understand all that has happened. The
individual draws on resources in the context of his or her lifestyle. Loss is
appreciated in this way and the expression of grief and mourning
commences. Walker's final stage of healing, forgiving and moving on does

not signal the closure of the resolution process. It is stressed that an individual may revisit any of these stages during the transformation process.

Parenting a child with a disability

The early emotional bonding between parent and child who has been newly diagnosed with a disability may be a vulnerable time. In the early stages, parental expectations of a normal infant who will fulfil his/her potential are challenged. Parental accounts by interview have revealed a range of emotions at the time of diagnostic disclosure, including sadness, disbelief, anger, sorrow, revulsion, inadequacy, helplessness and guilt (Ayer and Alaszewski, 1984; Byrne, Cunningham and Sloper, 1988; Lucas and Lucas, 1980; Rendall, 1997). The manner and timing of disclosure and the availability of relevant information are crucial factors in the parental experience. Even after the adaptation process has reached the stage of acceptance, it is thought that most parents experience feelings of grief and sorrow at different intervals during their child's life.

Several writers conclude that rather than working through a grieving process and resolving some feelings, parents of disabled children actually experience *chronic sorrow* (Lucas and Lucas, 1980; Quine and Rutter, 1994). Some parents react by refusing to accept the diagnosis, hoping there has been some mistake. Parents may elect to disregard the advice of the professional, carrying on as if nothing has happened, refusing all offers of help. This temporary coping strategy is considered a key stage in the process, unless it becomes prolonged, thereby delaying adaptation (Hornby in Mitchell and Brown, 1991). It is assumed that not all parents will experience *all* of the phases and that there may be 'oscillation' between several of them (Gompertz in Fawcus, 1997).

Resonance of early parenting experiences

Teresa describes her early experiences of having a child diagnosed with Down's syndrome. Both the pregnancy and birth had been uneventful, although Teresa recalls thinking something was not quite right immediately after giving birth to her daughter. Formal diagnosis 24 hours after the birth of her daughter left Teresa with juxtaposing feelings: she was aware that she should be enjoying her newly born child but at the same time was aware of negative feelings. Her husband Declan remembers experiencing similar internal discord that was augmented by a feeling of remoteness from what was happening. Both comment on the perceived inability of medical staff to cope with the situation, recalling the quick and clinical way that the diagnosis was communicated. Once Teresa and her baby returned home, contact with other parents in the local Down's syndrome association provided some much-needed support, empathy based on real experience, and useful information. Some years later, Teresa's early experiences resonate as her daughter grows up and life-course changes have to be addressed.

Implications for intervention

A carefully planned and executed intervention needs to be sensitive to the emotional state of the client and significant others. The psychological wellbeing of all concerned is dependent, in part, on recognizing possible factors that may feed in to anxiety levels, and making sure that a strategic response is in place.

Information about condition

Limited knowledge and incomplete understanding regarding the existing situation may compound the vulnerability of both clients and significant others. Ignorance or misplaced beliefs about what the problem is can only serve to fuel anxieties and concerns. Responding to and dealing with the disabling condition is dependent on individual understanding of what 'it' is.

Need for information

Parr et al. (1997: 88–89) identified a long list of things that people with aphasia want to know, ranging from the 'cause of the stroke' and 'prospect of recovery' in the immediate aftermath of a stroke, to the type and availability of 'services, aids and adaptations' in the coming-home-period, to 'how to maintain and monitor health and how to prevent another stroke' in the longer term. The therapist provides information that is accessible to the individual and seeks to fill the critical gaps in the person's knowledge base. For some people, obtaining information is crucial: '(it) can bring about a feeling of reassurance, a sense of being in control and able to understand and accept what has happened' (Parr et al., 1997: 89).

Not everyone requires the same level of detail, and information needs may change over time. There are a variety of reasons why a person experiences difficulty in taking in information as it is offered to them by professionals. It may be difficult for individuals and significant others to process what is being said when they are in a state of shock. Cunningham and Glenn in Lane and Stratford (1985) provide some useful advice. They observe that if the diagnosis (e.g. of Down's syndrome) is communicated in a sensitive and constructive manner, parents tend to adapt more quickly and establish a more positive relationship with the child, each other and with professionals. This is consistent with Parr et al. (1997: 90) who suggest that 'The amount and type of information offered needs to be determined with sensitivity to the needs and feelings of the individual.'

Communication style

The manner in which information is provided is, of course, very important to acceptance and adjustment in the long term. In 1996, Mencap reported the results of a large-scale survey of parental experiences of diagnostic disclosure. They found that only 15 per cent of parents described professionals as 'encouraging about the future', with most describing the disability in terms of what the child will *not* be able to do. The manner in which the professional communicates information has been identified as a source of dissatisfaction. Of the parents interviewed during the 50-year span of the Mencap study, only 23 per cent described the person diagnosing as 'knowledgeable'.

Reasons for dissatisfaction vary according to personal experience, but the most causes include: the professional not listening or not appearing to listen (Baron, 1985); the professional using jargon which confuses and alienates the parents, often leading to misunderstandings (Barnlund, 1976) and misinterpretation (Wilson, 1980); and the professional talking down to the patient.

Careful consideration of language and terminology used by professionals is a requirement. Where concepts and issues are difficult to grasp, a follow-up meeting to address any points of ambiguity or confusion should be offered. Rendall (1997) states that tact, truthfulness and empathetic guidance are basic requirements, with appropriate use of terminology and regular follow-up by a person with specialist knowledge.

Making sense of what has happened

Parr et al. (1997) provide the narrative account of 'Alf' to highlight the particular and diverse needs of people with aphasia. Alf recalls the difficult time he spent in hospital immediately after having had a stroke. His understandable confusion was compounded by the lack of information he needed to comprehend his altered circumstance. He recounts:

> I thought at first they were trying to put me in an asylum. That's what I actually thought – I didn't know the place. I always knew it as somewhere you died. I didn't know it was a rehabilitation place ... I thought they were putting me in there to give up the struggle. (Parr et al., 1997: 94)

It is recommended that the same information be presented in multiple ways, e.g. written copies, verbal presentation, pictures, etc. The same is true of almost any person who walks through the SLT door. Information should be handled in a flexible and imaginative way that is respectful of the skills, abilities, emotional state, values and cultural background of the individual.

Need for privacy

Another significant feature is 'privacy'. Diagnostic disclosure in an 'unsuitable' location is a frequently cited characteristic of the procedure experienced by the parent of the child with special needs (Ayer and Alaszewski, 1984; Cunningham, Morgan and McGucken, 1984; Rendall,

1997). Cases are illustrated where parents are told in a ward full of people, with only the curtains pulled round the bed for privacy. The exchange of critical information, sometimes of a highly sensitive nature, is best conducted in a secluded place that is conducive to the individual's expression of inner feelings (Rendall, 1997).

Timing of information giving

The aphasic people taking part in the Parr et al. (1997) study commented that information needs vary as circumstances change. This implies that checks on individual requirements should be an ongoing process. Cunningham, Morgan and McGucken (1984) were concerned with the disclosure of Down's syndrome. They identified some guiding principles for a model service based on published research and parental accounts. Parents wish to be told as soon as possible, together, in a private, direct, honest and sympathetic way, and to have immediate access to services that provide comprehensive and accurate support and guidance (Cunningham and Davis, 1985; Hornby in Mitchell and Brown, 1991). Evaluation of the policy in action revealed 100 per cent satisfaction from those parents receiving the model delivery compared with only 20 per cent satisfaction from the control group.

Relevant agencies

Once an adequate level of information has been established, it may be appropriate to access other relevant support agencies. It may mean a referral to another member of the multi-professional team or to a different agency, e.g. counselling. Waiting lists may compound the anxiety felt by individuals.

> Families of disabled children still face many barriers when they try to access social services. It is difficult for them to find out what services are available and support may only be offered when a situation has reached crisis point. Parents have to tell 'their story' to a range of professionals to receive all the support they need. (DoH, 1998: 1)

Threat of professional dominance

Primary relationships with the individual with a disability may be threatened by professional dominance. Those care functions that a parent or loved one naturally assumes, may be taken over by the 'experts'. Partnership working practice between professionals and family members, which involves sensitive negotiation, may avoid the pitfalls of professional dominance.

Consideration of identity and emotional state

The individual's identity and emotional state is central to the intervention process. Parr et al. (1997) describe the ongoing process whereby individuals navigate their unique life courses, reflecting on the past, digesting the present and anticipating forthcoming events on the horizon. The dynamic energy of the 'lived' biography means that new events are likely to affect its course. The advent of a speech, language or communication difficulty represents a new challenge to which an individual's life course is not immune. It follows that there are certain principles that guide the therapist's work.

Values and personal attributes

The therapist has a role in affirming the value, self-worth and -esteem of individuals. This is achieved by a heightened awareness of the person's social and cultural background, skills, abilities and potential, whilst not ignoring the difficulties and obstacles that need to be overcome. The intervention process is sensitive to the personal attributes and the unique value systems of the client and significant others:

- There is acknowledgement of individual entitlement to assert views and express feelings. Conversational floor is shared with the individual, and the therapist is an active and attentive listener.
- Each stage within the intervention cycle is negotiated between client and therapist, from referral, through assessment and therapy activities (including goal setting), to closure. The individual's role is one of valued partner and contributor in the intervention process. Each stage is subject to alteration based on the immediate needs and reactions of the client at the centre of the process.
- The therapeutic process is one of mutual social co-ordination. The SLT contributes professional knowledge and skills, whilst the individual also brings his or her own expertise to the situation.
- A wide range of learning opportunities and materials based on the individual's interests, strengths and life experiences are employed.

Milieu of communication

The nature of SLT means that the individual is brought into communicative contact with another human being. Expression of innermost thoughts and feelings is possible. The very process of communication will reveal something of the person's internal state and, as such, puts the therapist in the position of responsive listener. The therapist supports the individual's efforts to make sense of the situation they find themselves in by: (a) Identifying opportunities for the person to meet other people with similar experiences, both in therapy groups or else in support groups;

and (b) acknowledging and giving vent to the individual's cultural, personal and social interests through the types of activities selected.

Of course, there are some individuals who experience emotional struggle that requires special help that goes beyond the psychosocial support embedded in the speech and language therapy session. It is important that such needs are recognized by the therapist and a referral to an appropriate agency is made.

Chapter 4
Construction of intervention

Constructing intervention is a complicated process. It involves the on-going and timely appraisal of all the relevant information about an individual. This is then organized into a profile situated in the person's life course. Key decisions are taken for the appropriate design of an intervention plan that will build on the person's existing skills and related attributes, and address any areas of difficulty.

Bray, Ross and Todd (1999: 97) identify the main decision areas in a flowchart designed to channel the therapist's thinking (Figure 4.1). Aspects of therapy planning are demarcated in chronological order, e.g. from assessment to long-term aims, from short-term aims to objectives. A series of connecting arrows defines the relationship between the key aspects in the decision-making process, e.g. long-term aims relate to the outcomes/criteria for success.

Articulation of the therapy planning process means addressing many questions:

- What aspects of the individual profile are important to focus on?
- Where do I target the intervention?
- What informs my selection of a particular approach to intervention?
- How do I optimize therapeutic effectiveness and generalization of outcomes?
- Who needs to be involved in the therapy process and how should this be managed?
- Which facilitation techniques should I build into the intervention programme?
- How do I know where to go next?

Addressing these questions involves clinical reasoning that underpins key decision-making.

Clinical decisions

Decision-making provides the infrastructure for constructing intervention and has been described as 'an art based on data gathering and interpreting' (Gerard and Carson, 1990: 61). It involves the reasoned selection of

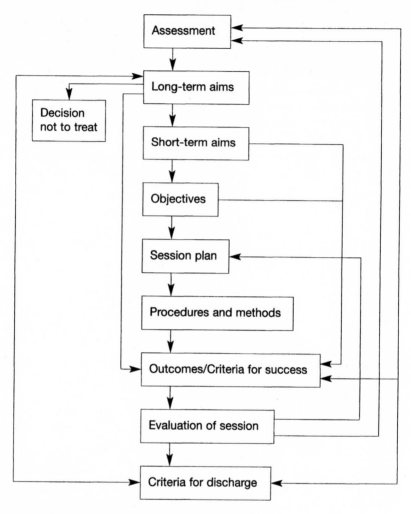

Figure 4.1 A flowchart of the therapy planning process
(Source: Bray, Ross and Todd, 1999: 97)

methods for collecting information, the systematic review of available data
from a wide range of sources, interpretation of data with reference to the
person and lifestyle, and prioritization of communication aspects that will
provide a focus for intervention activities. Williamson (2001: 4) places
judgement and decision-making at the centre of professional practice.
They are supported by knowledge and skills, and personal/professional
values and beliefs, thereby enabling the therapist to select the best course
of action and deal with each new situation as it arises.

Clinical reasoning

Clinical reasoning is about the organization of knowledge into patterns
that are both relevant and meaningful to client and therapist (Higgs,

1992). It involves the consideration of multiple factors (Ryan, 1995). In this way the therapist manipulates the available data (what is known about the individual at the precise point in time) and cross-refers to the broader store of theoretical and professional knowledge. Cultural bias and personal values will affect the stream of logic applied by a therapist to a given situation (Ryan, 1995; Williamson, 2001). This means that no one therapist is likely to reason exactly the same course of action with the same client.

Every intervention journey experienced by an individual should be underpinned by decisions that are the outcome of ongoing negotiation between client and therapist. This is why Higgs (1992) identifies not only data collection skills but also interpersonal skills as a critical part of the effective reasoning process. The contributions of the therapist are prompted by a professional knowledge base; the contributions of the client are informed by the expertise gathered from living with a communication disability. This combines what Schell and Cervero (1993) refer to as 'scientific reasoning' and 'narrative reasoning'. Appropriate use of interpersonal skills ensures that the two correspond and that co-operative decision-making between therapist and client is achieved. It is the conscious act of reasoning that ensures that the client is both listened to and has the opportunity to influence the intervention journey.

A systems view of decision-making

The frameworks offered by systems science have been used to capture and externalize decision-making processes in health care. Cramp and Carson (1985) defined the 'patient care loop' and identified the basic constituents as:

> ... the controlled process, that is the patient; the information system ... transmitting basic information concerning the controlled process; a control unit (the doctor, an element comparing information from the information system with the desired performance of the patient and taking corrective action if necessary); an activating unit (junior medical and nursing staff, who effect any changes required) (pp. 246–247).

Gerard and Carson (1990) adapted these elements describing the decision-making process in child language assessment, where the control unit is represented by the therapist and the activating unit comprises the people within the child's communication environment. Deutsch, Carson and Ludwig (1994: 5) depict the patient management process as a feedback loop 'whereby decisions are made based on a comparison of information concerning the actual state of the patient with the desired state' (Figure 4.2). Instead of control unit they refer to 'clinical decision-making'; for activation unit they use 'effecting the clinical decision'; for information system they use 'information gathering' which links the 'patient' into the therapeutic process.

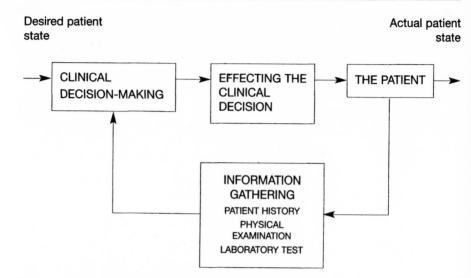

Figure 4.2 Depiction of the therapeutic process as a feedback loop
(Source: Deutsch, Carson and Ludwig, 1994: 4)

Based on the work of these authors, the decision-making process in SLT
is represented as a series of interconnecting components (Figure 4.3).
The *individual* (**A1**), i.e. person with a communication difficulty and/or
significant other(s), occupies a central place. The *environment* (**A2**) is
viewed in conjunction with the individual's characteristics and personal
attributes. The *individual profile* (**B**) represents the growing bank of
knowledge about the individual's communication skills, relevant medical,
developmental and psychosocial profile, and occupational, personal and
family background. It reflects aspects of the individual's identity and life
course. The *mediating role of therapist* (**C**) refers to the input of the
speech and language therapist here, but may also include other members
of the team as appropriate. Comparisons are made between the existing
state of the client (the individual profile) and the desired or targeted outcomes of the intervention. The *activation of change* (**D**) refers to the
process whereby change is brought about according to individual needs.
It is variously focused on prevention, promotion and/or maintenance.

Levels of decision-making

Two levels are defined within the SLT decision-making system. These are
viewed as distinct but overlapping cycles of movement where information
is passed from component to component in a constant process of appraisal and review. The first level is referred to as the *information flow* (see
Figure 4.4) and the second as the *activation process* (see Figure 4.6; p. 88).

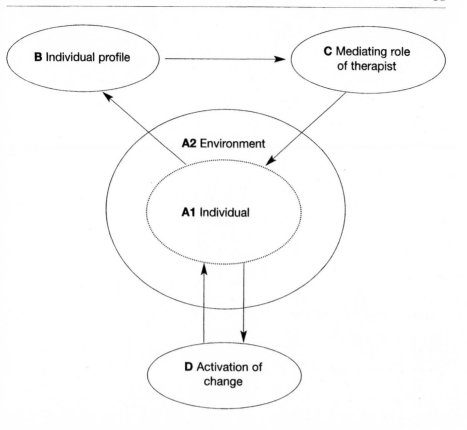

Figure 4.3 Interconnecting elements of the decision-making system in SLT

Level 1: Information flow

The information flow is depicted in the **A B C** cycle shown in Figure 4.4. The cycle has no fixed starting point and no terminus: the correspondence is from therapist to individual or individual to therapist, and then to the individual profile and so on. Implicit in the process is:

- The release of information from and by the individual and/or significant other(s), either as part of an intentional act or revealed unintentionally through the interaction process. It contributes to the growing bank of information that is the individual profile.
- The therapist analyses this information and interprets it for unbiased presentation to the client.
- The individual reviews the information and may challenge, modify, reject or concur with different aspects. Further information is therefore released into the system, and the flow of information continues.

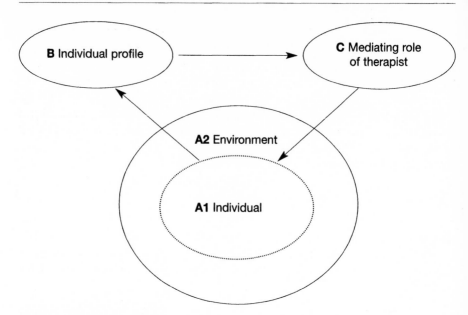

Figure 4.4 Information flow

Individual and environment

Consistent with Bronfenbrenner's (1979) ecological model of human development cited in Chapter 1, the reciprocal influence of environment and individual is considered. Appraisal of the family context, the value system of the immediate and wider community, and 'the impact of political resource factors' are all important (Ballard in Mitchell and Brown, 1991: 142). Dockrell and Messer (1999) identify two reasons for looking at the individual in context: first, the type and quality of experiences a child has can affect the way their language skills develop; and, second, there may be considerable variation in the ways a child's difficulties are interpreted across contexts. This is applicable across the range of client groups, for example, the experiences of an adult with acquired language impairment may vary with context, and affect recovery and use of residual skills over time; living in a poor-quality environment with a low level of stimulation will affect the engagement skills of the person with a learning disability.

Transactional approach

Development and functioning are seen as the outcomes of reciprocal interaction between the individual and environment. In keeping with a transactional approach, the underlying impairment is not viewed as an ever-present obstacle to progress: both the person and the environment change because of the mutuality of influences (Ballard in Mitchell and Brown, 1991). There is 'the ongoing interplay between a changing individual and a changing environment' (McCool, citing Bell, 1968, in McCartney, 1999: 155).

The social environments that any one individual moves in are defined by the distinct nature and stage of life course. Generally, as the life course progresses, so the social horizons broaden. The pre-school child's main social context exists within the family, and gradually moves outwards in correspondence with maturation and a broadening of human relationships, through the primary and secondary education systems, to the adult world of further or higher education and employment. At the other end of the spectrum, retirement may bring a narrowing of horizons as occupational and recreational networks recede.

Individual characteristics

Naturally, individual characteristics such as the age of the person, the nature and severity of the communication difficulty, and any causal and/or maintaining factors must be considered (Dodd, 1995); however, attention should also be given to the following aspects in relation to client and significant others:

- The degree of awareness, understanding and acknowledgement that a problem exists.
- The psychological or emotional state of all those concerned.
- The levels of general stimulation in the environment, including current communication practice, which may alternately inhibit or ameliorate development (Horowitz and Haritos, 1998).
- Motivational factors or the desire to participate in therapy.
- The philosophical orientation of the client's main context or 'informal culture' and any values that may influence practice (Hastings and Remington, 1994).
- The infrastructure of the client's context and relevant accountability procedures (McCartney, 1999).

Individual profile

The individual profile is an information system that has been derived from a range of sources. Its size and density will vary across time and as the cycle of intervention progresses. Release of information about and from the individual is dependent on the following variables.

Emotional state

The emotional state of the person contributing information will variously affect their confidence and willingness to share experiences and knowledge. The parent who is in a high state of anxiety about his or her child's development may find it difficult to voice concerns. The adult with acquired language impairment, who is also depressed, may feel disinclined to share their own experiences or to participate in assessment activities that might expose any communication difficulties. The paid carer who has a lack of formal training and/or limited experience of working with the client may be nervous about expressing his or her views and observations to the professional.

Relationship

The relationship between therapist and client/significant others is crucial to the timely release of relevant information. A positive rapport provides a fertile backdrop for the exchange of confidences and relevant details. Many therapists use planned informality in initial interviews, where active listening and sensitive responding to the person's narrative occur (see Pound et al., 2000). This is designed to put the person at ease and to encourage disclosure of real experiences.

Conversely, an initial contact in which the therapist moves through a battery of formal, structured assessments carries the risk of constraining the flow of information. This is not to say that structured assessments do not contribute to the information system – they do. They are tools that help the therapist to extend what is known about an individual by focusing on a particular aspect of their communication skills and functioning; however, the mistimed use of such tools may compromise the information system because the client is not in an appropriate state to respond optimally. Familiarity with a situation and the other players is likely to affect responding behaviours.

Setting variables

Clearly, there are some general setting variables that will influence the course of interaction between therapist and client. With reference to Hargie (1997), the factors of influence include:

- The goal structure or the reason why the interactants find themselves in that situation and any personal beliefs, e.g. the client who is there for a 'cure', the therapist who believes she holds 'the answer'!
- The different roles that are played by the participants: the service provider and the person who requires something from that service; the professional and the client; the therapist and the person who is an expert based on their own experience of communication disability.
- The implicit rules of the situation that determine the focus of the interaction and associated use of communication skills.
- The repertoire of communication behaviours that are acceptable or appropriate for the situation.
- The nature of the physical environment in terms of its attributes: the degree of comfort offered by the setting and furnishings, the physical orientation of client to therapist.
- The language and concepts that are part of the situation, e.g. the therapist who uses technical language risks ostracizing the client by the introduction of such a barrier.
- The cultural milieu of the situation and whether it reflects the client's own culture (see Chapter 2).

Interpersonal communication

The individual contributions and communication styles of therapist and client will have a mutual effect. Each brings different knowledge, experience, attitudes and expectations to the situation. The therapist picks up verbal and non-verbal information about the individual by actively observing and listening, and shapes responses accordingly. Becker, Heimberg and Bellack (1987), discussing social skills training, might have been writing about the interaction requirements of the SLT: 'To perform skilfully, the individual must be able to identify the emotions or intent expressed by the other person and make sophisticated judgements about the form and timing of the appropriate response' (p. 9).

Hargie in Hargie (1997: 32) presents an extended model of interpersonal interaction that demonstrates the mutuality of the social communication process. It illustrates the multiple pathways of feedback: how we receive feedback not only through our own actions on the environment but also through the perceived actions of others. In this way the individual goals of one interactant are modified by the actions of the other. The model is reproduced in Figure 4.5, focusing specifically on the relationship between therapist and client/significant other(s). Annotations have been added to define the routes of feedback.

Person–intervention context

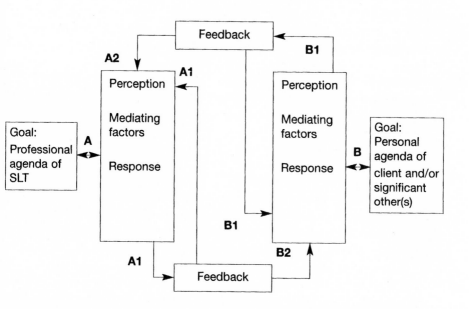

Figure 4.5 Interpersonal communication in the intervention context (Adapted from the extended model of interpersonal communication: Hargie in Hargie, 1997)

Underlying goals

Each interactant enters the intervention context with an underlying purpose or goal (A/B). The goals may not be obvious to the interactants initially, but become clearer through the process of interaction and feedback. The therapist enters the situation with a professional agenda that is supported by theoretical knowledge, clinical skills and experience. The client and/or significant other enters the situation with personal expertise in relation to communication difficulty, self-knowledge and life skills, and personal experience. This is regardless of age, maturity or ability. Just as an adult with aphasia is the authority on their communication skills because it is part of their life-course experience, so the child brings expert knowledge of what it is like to be a child, to play and learn, and to go to school.

Mediating factors

The perceptions of each interactant are subject to mediating factors such as past experience, acquired knowledge, and current psychological state. These will affect individual perceptions of the situation and consequential responses.

Feedback

Feedback occurs simultaneously and at different levels in an interaction. It arises from our own contributions to the situation as well as the responses of the other person.

The feedback loop **A1/B1** provides information about our own performance. It is a form of self-monitoring. This enables a poorly worded utterance to be amended before the other person has a chance to respond;

The feedback loop **A1–B2/B1–A2** represents the feedback gained from the responses of the other interactant. Information about the effects of our contribution is gauged in terms of how we perceive the other person's reaction;

In this way, each person monitors his/her own responses *and* the concomitant responses of the other person. Self-monitoring may be difficult for the person with a communication difficulty. It is incumbent on the therapist to use a skilful communication style that is sensitive, encouraging and responsive. Faulty management of the feedback loops will lead to insecurities in the interaction process and may inhibit the build-up of the information system.

Communication parameters

The linguistic demands that are placed on the client and the timing of those demands are relevant to compiling the information system. There may be natural constraints in the set demands of a structured assessment procedure. Furthermore, standard use of verbal and non-verbal stimuli with an emphasis on the person's successful and failed responses has the potential to dishearten and even discourage the person's attempts (Lund and Duchan, 1988; Pound et al., 2000).

Dynamic assessment overcomes these difficulties to a certain extent by focusing on the individual's *potential* for improving speech and language functioning. It is based on the work of Vygotsky (1896–1934), who observed that human behaviour is never static but is in a constant process of transformation. Dynamic assessment takes a forward-looking perspective on the individual's skills by exploring the interaction between the person's communicative competence and the mediation offered by others, i.e. What new responses emerge as a result of mediation? This focuses on the learning potential of the individual, or what Vygotsky (1978: 86) referred to as the *zone of proximal development*. Information about an individual is gathered in a context of positive and supportive interaction. The communication repertoire of the person is opened up so that assessment activities become therapeutic in themselves.

Mediating role of therapist

Byng (1995) questions the contribution 'clinical intuition' makes to the decision-making process in speech and language therapy. If effective intervention owes its success to something that is inborn, the implication is: 'There is nothing that can be done to make a good (aphasia) therapist, you either have to "have it" or to be told' (p. 5).

Bray, Ross and Todd (1999) stress the importance of knowledge coupled with range and depth of experience. Certainly these factors provide a valuable frame of reference for exploring and making sense of the client's needs; but it is the *mechanism* whereby the individual and environment are represented in the information system that is so crucial to good decision-making. The individual profile is made up of positive factors in the individual and environment that can be drawn on, and difficulties that need to be addressed. Consideration is given to the potential of the client and environment to learn new ways of communicating, to maintain skill use or to achieve more frequent use of an existing repertoire (Gerard and Carson, 1990). The energies and analytical skills of the therapist are directed at the information system throughout the cycle of intervention. There is an ordering of the available data in response to some key questions:

* What is the priority for enhancing the client's functioning?
* Is working on communication skills the priority?
* What strengths can be built on?
* What positive factors in the person's life can be drawn on?
* What difficulties need to be addressed, or what barriers need to be overcome?

Level 2: Activation process

The second level of decision-making concentrates on the *activation process*, which is depicted in Figure 4.6. It includes the different centres of influence and significant others who are potential agents within the intervention process. The individual occupies a pivotal role between the *information flow* and *activation process*. New information arises from the activation process and is passed to the information flow, which in turn influences the way the intervention progresses.

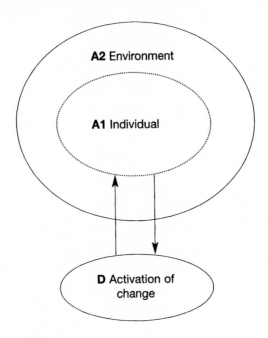

Figure 4.6 Activation process

Activation of change

The final component in the decision-making system is concerned with how a desired outcome will be brought about. It focuses on the content, process and context of intervention which correspond to the nature of individual need. Additionally, organization-based interventions, e.g. mainstream school, residential care home, acute hospital site, etc., need to consider the structure of the host organization, its value system and the practice of staff/significant others.

Impeded intervention

There are factors that may challenge the activation process and interrupt the progress of intervention. The therapist needs to be alert to their possibility and address them as they arise. Potential obstacles include the following.

- Fear of failure or of 'looking stupid' may make the client and significant others reluctant to experiment with skills in pursuit of change. It may give rise to feelings of insecurity, as usual and familiar patterns of communication are subject to change, e.g. the person with a stammer who is wary of how listeners will respond to a new, more fluent way of speaking, the aphasic person who does not know how family and friends will respond to 'drawing' as a primary mode of communication.
- The intervention of the therapist may threaten the core skills and competencies of client and significant others, or even challenge their status and power base, e.g. the parents who are required to talk differently to their language-delayed child.
- A lack of perceived benefits in attending SLT may lead to the detachment of the main players. When the need for intervention is not clear or the intended effects of the intervention remain elusive to the client and significant others, engagement in the therapy process is made difficult.
- Historical factors and custom-bound practice may inhibit new ways of dealing with a problem, e.g. a recent diagnosis of a moderate to severe hearing impairment in a 40-year-old woman with learning disabilities was refuted by her key worker, who for 15 years had known the client as a 'hearing' person.

Collaborative decision-making

How are these difficulties pre-empted or overcome when they do arise? Collaboration provides the way forward. Joint decision-making is not a new idea in the working practice of SLTs with other professionals. Van der Gaag and Dormandy (1993) advocate co-operative working practice between therapist and support staff in learning disability services. In the educational context, successful collaboration between therapist and teacher demands joint planning early on in the intervention process (Rinaldi, 2000), shared selection and prioritization of children (McCartney, 1999; Wright and Kersner, 1998) and consciously involving parents in this collaboration (McCool in McCartney, 1999).

The public agenda is very much about involving and promoting the participation of consumers in the provision of health care (DoH, 2001c). The importance of partnership practice with parents of young children has been stressed because they will be instrumental in carrying out the therapy: 'The parent should ... be closely involved in the decision-making process, and aims and objectives for intervention should be negotiated and agreed with them (and the child where this is appropriate)' (Bray, Ross and Todd, 1999: 128).

A negotiated process

Communicating Quality 2 (RCSLT, 1996) advises that 'All episodes of care will be negotiated and agreed between client and carer and the speech and language therapist' (p. 22).

What exactly does a *negotiated* process mean? It is a working partnership of openness, whereby individual agendas are shared; personal and ideological differences are exposed; differences in knowledge, skill and role are uncovered, and the perspective of each contributor is established. The question of 'Who is the expert?' must also be addressed. A balanced partnership assumes the equal status and value of the contributors; however, this balance may be disrupted when one half of the partnership is viewed as 'expert'. It is perhaps more useful to talk about the varying expertise that each participant brings to the partnership, as a way of acknowledging difference and resolving areas of potential conflict. The realities of the client provide a check on the professional's viewpoint. Pound et al. (2000) stress the importance of 'redressing the balance of power between therapist and client, as well as in identifying therapeutic aims which have genuine relevance and meaning to the person' (p. 48).

Partnership practice is characterized by:

- respect for individuality and acknowledgement of the intrinsic value of the other person's contributions;
- balanced communication that avoids professional dominance and where shared linguistic code and mutual access to conversation floor are features;
- open access to an unbiased information system so that each participant is acquainted with the relevant facts, and agreement is not an outcome of pressure from one party;
- joint identification and appraisal of the relevant options at any stage in the therapy process, with opportunities to reject, modify or affirm;
- decisions that are an outcome of a negotiated process between the therapist and client or significant others.

Negotiating with Shaun, a man with learning disabilities

Shaun was a 27-year-old man with moderate learning disabilities. He lived in the family home with his widowed father. Shaun attended a social education centre on five days of the week. He was involved in an employment opportunities project, which included various work placements in the community. He was an active member of the day centre's self-advocacy group and attended classes at the local further education (FE) college, learning basic computer skills, literacy and numeracy. Shaun had a girlfriend who followed the same weekly programme.

Shaun was referred to SLT because of a severe fluency disorder that was felt to limit his participation on work placement and at the FE college. An initial contact was made with Shaun and he was asked if he would like an appointment to explore some of the difficulties he was experiencing. Shaun was given some 'easy to read' information about SLT supported by pictures so that he could consider it as a possible option.

The therapist met him the following week, as agreed, to explore the option of SLT further. Shaun revealed that he would like to 'do something' as he was 'having a hard time at college'. He stated that his girlfriend was unhappy about him coming to SLT, which was making him uncertain. It was suggested that a three-way meeting between Shaun, his girlfriend and the therapist take place. At the meeting, it became clear that Shaun's girlfriend was suspicious of the female therapist spending time with her boyfriend. The therapist reassured her that this was not a competition for Shaun's affections and proposed that the girlfriend also come to the SLT sessions. Shaun and his girlfriend approved this arrangement.

The pattern of negotiation that took place in the initial stages of the intervention process set the tone for later. Assessment activities, therapy goals and communication opportunities were devised through the contributions of the three players. The dominant tendency of the girlfriend was easily managed when she felt that she was involved in her partner's therapy. Shaun felt more confident about expressing his views to his girlfriend when a third party was present.

Framework for constructing intervention

With reference to Gerard and Carson's (1990) decision-making procedures and based on the work of Sally Byng (Connect – the communication disability network), a framework for guiding the construction of intervention is proposed. There are three stages comprising a number of steps where the therapist, in negotiation with client and/or significant other(s), addresses key questions.

Stage 1: Appraisal of individual profile

The individual profile is ordered in terms of positive factors and factors that challenge. Positive factors are defined as those aspects of the person's functioning and lifestyle that may provide useful supports for a particular approach to therapy or else offer a basis for therapy activities. Skills, attributes, experiences, knowledge, attitudes, situational dynamics and other resources may be drawn on, including:

Individual factors:

- Using residual or emergent skills; emergence of natural strategies or ways of dealing with difficulties such as drawing, pointing and writing. This may include non-conventional ways of communicating such as eye gaze, body language, gesture and facial expression.
- Personal characteristics or attributes of identity that may support the process of change, e.g. individual persistence and determination, creativity, humour in adversity.
- Small behaviours or aspects of functioning that provide natural bases for building and extending communication skills, e.g. ability to write in the letters of words, interest in touching objects.

Partnership factors:

- Relationship that supports individual interests and shared characteristics.
- Interest in developing and progressing communication and developing relationship.

Environmental factors:

- Local commitment to support intervention evidenced by relevant policies and procedures that are already in place, e.g. a total communication approach in the environment.
- Interest in providing a positive environment with a wide range of opportunities for participation.

Societal factors:

- Current and relevant social policy and legislation that support the intervention approach, e.g. acts of Parliament to do with community care, valuing people.
- Activities and campaigns of voluntary groups and pressure movements.

Challenging factors are defined as difficulties or complicating barriers. They are located in all centres of influence and may include impaired knowledge, skills, limited experience, attitudinal barriers, behavioural or attention problems, associated sensory and/or motor impairments, emotional difficulties, and personal attributes that appear to be in conflict with the situation. They are identified so that appropriate contingencies may be put in place to address the difficulties or overcome the barriers.

Appraisal of the individual profile consists of two basic steps.

Step 1: Characteristics of individual and environment

- Look at the overall profile of the individual(s): What are the strengths, including positive factors or resources that can be drawn on, and what are the difficulties or barriers that need to be addressed?
- Make a judgement about the contribution of those around the client: Does the environment need to be modified in any way?

Step 2: Focal aspect of profile

- Talk to the key players in the intervention process about their priorities, e.g. individual client, group of service users, parent, carer, teacher, support staff, etc.: What would they like to see happen in this situation?
- Make a judgement about the aspect(s) of the individual's profile that might be most amenable to change: What *small* aspect of the client's functioning can be used as a basis for intervention?
- Establish a rationale for the selected starting point: How can I use that small aspect to make what I do relevant to the areas I am trying to change?

Profile factors are ordered and numbered for easy reference in the next stage of activity planning.

Case examples

Three contrasting case examples are profiled here.

Case study 1: Individual profile of Lee, a man with profound and multiple learning disabilities (PMLD)

Lee was a 23-year-old man with severe to profound and multiple learning disabilities. He was referred to SLT by his keyworker, who was concerned at Lee's poor level of engagement with people in his residential home and day centre. Assessment activities included: interviews conducted with Lee's keyworkers, at the day centre and his home, and the use of systematic observation techniques, i.e. momentary time sampling, for the structured exploration of Lee's interactions across a range of natural contexts. A classification system for coding subject activity that is broadly similar was used.

A: Positive factors – e.g. What can this person do communicatively, or what resources can they draw on?

A.1 Uses unconventional communication and interaction behaviours, e.g. person contact includes hand-arm reach, gesture (requestive), touch, vocalization, body movement, relating to self, refusal; object contact includes reach, touch, manipulating, relating to self; occasional vocal behaviour with person and object.

A.2 Visual and tactile exploration of environment.

A.3 Good use of fine motor skills for picking up and manipulating objects.

A.4 Responds to his name being called accompanied by a demonstration of a favoured activity.

A.5 Fully mobile within home and day centre environments.

A.6 Both staff teams, at home and in the day centre, express a desire to work with Lee and the SLT service.

B: Difficulties – e.g. What does this person have difficulty doing, or what are the complications and barriers to overcome?

B.1 Dependence on unconventional communication behaviours makes interpretation of meaning difficult.

B.2 Engages in a high level of stereotypic behaviour characterized by repetition and a lack of obvious function, e.g. rocking, bizarre hand-arm movements, face slapping, etc.

B.3 Does not maintain communicative position for very long; tendency to wander.

B.4 Applies pressure to laryngeal area, inducing vomiting and substance play.

B.5 Tendency to solitary behaviour.
B.6 Limited interactions between staff and client.
B.7 Limited interactions with peers.
B.8 Low level of stimulation in home and day centre environments.
B.9 Staff have a heavy reliance on verbal communication with Lee.
B.10 Recently diagnosed as having a moderate-to-severe hearing impairment.

Case study 2: Individual profile of Michael, a man with severe aphasia

Michael was a 55-year-old man with aphasia. He was referred to an SLT group held at a community rehabilitation centre approximately two years post-onset. Previously involved in a drawing project, he was referred by the SLT researcher for development of total communication skills. Assessment activities included:

- interviews conducted with Michael and his wife at initial visits to the centre;
- structured assessment of language skills using PALPA subtests plus a battery of non-verbal assessments, e.g. Pyramids and Palm Trees, generative drawing tests, etc.;
- informal exploration of Michael's use of communication skills within one of the therapy groups he attended.

A: Positive factors – e.g. What can this person do communicatively, or what resources can they draw on?
A.1 Able to use a fairly reliable 'yes' and 'no' – can be verified at least.
A.2 Able to recognize pictures.
A.3 Can draw interpretably some of the time if context known.
A.4 Can follow simple instructions and conversation.
A.5 Can write some numbers and first letters.
A.6 Can use single letters.
A.7 Attempts gesture but often not interpretable.
A.8 Partner willing to join therapy sessions to learn how to interpret and facilitate drawing, although sceptical.
A.9 Motivated to communicate.
A.10 Retained memory from one session to the next.

B: Difficulties – e.g. What does this person have difficulty doing, or what are the complications and barriers to overcome?
B.1 Somewhat passive in social situations.
B.2 Flat affect.
B.3 Attempts gesture but often not interpretable.
B.4 Little or no speech except for 'aye' for yes and occasional repeated syllables.
B.5 Speech has been tried before with no success.

B.6 Much struggle, little communication.
B.7 Doesn't initiate or think to use drawing.
B.8 Doesn't initiate much communication.

Case study 3: Individual profile of Jenny, a child with expressive language and phonological difficulties

Jenny was a seven-year-old girl with severe expressive language and phonological disorder attending a language unit attached to a mainstream school in an inner city area. She had a history of delayed and disordered speech and language development and had been known to speech and language therapy services since referral by her health visitor at the age of two. On arrival at the language unit a number of assessments were carried out, including the following:

- assessments of language comprehension at single word and sentence levels;
- assessments of expressive language – both formal assessments and elicitation of language samples for qualitative analysis;
- analysis of elicited speech samples in respect of Jenny's phonological system;
- a battery of psycholinguistic language processing tasks at a single word level aimed at exploring her auditory and semantic processing skills;
- classroom observation of her interaction with peers, listening and attention skills in a teaching and learning situation, and ability to work independently.

A: Positive factors – e.g. What can this person do communicatively, or what resources can they draw on?

A.1 Active contributor in communication situations.
A.2 Excellent non-verbal communication skills, e.g. gestures to supplement speech.
A.3 Excellent social communication skills – engages readily in interactions, makes appropriate eye-contact, takes turns, etc.
A.4 Single word comprehension within the range expected for her age.
A.5 Sentence level comprehension at the lower borderline of the range expected for her age but a strength in relation to expressive skills.
A.6 Able to produce intelligible single words expressively with effort.
A.7 Age-appropriate non-verbal problem-solving skills as assessed by the educational psychologist.
A.8 Reading and writing skills emerging although not age-appropriate.
A.9 Able to maintain attention to a task appropriately – a tenacious personality.
A.10 Well integrated within her peer group.
A.11 Staff enjoy working with her.
A.12 Very supportive home environment.

B: Difficulties – e.g. What does this person have difficulty doing, or what are the complications and barriers to overcome?

B.1   Expressive language limited in form and content.
B.2   Word-finding difficulties.
B.3   Speech often unintelligible in continuous speech or narrative.
B.4   Auditory input skills limited – e.g. auditory discrimination, lexical decision.
B.5   Some errors in comprehension due to poor auditory discrimination skills.
B.6   Reading and spelling skills are affected by her processing difficulties.
B.7   Jenny becomes frustrated when she is unsuccessful in communicating her message – this leads to either withdrawal or occasionally an angry outburst.

Stage 2: Activity planning

The second stage is where activities on the assessment–therapy continuum are defined. It is subdivided into three sections that correspond with one another:

1) Content decisions
2) Process decisions
3) Context decisions.

The therapist thinks through WHAT will be done in therapy (the *content*), HOW it will be done (the *process*), and HOW the *context* will be manipulated or the conditions of therapy created.

Content decisions

Content decisions relate to the focus of the intervention activities. These decisions revolve around two main components:

Goals of intervention	critical aspect of functioning relevant to the individual's lifestyle and available skills.
Focus of activity	activity or activities that will support the goals of intervention.

Step 1: Goals of intervention

- Identify the goals or targets of the intervention in relation to the focal aspect of the person's functioning and the located centre of influence: What is the primary domain(s) that should benefit from the intervention process?
- Consider the interdependence of intervention goals: Are there any subsidiary domains where collateral effects of the intervention are likely or desirable?

Step 2: Focus of approach

- Devise activities or opportunities that support the intervention goals and are appropriate to the centre of influence: What are the dimensions of the activity in terms of the demands presented to the individual and how do they build on factors in the individual profile?
- Select and adapt materials to correspond with the positive factors and difficulties identified in the individual's profile: What are the critical features to promote optimal responding in the individual?

Case study 1 (Lee, adult with PMLD)

Step 1: Goals of intervention	• Promote the use and development of unconventional communication behaviours by Lee and the staff. • Promote access to choice in everyday life. • Reveal the positive aspects of Lee's identity.
Step 2: Focus of approach	Social interaction opportunities characterized by sensory stimulation, e.g. tactile and vestibular.

Building on positive factors – A.1, A.2, A.3

Addressing difficulties – B.1, B.2, B.6, B.9, B.10

Case study 2 (Michael, adult with aphasia)

Step 1: Goals of intervention	• Promote the use and development of total communication skills with a particular focus on drawing. • Promote access to lifestyle choices and opportunities that are important to Michael. • Develop a communication book to express identity.
Step 2: Focus of approach	Social interaction opportunities and informal conversation characterized by communicative drawing and use of a communication book.

Considering positive factors – A.2, A.3, A.5, A.6, A.9

Addressing difficulties – B.1, B.2, B.3, B.4, B.5, B.6, B.8

Case study 3 (Jenny, child with expressive language and phonological disorder)

Step 1: Goals of intervention	• Promote use of semantic–phonological communication therapy to develop language processing skills. • Promote use and development of functional social communication strategies to supplement verbal communication. • Develop resilience strategies for dealing with frustration that leads to social withdrawal.
Step 2: Focus of approach	Social interaction in curriculum learning opportunities characterized by use of multimodal strategies for communication as well as specific rehearsal of verbal skills.

Considering positive factors – A.1, A.2, A.3, A.6, A.8, A.9

Addressing difficulties – B.1, B.2, B.3, B.4, B.5, B.6, B.7

Process decisions

Process decisions relate to the mechanisms or routes for the realization of intervention goals in relation to the targeted centre of influence. Included in this definition are:

Centre of influence	The primary location for the intervention where assessment or therapy activities are targeted.
Role of SLT	The behaviour and interaction style of the therapist as a factor in creating the conditions of effective intervention.
Enactment processes	The main techniques that will be used to carry out the intervention.

Step 3: Centre of influence

• Make a judgement about where to locate the intervention's centre of influence for maximum impact on the individual(s) and significant others: Which centre of influence is ideally suited to the focal aspect of communication that is being targeted, e.g. individual, partnership, environment or society?

- Map out the planned trajectory from the primary centre of influence that considers how generalization will occur: What other sources of influence will emanate from the selected centre of the intervention and what contingencies are needed to be in place to support the planned trajectory?
- Identify the key players or agents of change within the planned trajectory and work out their involvement: What is the role of the client, parent, partner, teacher and support staff in relation to the goal(s) of intervention?

Step 4: Role of SLT

Define the role of the speech and language therapist under the established implementation arrangements: What are the contributions of the therapist in relation to the centre of influence?

- Working with the individual client as a direct facilitator of the client's communication – intervention takes place with one or more individual clients, where the therapist actively facilitates the therapist–client interaction.
- Working with the client and significant other(s) as a facilitator of the communication partnership – intervention takes place with one or more clients with their significant others, where the therapist models and actively facilitates the partnership interaction.
- Working with significant others and/or the environment as a facilitator of the social environment – intervention takes place with one or more aspects of the environment, where the therapist actively facilitates change and development in the communication skills of significant others and the techniques and materials used to support communication.
- Working with societal systems as a facilitator of change – intervention is focused on the wider agenda, where the therapist may be involved in a particular interest group activity to support the generation of ideas, strategy planning and the actual process of negotiation with other people and organizations.

Step 5: Enactment processes

- Select and identify the key enactment processes that correspond to the theoretical underpinning for the selected approach: What will happen at the interface between the therapist and client/significant other(s) so that the goals of intervention are realized? What are the key strategies and therapy techniques that are relevant to this approach?
- Define the mechanism for change and maintenance as relevant to the intervention: How will the intervention affect the behaviour of the key players involved in the intervention process?

Case study 1 (Lee, adult with PMLD)

Step 3: Centre of influence	Partnership practice between SLT and key worker/significant others within a small group setting. Change in the communication environment is desirable.
Step 4: Role of SLT	Therapist assumes role of group manager, organizing equipment and the general context; skilful demonstrator of interaction techniques to staff; observes staff and client interactions and provides qualitative feedback.
Step 5: Enactment processes	Therapeutic techniques include: *For Lee* • using clear and meaningful attention calls for accessing interaction opportunities; • using a hierarchy of facilitation cues to help him use available skills; • observing closely and responding sensitively to his small communication behaviours; • controlling the dimensions of interaction opportunities in terms of the sensory stimuli, so that he is not required to attend to person and object at the same time; • adapting communicative input by use of minimal verbal code; • providing feedback in terms of sensory stimulation. *For communication partner* • providing information and negotiating rationales for the way forward; • modelling interactions with Lee; • giving feedback about interactions with Lee.

Building on positive factors – A.6

Addressing difficulties – B.1, B.3, B.4, B.6, B.7, B.9, B.10

Case study 2 (Michael, adult with aphasia)

Step 3: Centre of influence	Individual with Michael and partnership practice involving Michael's partner.
Step 4: Role of SLT	Therapist assumes role of communication book 'publisher' – listening, exploring, recording client's ideas and advising on index; provides a model for use of inclusive communication skills with Michael and his partner.
Step 5: Enactment processes	Therapeutic techniques include: • using modified forms of communication, e.g. drawing and interpretation strategies to support inclusive communication; • facilitating attempts at communicative drawing as appropriate to the construction of meaning; • providing relevant and differential feedback for Michael's contributions; • demonstrating sensitivity and acknowledging Michael's emotional state and sense of self when exploring life-course information to include in his communication book; • providing information and clearly worked rationales for the way forward using augmentative communication forms.

Considering positive factors – A.1, A.8, A.10

Addressing difficulties – B.1, B.3, B.6

Case study 3 (Jenny, child with expressive language and phonological disorder)

Step 3: Centre of influence	• Individual with Jenny and partnership practice involving a peer for semantic–phonological therapy. • Partnership practice in small group for social communication therapy.
Step 4: Role of SLT	• Direct facilitator in terms of semantic–phonological therapy. • Group facilitator/group manager in terms of social communication therapy.

	Therapeutic techniques include:
Step 5: Enactment processes	• use of modelling, reflection, direct facilitation in semantic–phonological therapy; • acknowledging frustrations and providing emotional support as appropriate; • use of differential feedback to refine responses; • use of gesture, pictures and written words to support social communication in peer partnerships.

Considering positive factors – A.6, A.7, A.8, A.9

Addressing difficulties – B.1, B.2, B.3, B.4, B.5, B.7

Context decisions

Context decisions relate to the philosophical and cultural backdrop for intervention activities to take place. Usually encased within a set of core values, context decisions create the conditions for the content and process of therapy. Context decisions deal with the following:

Implementation arrangements	The conditions for the intervention to take place.
Physical and social setting	The attributes of the location in which the intervention takes place.
Individual maintenance	The adaptations and special arrangements that are put in place to meet the individual's needs and to maintain their participation in the intervention process.

Step 6: Implementation arrangements

• Specify how the intervention will be carried out: What are the implementation arrangements that are relevant to the identified aspect of communication and the centre of influence, e.g.:
  – The pattern of delivery in terms of frequency of contact?
  – The mode of delivery, whether individual, small or large group?
  – The duration of the intervention episode or the estimated period of contact?

Step 7: Physical and social setting

- Consideration is given to the physical location and social setting of the main environments where the intervention will take place: What physical or social adjustments to the location are needed in terms of:
  - The physical attributes of the setting?
  - The values that are apparent in the physical and social environment?
  - The ambient level of sound and luminescence?
  - The other people in that location?

Step 8: Individual maintenance

- Consideration is given to attributes that are known to be present in the individual(s): What personal maintenance strategies need to be invoked in order to maintain the content and process of therapy in terms of:
  - The individual's emotional and behavioural needs?
  - The individual's state of consciousness and alertness?
  - The individual's level of stimulation and interest?
  - The individual's level of insight and self-awareness?

Case study 1 (Lee, adult with PMLD)

Step 6: Implementation arrangements	Intervention takes place in a small group of four clients, SLT and keyworker; twice a week for one hour, for a period of four weeks. Regular liaison with support staff at home.
Step 7: Physical and social setting	Work in a familiar but closed environment in the day centre for addressing Lee's high level of distraction and wandering behaviour.
Step 8: Individual maintenance	Break up Lee's physical position, when he is about to apply pressure to laryngeal area, by encouraging hands to table and feet to floor.

Considering positive factors – A.6

Addressing difficulties – B.3, B.4, B.6, B.7, B.8

Case study 2 (Michael, adult with aphasia)

Step 6: Implementation arrangements	Intervention takes place in individual sessions (once a week), and shared sessions with partner (once a fortnight).

| Step 7: Physical and social setting | Work in a closed environment within the clinic setting to give Michael and his partner confidence and security in experimenting with new communication strategies. |
| Step 8: Individual maintenance | Real communication opportunities that reflect Michael's interests and lifestyle. |

Considering positive factors – A.8, A.10

Addressing difficulties – B.1, B.7

Case study 3 (Jenny, child with expressive language and phonological disorder)

Step 6: Implementation arrangements	Intervention takes place in individual or paired sessions in respect of semantic–phonological therapy, and within the language unit class group (seven children) in respect of the social communication therapy.
Step 7: Physical setting	The language unit classroom with carry-over activities for parents to use at home.
Step 8: Individual maintenance	Group sessions allow Jenny to implement strategies developed through individual and paired sessions, building confidence and engendering feelings of success.

Considering positive factors – A.1, A.2, A.3, A.9, A.10, A.12

Addressing difficulties – B.1, B.2, B.3, B.4, B.5, B.7

Stage 3: Evaluation activities

The effectiveness of any intervention is measured against what it sets out to achieve. Consideration is given to the presence of factors that may influence change, such as natural maturation, changes in personal circumstances and life-course events. Comprehensive evaluation is concerned not only with the individual's performance, but also with the effectiveness of the intervention. Dockrell and Messer (1999: 136) recommend that 'The intervention process should be viewed as cyclical and requiring constant evaluation.'

Levels of outcome

There are different levels at which therapy is monitored. Frattali (1998a) uses the terms originally coined by Rosen and Proctor (1981):

intermediate, *instrumental* and *ultimate* outcomes. *Intermediate* outcomes allow ongoing evaluation of the intervention process, e.g. during and at the end of a session. In this way, individual objectives can be measured against the client's performance (Kersner in Kersner and Wright, 2001) and internal adjustments to the therapy plan made as required. *Instrumental* outcomes 'activate the learning process ... when reached, [they] trigger the ultimate outcome' (p. 9). This level of outcome indicates whether to continue or close an episode of intervention. Once instrumental outcomes are achieved, it is assumed that the individual's progress will continue beyond the intervention episode. *Ultimate* outcomes examine the 'social or ecological validity' of the intervention (p. 10). The focus is on outcomes that are meaningful, accessible and relevant for individuals (Byng, van der Gaag and Parr in Frattali, 1998), such as functional communication, access to learning opportunities in the classroom, employability and participation in social events of personal value.

Roulstone in Kersner and Wright (2001) distinguishes between primary and secondary outcomes. Primary outcomes focus on aspects of the individual's communication behaviour, whilst secondary outcomes measure related aspects, such as the communication behaviour of significant others. The latter would be of interest in intervention approaches that involve significant others at the level of communication partnership, e.g. parent–child interaction (Cummins and Hulme in Kersner and Wright, 2001), teacher and child (Bray in Kersner and Wright, 2001), and keyworker and person with a learning disability (Dobson, 2001).

Challenge of attribution

Outcomes measurement is critical in determining the effectiveness of an intervention. It is about demonstrating that change has taken place and is related to 'identifiable actions, resources or events' (Health of the Nation, 1991: 43). In order to understand *why* change has occurred, it follows that there must be a clear definition of the intervention that has taken place. Byng, van der Gaag and Parr in Frattali (1998: 565) comment on the lack of specificity of speech and language therapy, stating that 'it typically uses a portfolio of therapeutic techniques integrated into one therapy program'.

There are many factors that influence change in communication skills, including age, the nature and severity of the condition, motivation and demonstrable commitment, degree of support from significant others, personality traits and associated skills (Byng, van der Gaag and Parr in Frattali, 1998). Causal factors are not necessarily restricted to the client but may be linked to individual characteristics of the clinician, the service and various processes of care (Frattali, 1998a). Out of the multiple causal factors and components of the intervention, which aspect(s) is primarily responsible for bringing about change?

Attributing change is further complicated where there is inter-disciplinary collaboration. Centring the intervention on the individual encourages the use of a unified monitoring schedule, which reflects the various dimensions of the intervention. In the educational context, McCartney in McCartney (1999) recommends evaluation of the 'total learning experience', which implies a multi-faceted assessment framework, combining educational and therapy measures.

Outcomes measurement in a climate of change

Speech and language therapy draws increasingly on the work of the disability movement, utilizing the social model to promote understanding of communication disability. This has brought about a shift in the culture of SLT practice. Identification of communication barriers is a feature of intervention with some client groups, e.g. people with aphasia (Parr et al., 1997) with learning disabilities (Money in Abudarham and Hurd, 2002) and with a hearing impairment (Beazeley, Frost and Halden in Kersner and Wright, 2001). Byng, van der Gaag and Parr in Frattali (1998: 574) identify three elements that contribute to this changing culture of SLT: (1) the increasing use of qualitative methods for measuring and interpreting change in a way that is relevant to the service user(s) (Frattali, 1998b); (2) the recent focus on negotiation and collaboration between therapist and service user(s) in designing and implementing intervention (citing French, 1994); (3) the 'ongoing analysis of components of intervention provided by speech and language therapists to make more explicit what we are doing and what motivates our actions' (citing Byng, 1995).

Deciding what and how to evaluate

RCSLT (1996) recommends a combination of clinical measurement and service user evaluation. The type of condition and the nature of the intervention determine the choice of outcome measurement (RCSLT, 1993). Implicit in *type of condition* are the various levels of representation. Enderby's Therapy Outcomes Measures (TOM) (Enderby, 1997) referred to in Chapter 1, uses the WHO definitions of 'Impairment, Disability, Handicap' with the addition of 'Well-being'. Usually, the *nature of the intervention* will correspond to the context and therefore define the locus of interest. For instance, learning ability is of interest in the educational context, and quality of life is high on the agenda of client and family (Frattali, 1998b). For people living with communication disability, functional gains determined in the context of daily life activities are relevant, e.g. people with learning disabilities (Hickman in Abudarham and Hurd, 2002), and people with aphasia (Pound et al., 2001).

In the field of aphasia, Holland and Thompson in Frattali (1998) emphasize the importance of looking at not only language and communication skills but also psychosocial issues. The experience and opinions of people with communication disabilities provide crucial insights to intervention effectiveness. Pound et al. (2000) describe a range of evaluation tools that are used at the London Centre of Connect. Their approach is user-centred and includes: in-depth interview of individual clients before, during and after an episode of intervention; focus group interviews; recording personal narratives; observing focal communication behaviours as they occur in context; accessible rating scales that focus variously on degrees of consumer satisfaction and personal feelings; and regular monitoring of individuals and groups in relation to the defined goals.

In the educational context, McCartney in McCartney (1999) proposes a service evaluation framework using the four quadrants of Banathy's model (1992): (i) 'Structure' is concerned with the specification, allocation and use of resources. An analytical account of organizational structures is completed by review of decision-making procedures and relevant policy documents, e.g. managerial allocation of SLT resources and teacher time in collaborative practice. (ii) 'Function' evaluates the aims and minimum standards of service provision. The reliability of implementation is measured by checking for evidence of what actually happened against any agreed service-level plans. Timetables, therapy plans, notes of teacher–therapist meetings, professional logs and other relevant documentation may be used as evidence. The child's progress is measured against the Individual Education Plan (IEP). (iii) 'Process' measures are taken alongside the 'function' where 'event sequence concerned with a child's contact with a service – entry to it, interaction within it and leaving it' is tracked (McCartney in McCartney, 1999: 168). The child's progress is checked against joint record keeping (Wright and Kersner, 1998) and attainments documented in IEPs (Gascoigne in Kersner and Wright, 2001). (iv) 'Systems-environment' measures focus on related contexts such as the home environment. Methods include the use of parent questionnaires, discussion groups and reports.

Steps to evaluation

Two basic steps guide the design of evaluation activities. Unlike previous stages, evaluation measures do not build on specific positive factors or attempt to address difficulties, although the individual profile is a constant frame of reference.

Step 1: Different perspectives
• Identify the relevant perspectives of stakeholders in the therapy process (client, significant other, therapist, and others) as well as the critical aspects of communication in relation to the planned goals of therapy, where change is anticipated: What type of change is expected by, and is meaningful, to the different stakeholders in relation to the goals of intervention?

Step 2: Evaluation tools
• Select the most appropriate method for measuring the effects of the intervention in relation to the different perspectives of the stakehold-

ers, the content, process and context of the intervention, and the individual's lifestyle and occupations: How will any effects be measured, what tools are recommended and who needs to be involved in the administration? For example, client completes self-rating questionnaire, SLT re- administers a structured assessment, significant other completes a defined rating scale, etc.

Rosen and Proctor's (1981) levels of outcome measure cited by Frattali in Frattali (1998), discussed earlier in this section, provide a frame of reference for the individual cases illustrated here.

Case study 1 (Lee, adult with PMLD)

Step 1: Different perspectives	The key players in Lee's intervention are Lee, his keyworking staff in the day centre/home and the SLT.
Step 2: Evaluation tools	Evaluation tools include: • systematic observation of Lee's interactive behaviours across a range of contexts and at different times (ultimate); • interview of keyworking staff at home and in the day centre (ultimate); • joint record-keeping of intermediate outcomes between therapist and staff (intermediate); • micro-analysis of communication partnerships in action (instrumental).

Case study 2 (Michael, adult with aphasia)

Step 1: Different perspectives	The key players in Michael's intervention are Michael, his wife, other group members and the therapist.
Step 2: Evaluation tools	Evaluation tools include: • video recording and observation of Michael's inclusive communication style in the group setting (instrumental); • comparison of topics in communication book with Michael's life course (intermediate); • in-depth interview of Michael and his wife before, during and after the intervention episode (ultimate); • rating scale of feelings completed by Michael (intermediate and ultimate).

Case study 3 (Jenny, child with expressive language and phonological disorder)

Step 1: Different perspectives	The key players in Jenny's intervention are Jenny, her parents, her peers, the language unit teacher and the therapist.
Step 2: Evaluation tools	Evaluation tools include:

- psycholinguistic assessment of processing skills (instrumental);
- joint record-keeping between therapist and teacher (intermediate);
- analysis of language samples in terms of content and form (instrumental);
- video samples before and after of Jenny interacting with peers (ultimate);
- rating scales of communication skills completed by parents and language unit teacher before and after intervention (ultimate);
- checking attainments against IEP goals achieved (intermediate and ultimate);
- rating scales (visual) of feelings about communication completed by Jenny before and after intervention (ultimate).

Constructing intervention

The construction of intervention reflects its organic nature. The ground shifts continuously because of the interaction between individual and contextual factors. Clinically reasoned decisions are the outcome of ongoing negotiation. It is this process of mutually co-ordinated decision-making to which both service user(s) and therapist contribute their expertise, which makes for a relevant, timely and meaningful intervention.

Chapter 5
Enactment of intervention

The enactment of intervention is concerned with what happens at the interface between therapist and service user, e.g. client(s) and/or significant other(s). Described as the mechanisms or routes whereby the intervention will take place, it refers to the *how* of intervention practice. Ferguson (1999) points out that such detail is often missing in descriptions of therapy. It is how the goals of intervention are realized in terms of: the centre(s) of influence targeted for the intervention activity; the role of the therapist as defined by behaviour and interaction style; and the enactment processes, which are the main therapeutic techniques that are used to effect change in the existing situation.

Relationship between theory and process

The first stage in examining the process of intervention looks at the influence of theory. Exploration of the relationship between theory and process give rise to a number of questions:

1) What is the place of theory in promoting understanding of the *nature of the communication difficulty*?
2) How does theory provide an explanation of the *mechanistic processes of intervention* as defined by the centre of influence and the role of the therapist, i.e. how will change or maintenance of communication skills be brought about?
3) What is the place of theory in the therapist's *selection and use of enactment processes* and how does it relate to what is understood about the nature of the communication difficulty?

How intervention is enacted is influenced by the knowledge base of the therapist. The relationship between theory and process is illustrated in Figure 5.1.

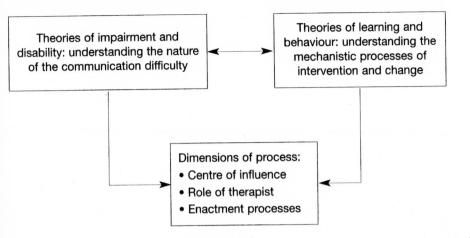

Figure 5.1 Influence of theory on process

Theories of impairment and disability

Theory provides an explanatory framework for understanding particular phenomena of interest where causal factors and relevant hypotheses are identified. There may be different theoretical perspectives or alternative explanations of the same happening. Howard (1999) asserts that the quality of a theory lies in its capacity to predict. Therefore, a clear explanation of a communication problem should be able to forecast the effectiveness of different approaches to intervention. The difference between language acquisition and the recovery process in aphasia is important to our understanding of communication difficulties, clinical decision-making and intervention enactment. For example, knowledge of language development in relation to the child's chronological age, environmental background and presentation of communication skills may prompt the timing of a decision on whether to intervene or not. This may affect the definition of the specific target of intervention as well as recommending a therapy approach that is in line with the explanatory framework. Gordon (1999: 136) argues that in order to attribute the positive change in an individual's communication impairment to the particular therapy approach, there needs to be a 'thorough understanding' of the impairment *and* the therapy.

Theories of impairment and disability help us to understand the individual's communication difficulties. Hypotheses are formulated in relation to the genetic, neurological and environmental bases that underlie the communication difficulty. They provide a frame of reference for explaining any problems or unusual processes in the existing communication situation, in terms of:

- The development of speech, language and communication skills:
  - the delay or disorder of any aspects of communication development and the process of natural progression;
  - the arrest or deterioration of skills already acquired.

- The effective use of speech, language and communication skills:
  - the disruption of skills for whatever reason and the process of spontaneous recovery;
  - the progressive deterioration of skills and any aspects of natural maintenance.

With regard to acquired language impairment, Howard and Hatfield (1987) point out that being able to explain the nature of a communication difficulty does not in itself determine the course of action to be taken. Howard (1999) later states that theories of impairment might support the selection of relevant intervention goals, i.e. in defining the 'what' of intervention: 'The vehicle of the therapy is, in a sense, learning, but what determines what is to be learned is the theoretical analysis of the disorder' (p. 142).

Cognitive neuropsychological theory

Cognitive neuropsychological theory provides an example of how theory can support understanding of the nature of the communication problem and guide the way forward in terms of intervention. It provides a basis for a range of interventions, e.g. children with speech and literacy difficulties (Stackhouse and Wells, 1997; 2001) and language disorders in children and adults (see Chiat, Law and Marshall, 1997). It is based on the assumption that different cognitive functions 'involve a number of different processes each of which is carried out by a specialized processing component or module' (Edmundson and McIntosh in Code and Muller, 1995: 138).

The individual's 'damaged' or 'atypical' language processing ability is analysed according to what is hypothesized to be the 'normal' processing system. Assessment has been likened to detective work whereby 'the source of the deficit' is identified (Jones and Byng, 1989: 2). A rational explanation for the child or adult's difficulties is proposed by locating the deficit on the normal processing model. In this way, the therapist is able to establish a causal relationship between the individual's impaired processing system and their resulting communication difficulties. The resultant hypothesis is the driver of the therapy programme. Howard and Hatfield (1987) identify three approaches to therapy, directed variously at: (1) enabling or improving access to intact information where access is flawed, i.e. *facilitation*; (2) bypassing the processing deficit by promoting alternative routes that remain intact, i.e. *reorganization*; (3) re-establishing information and items that have been affected, and learning rules and procedures to replace damaged ones.

Social constructivist view of language development

A social constructivist theory of language development might aid the therapist's understanding of any difficulties experienced by a child. For example, the interaction between developing infant and parent is based on the premise 'that intentional communication arises from the interaction of the cognitive development of the child and a responsive carer' (Goldbart, 1996 cited by Grove, Bunning and Porter in Columbus, 2001: 94).

It is understood that the infant expresses affective states from birth (Trevarthen, 1993). The carer is an acute observer of and sensitive respondent to expressive acts emitted by the infant. Meaning is ascribed to the observed act, which prompts a certain type of response by the carer. Thus, the expressive act gradually and over time acquires meaning for the infant by virtue of the interactions that have taken place. Goldbart (1996) highlights some of the difficulties that may be experienced by parents of infants with developmental disabilities. Recognition of expressive acts frequently requires greater caregiver sensitivity. It may be harder to differentiate between acts because 'extended experience of interactions at very basic developmental levels may reduce sensitivity to and expectation of change in the non-verbal individual. Thus developments of progressions in caregiver–nonverbal person interaction strategies become ever less likely' (Goldbart, 1996 cited by Grove, Bunning and Porter in Columbus, 2001: 94).

A child's delayed communication skills development may be explained by a lack of stimulation in the environment. The importance of a responsive communication environment becomes the driver of subsequent intervention activities. The 'Hanen Early Language Parent Programme' (Manolson, 1983) is based on a social constructivist model of language development. It aims to develop the partnership skills of parent and child by promoting sensitive responding: 'an approach to overcome the(se) barriers to good communication – our child's limited ability to communicate, his negative emotions, his perceived lack of power, his scepticism about the benefits of communicating' (p. v).

Theories of learning and behaviour

The mechanistic process of intervention, or how change is brought about in an existing situation, is underpinned by theories of learning and behaviour. They influence the design of particular therapy activities and the selection of enactment processes (Ferguson, 1999). Furthermore, understanding the process of learning and of behaviour change helps to rationalize change as it occurs.

Theories of learning and behaviour provide a frame of reference for the operational procedures of intervention. Ferguson (1999) argues that a theory of learning is needed to steer the implementation of therapy: 'Learning methodologies exist which allow for the integration of affective, cognitive and behavioural learning' (p. 129).

Learning methodologies prompt the use of practical strategies that enable the therapist to manipulate or alter an existing situation and for realizing the specified goals of intervention. For instance, positive reinforcement is derived from learning theory (instrumental or operant conditioning – work of Skinner, 1904–1991, cited by Schwartz and Robbins, 1995). It is used in SLT to support and encourage an individual's use of certain desirable behaviours. Ferguson (1999) suggests that alternative methods of adult learning such as problem-based and experiential learning provide useful adjuncts to more traditional methods, e.g. didactic teaching approaches.

Relationship between theories of impairment/disability and theories of learning/behaviour

There is not a direct one-to-one mapping between theories of impairment/disability and theories of learning/behaviour (Gordon, 1999). Individual characteristics of therapist and client as well as contextual factors will have an influence over the situation. In an effort to devise an intervention that will have maximum effect, the therapist draws on different theoretical perspectives, i.e. what is known about a particular communication difficulty and approaches to intervention that either have a proven track record or are appropriate to the formulated clinical hypothesis. In addition to these important components of clinical reasoning, Williamson (2001: 22) identifies a critical understanding of 'the broad contextual issues (e.g. related to healthcare policy and philosophy, local context, client's linguistic/cultural background)'. Van der Gaag and Davies (1994: 215) describe this multi-faceted process as the 'complex integration of knowledge and skills'.

Dimensions of process

With dual reference to the communication difficulty and the process of learning, a course of intervention is enacted that is likely to bring about the desired outcome of prevention, change or maintenance as appropriate to the given situation. Howard (1999: 142), talking about aphasia, asserts that the theoretical bases of intervention practice go beyond the learning process and should clarify the relationship between 'the processes of effective therapy' and the nature of the communication difficulty.

The dimensions of process were delineated in the previous chapter with regard to the construction of intervention: the centre of influence, role of therapist and enactment processes. The *role of the therapist* should correspond to the targeted *centre of influence*. For instance, the therapist may change from direct facilitator of the individual to trainer of significant others in the communication environment. The mechanism for change is implied, to a certain extent, by this relationship together with the defined *content* of intervention (see Chapter 4). For example, the intervention that targets the partnership might bring about change through altering the communication opportunities and contributions offered by the non-disabled partner so that the individual is able to reveal their true competence. *Enactment processes*, or the technical skills of therapy, are selected as appropriate to the identified mechanism for change and in relation to the contributions and presenting needs of the other person (Byng and Black, 1995).

Relationship between centre of influence and role of therapist

Different centres of influence are involved according to presenting needs and the goals of the intervention: the *individual* with a communication difficulty, the *partnership* of client and significant other, the social *environment* and *society*. Accordingly, each centre involves different people in different relationships to the client(s), e.g. parent, partner, support staff, nurse, keyworker, teacher, etc. It therefore follows that the role of the therapist will change according to the dynamic that is present in the targeted centre of influence. Within any one cycle of intervention there may be several centres of influence that are specifically targeted, either concurrently or chronologically.

Introducing strategies to circumvent an area of difficulty

Vida was a young woman with aphasia as a result of a stroke approximately 12 months earlier. Previously a full-time university student, she experienced a huge loss in relation to her peer group. She was very aware of her difficulties and this undermined her self-confidence. Although willing to try different approaches in therapy, she was naturally a perfectionist, and not prepared to make mistakes.

Intervention aimed to build on such positive factors as her interest in language changes and her ability to reflect on her own performance. Her own language skills allowed for in-depth discussion about complex and subtle ideas. Vida had strong non-language cognitive skills. She also derived much pleasure from writing before her stroke. Discussion with Vida revealed her readiness to take ownership of her therapy programme and therefore therapy activities were centred on her as the primary agent of change.

Therapy activities involved introducing Vida to a new way of planning an essay. In the first instance, mind maps were used to help Vida generate her ideas and to put them in an accessible order. The role of the therapist in the sessions was to support Vida in decision-making, initiating and recording of ideas. Enactment processes (therapeutic skills) were used with Vida as the agent for change, i.e. she was learning new ways of overcoming some of her particular difficulties. Change was not restricted to the clinical environment, however, because Vida was being prepared to carry forward the use of strategies to a broader learning environment.

Learning to use alternative communication together
Jadine was six years old. She had severe cerebral palsy, making verbal communication effortful and largely unsuccessful. After a period of assessment involving both Jadine and her mother, a technical communication device was recommended, funding was accessed and the device was purchased.

In the initial stages, therapy activities concentrated on use of the communication device within the partnership of mother and child. This is in keeping with the multiple agency approach to intervention recommended by Bjorck-Akesson, Granlund and Olsson in von Tetzchner and Jensen (1996: 331):

> ... actions by people, adaptation of the physical environment and provision of assistive technology. The expertise of the professionals is used to generate ideas about what the important elements of the strategy are. The person in question and/or significant others provide information about how and when the method can be implemented.

It was felt important to introduce the device into the most familiar partnership in Jadine's life right from the word 'go'. The main focus was on the desirable attributes that make for a 'good' communication partner with the aim of establishing ease in contributing to real conversations (Blackstone, 1999). Therapy concentrated on:

* proficient use of the communication device, including storage of vocabulary, operation and maintenance of device and accessing technical support as required;
* mutual development of conversational style with introduction of AAC, including use of eye contact (switching between visual display and other person), other forms of communication and timing of exchanges;
* establishing clear conversational opportunities for developing a shared communication style in the home setting.

Intervention centred on the partnership of Jadine and her mother drew on a similar pool of enactment processes to that of the previous case exemplar (Vida), although they were not directed exclusively at Jadine as the primary user. Instead, technical skills were invoked to manage the introduction of a computer-aided device for Jadine's expression of ideas, to support its usage, and to develop and maintain the contributions of both participants in social interaction.

Creating a responsive environment for people with a
hearing impairment
A number of people with learning disabilities, who lived in the same community residential facility, had been identified as having hearing problems. The attitudes of individuals and their support staff towards hearing impairment were considered to be key determinants in the adoption of a positive communication environment (MacMillan, Bunning and Pring, 2000).

A local training initiative was developed in response to this need. The overall aim was to establish a relevant and skilful communication environment to meet the needs of individuals with a hearing impairment. A series of practical workshop sessions was carried out in the home with the staff team, focusing on:

- Tactics for a positive communication environment:
  - systematic organization of the physical environment including relevant adaptations as appropriate, e.g. checking the light source, furnishings, positioning, etc.
  - selection, definition and practice in the use of communication support based on individual needs, e.g. communication distance, use of visual forms of communication, etc.
  - observation of and sensitive responding to communication attempts of individuals.

- Strategies to support use and maintenance of hearing aid(s):
  - meeting the individual support needs of the person in the practical use and maintenance of the hearing aid, e.g. fitting the hearing aid, cleaning and operating the device, re-tubing and changing the battery.
  - identifying positive environments or circumstances for wearing of hearing aid.
  - establishing effective channels of communication with relevant agencies to support the communication environment, e.g. local hearing aid centre.

The therapist and significant others worked towards the establishment of a responsive environment through identifying and addressing possible communication barriers (Beukelman and Mirenda, 1998). The therapist was concerned with the key constituents in the communication environment, e.g. the skills of significant others, the communication opportunities, social routines, etc. Significant others were coached in the use of enactment processes relevant to the needs of hearing-impaired residents.

Working together to influence outside agencies
As part of a nationally funded research project investigating the communication process in primary health care, a working group was formed comprising two people with aphasia and three adults with learning disabilities ('Making sense in primary care', Law et al., 2002/3). A researcher and therapist co-facilitated the group. The participants had a shared concern about health issues coupled with a desire to make communication in primary care better. The group met at approximately monthly intervals over an eight-month period. Although the overall focus of the group was prescribed by the project, i.e. use of primary care facilities, the group's

discussions of health and sharing of personal experiences helped to construct the agenda. In this way, the group was able to influence the direction of the research and to participate in the development of proto-type materials to facilitate communication in primary care. The therapist and the researcher had a role in creating suitable opportunities for people to address concerns and in supporting them through this process.

In a way, society as a centre of influence is not as tangible as the other three. It is about the individual or a group of people making their mark on the structures of society. At its highest level, action moves beyond the intervention cycle, e.g. it may involve influencing government policy. More usually it involves individuals tackling issues that affect daily life on a local basis. At this level, people engage in a range of advocacy activities that equip them to ask questions, challenge authority and communicate needs.

Moving across the centres of influence

A speech and language therapy service for children with fluency problems is provided at a community centre. Intensive courses are run for teenagers during the school holiday period. The participants engage in a range of therapy activities within small therapy groups, aimed at:

- reducing the severity of the stammer to a more comfortable level for both speaker and listener;
- reducing the anxiety and embarrassment associated with stammering;
- encouraging the participants to be more confident about tackling the speech situations which they normally fear or avoid;
- establishing effective problem solving strategies to address personal goals.

Because stammering has such a different personal meaning for each person, flexibility is built into the therapy methods used. For example, some individuals may spend considerable time on modifying the stutter itself, some place a greater emphasis on general communication skills, and others address the problem of avoidance methodically through discussion and experimentation, also known as assignments. Behavioural and psychological frameworks are employed, sometimes in combination, e.g. block modification (van Riper, 1973) and personal construct therapy (Kelly, 1963). Active consideration is given to the life-course stage of the individual and any relevant external events, e.g. a participant may seek help with a looming French Oral GCSE examination in the intensive course of the summer term.

In the initial stages, contact is made with three main centres of influence so that the change and generalization is built in from the start:

1) The *individual* who experiences fluency difficulties and is the primary agent of change.
2) The *partnerships* that are significant in the individual's lifestyle and relevant to the support and maintenance of therapeutic change, e.g. parents and immediate family members.

3) The *social environments* that are relevant to the individual's lifestyle, e.g. peer group, particular classroom activities, general communication in the classroom, etc.

The primary centre of influence is the *individual* who experiences fluency difficulties. The goal of therapy activities is for each participant to develop strategies that support a communication style that is acceptable and comfortable to the individual. In order that there should be generalization of therapy effects, there is a planned shift in the centre of influence to the *partnership*, where parents and/or other family members are involved in the development of support mechanisms for the maintenance of gains. Communication in the school *environment* is tackled through the use of simulated role-play and group discussion that addresses daily communication issues.

The intervention process may target a primary centre of influence, but this is not to the exclusion of all other centres. As shifts occur, so the role of the therapist changes, which in turn will affect the use of enactment processes.

Enactment processes

Enactment processes are described as the technical aspects of the therapeutic interaction (Horton and Byng, 2000: 356): 'Verbal and non-verbal components of the discourse structure oriented to the completion of language tasks, or "language-work together", rather than the pragmatic abilities per se of the interactants.'

This is akin to what Bray, Ross and Todd (1999) refer to as interpersonal skills (after Stengelhofen, 1993), which are critical to the development of the therapeutic relationship. A process of mutual social co-ordination occurs at the interface between therapist and the client and/or significant others. It is characterized by the therapist's use of particular technical skills in relation to the contributions of the service user(s). Creating the circumstances and providing support for the client to use available skills is part of the therapist's role as an interactant.

Describing enactment processes

Detailed and explicit descriptions of technical skills and their usage remain fairly elusive, although, as Horton and Byng (2000: 356) point out, 'Interest in "cues" and "feedback" is clearly far from new in therapy.'

A few authors, in particular Byng and Black (1995) and Horton and Byng (2000), have grappled with the problem of detecting and defining the specific skills that are used in the enactment of therapy with adults with aphasia. Horton and Byng (2000: 356) were specifically concerned with looking in detail at the technical features of the therapeutic interaction. They ask an important question:

There is an abundance of anecdotal evidence for what goes on in language therapy in clinical practice ... there are some fundamental issues about therapy that remain opaque. For example, do any two therapists with the same level of experience, and given the same language therapy tasks to carry out with the same aphasic person, actually enact therapy in the same way? (p. 356)

Horton and Byng (2000) point out the methodological difficulties in attempting to observe and analyse the therapist's use of enactment processes. There must be some agreement on what these so-called enactment processes are, supported by clear, unambiguous descriptions. Their paper introduces a categorical coding framework for analysing the client–therapist interaction, called the *aphasia therapy interaction coding system* (ATICS). This is described as 'a top-down hierarchical system with mutually exhaustive codes' (Horton and Byng, 2000: 263).

The categories were derived from transcriptions of routine language therapy sessions between eight client–therapist dyads across 13 different sessions, where recurring patterns were identified from repeated examination of the data. Two levels were defined: content of therapy and interaction, each level comprising separate items arranged in hierarchical order. ATICS provides a systematic approach to examining therapeutic discourse that is concerned with the 'complex interaction between task demands and interaction' (Horton and Byng, 2000: 372).

Function of enactment processes

Exploring the therapy process with aphasic adults, Kagan (1995) identifies two aspects of conversation: transaction and interaction. Transaction is defined as the giving and receiving of information, the exchange of ideas, and the sharing of internal judgements and feelings. Interaction refers to the process whereby a social connection is established between therapist and service user. The use of enactment processes is embedded in a communication relationship between client and therapist that aims to be balanced. This implies a process of mutual social co-ordination to which each person contributes (Alm and Newell, 1996).

Transaction

The process of formal transaction helps to define the goals and responsibilities of the participants. Therapist and client orient to a turn-taking format that is conducive to the clinical focus. There is the implicit understanding of each other's roles, which influences the content of the interaction. The focus of therapy and the boundaries of each encounter are established by the use of particular rituals that act to inform the participants.

Openings and closures

Hargie, Saunders and Dickson (1994) emphasize the roles of opening and closing in social interaction. They refer to the opening sequence as 'set induction', which helps to establish the frame of reference for both therapist and client. It brings about a state of readiness in the participants. The expectations of the encounter are articulated and objectives shared. In SLT, the function is made clear and links to previous interactions/ sessions are highlighted. Through this induction process, the therapist is able to gauge the person's knowledge and understanding of the situation, which in turn may prompt the use of facilitation strategies.

Closure involves the use of 'interaction rituals' (Hargie, Saunders and Dickson, 1994: 161). Closings operate to segment talk (Button and Casey in Atkinson and Heritage, 1984). As well as demarcating shifts in activity or topic within the session, closing actions serve to draw a session or episode of intervention to a close. Hargie, Saunders and Dickson (1994) argue that effective closure is usually planned and is characterized by overt completion of a topic, mutual check on what has been addressed, acknowledgement of the individual's sense of achievements and an indication about where therapy will go next if appropriate. The latter is said to be important to the individual's motivation so that the next encounter can be anticipated positively, or 'moving on' can be achieved.

Exchanging information

Clearly, the exchange of information is a relevant part of the intervention process and the therapist uses certain techniques to facilitate the information flow with the service user (Bray, Ross and Todd, 1999). The therapist performs an action with the specific aim of soliciting a response from the individual. Diverse question forms are used in order to access the necessary information (Dillon in Hargie, 1997), e.g. conducting a case history interview, or reviewing an activity that has been carried out in another setting. Where a question is unsuccessful, the therapist pursues a response by various means, including clarifying what is known about the individual's situation, reviewing any commonly held knowledge and rephrasing the question form (Pomerantz in Atkinson and Heritage, 1984). The idea is to increase the store of common knowledge shared by therapist and client, i.e. the 'individual profile' (see Chapter 4).

Giving instructions and explanations

Providing the individual with prior instructions helps prepare the person for the task or activity requirements. The rules of engagement are understood so that the person knows what to expect and what skills to focus on. This type of preparation may serve to promote the client's performance. Usually, a common ground of knowledge is established, i.e. identification of the skills that the individual possesses, which is then linked with novel material (Hargie, Saunders and Dickson, 1994, citing Novak et al., 1971).

Providing explanations is also identified as a 'core skill in most professions' (Brown and Atkins in Hargie, 1997: 181). The *what*, *how* and *why* are relevant to individual understanding of the current situation and any proposed changes. It involves the organization and presentation of ideas in an accessible way, avoiding professional terminology and using linguistic code that is shared by client and therapist. Concrete examples and use of multiple media may facilitate linguistic accessibility. As Hargie, Saunders and Dickson (1994: 175) state, it is about getting to the 'heart of the matter'. Defining the rationale for intervention activities helps to establish the scope of the intervention whilst also addressing any false or misleading assumptions held by an individual. Mutual articulation of therapy goals helps to structure therapy encounters.

Engaging with the person

Heath in Atkinson and Heritage (1984: 247) describes the demands of social interaction: '(it) requires participants to establish and sustain mutual involvement in the business or topic at hand and to co-ordinate systematically their actions and activities'.

Interaction in the therapy setting is concerned with how the therapist and client/significant other orient to each other or 'direct communicative or social actions toward one another' (Nofsinger, 1991: 13). The context and the situational rules that are implicit help to define particular speech acts (Nofsinger, 1991). The participants make moves to satisfy a range of communicative functions that relate to the clinical situation, e.g. to solicit information, disclose knowledge about self, express internal ideas and judgements and display recognition of one another.

In the professional–client, service provider–service user relationship, asymmetrical communication is always a potential by-product. Power is often conferred on the person of professional status. The communication difficulty of the individual is a further aspect that compounds the situation, which may leave that person vulnerable to the suggestions and ideas of the person with a full communication skill set, i.e. the therapist. Therapist contributions to the interaction are driven by a desire to reveal the individual's competence (Kagan, 1995) and to achieve a balanced interaction. Accordingly, the therapist has 'the ability to focus on and remain focused on salient features of the situation in order for learning to take place' (Bray, Ross and Todd, 1999: 47).

Modifying language

The discipline of conversation analysis (CA) describes language primarily as 'a vehicle for communicative interaction' (Hutchby and Wooffitt, 1998: 37). The therapist, as a skilled communicator equipped with knowledge about communication disability, suspends the usual use of communication skills. On the basis of what is known about a particular disorder and what is observed in the individual client, the therapist selects and modifies the form, content and function of her/his conversation turns so that any potential asymmetries are addressed. Weismer in Bishop and Leonard (2000) identifies three factors that are hypothesized to affect lexical processing in children with specific language impairment (SLI):

(i) Rate of speech – the act of 'slow speaking' may serve to provide the child with 'additional processing time', thereby facilitating 'linguistic computation and storage of lexical items' (p. 163). This may be particularly important in instructional situations.

(ii) Vocal stress – the use of emphatic stress may highlight the salient points of an utterance, thereby reducing the processing demands on the individual.

(iii) Use of visual cues – the use of gesture, environmental reference points and pictures may also reduce the processing load as well as enhancing attention and memory.

Turn organization

The organization of turns is crucial to the balanced participation of the interactants. In CA terms this is described as 'how one *gets the floor*', which 'depends on some way of changing and alternating speakers' (Nofsinger, 1991: 78–79). It is about recognizing the potential end of a turn, which Sacks, Schegloff and Jefferson (1978) call 'transition relevance place'. Various methods are employed to demarcate turns and to support the person with a communication disability taking conversational floor during an encounter, including altering pitch or volume of voice, nonverbal signal and change in verbal emphasis.

In naturally occurring conversation, turn-taking is viewed as *locally managed* and *interactionally managed* (Sacks, Schegloff and Jefferson, 1978). That is, the acts of the participants determine characteristics of the turns and who shall make the next contribution (Nofsinger, 1991). There is no fixed ordering or allocation of turns. The individual characteristics of the participants (personality, knowledge base, motivation for turns, cultural and ethnic background, etc.), the goals of the interaction and contextual features suggest that considerable variation is to be expected. The nature of SLT – an interaction between therapist and person with a communication disability, or professional or significant other – demands sensitive negotiation of the conversational floor. Therapist awareness of the knowledge base, lived experience and skill set of the individual shapes the content and use of language in turns and the way 'transition relevance places' are indicated. For instance, the therapist may use silence to encourage initiation in the person with a learning disability or to provide extra processing time for the person with a language disorder.

Waiting time

The use of pause or 'waiting time' not only separates the turns of speakers but also may have a beneficial effect on language processing. Weismer in Bishop and Leonard (2001) observes that when teachers were trained to insert extended pauses (three seconds or longer) after posing questions to pupils in the classroom reviews, there was a resulting increase in the retention of information and the complexity of responses (citing a study conducted by Weismer and Schraeder, 1993). Weismer also recommends the use of linguistic routines and scripts that are already in use by the child. Processing demands are reduced 'by embedding language targets within highly familiar routines or scripts' (p. 171).

Being a responsive listener
How the therapist indicates recipiency of the client's contributions is important to the progress of the interaction. It lets the client know that his/her contribution is not only valued but also relevant. This is an integral part of the feedback loop depicted in the model of 'interpersonal communication in the intervention context' (Figure 4:3), illustrated in the previous chapter. The therapist indicates recipiency through verbal and non-verbal behaviour (Heath in Atkinson and Heritage, 1984). Non-verbal signals include body posture, eye gaze and facial expression. Verbal signals include vocal expression and phrases of acknowledgement and encouragement.

Gaining and maintaining attention

Attention is a prerequisite for accessing the social opportunities and tasks presented by the therapist; however, the very nature of the individual's difficulties may make it hard to channel and maintain attention. The therapist is concerned with arousing the person into a 'state of readiness appropriate to the task to follow' (Hargie, Saunders and Dickson, 1994: 144). Different attention call strategies may be employed according to the age and individual characteristics of the person. Gaining the attention of a child with language delay may involve augmenting the visual and auditory features of materials and activities, e.g. slowly revealing a play item to increase the child's anticipation, using exaggerated intonation patterns or facial expressions to attract the child's interest. The therapist working with an adult with aphasia may use discreet gestures and verbal prompts to secure and maintain attention.

Facilitation and feedback

The business of speech and language therapy requires that problems in communication are identified and addressed appropriately. In the field of CA, the occurrence of such a difficulty is referred to as 'trouble'. The analyst identifies the conversational turn which is the source of the problem (Hutchby and Wooffitt, 1998). In correspondence with locating the trouble source is the organization of repair. Schegloff, Jefferson and Sacks (1977) describe a repair system that defines the properties of the different types of repair. A distinction is made between repair initiated by 'self', i.e. the person whose conversational turn is the source of trouble, and that initiated by 'other'.

Addressing sources of trouble

The therapist uses facilitation and feedback to address trouble sources. They are common features within the therapy process (Davies and van der Gaag, 1992; Schubert, Miner and Till, 1973; Simmons-Mackie, Damico and Damico, 1999). Although related in terms of their function in supporting the individual to resolve any difficulties experienced, facilitation and feedback are distinctive in application. Cairns in Hargie (1997: 140) states that the idea of feedback 'leads to continuation of the communication or some modification'. Nickels (1997) asserts the importance of giving feedback on the quality and accuracy of a client's response. Facilitation is somewhat similar in that it too is designed to support the continuation of the client's contribution to the interaction and involves the use of cues, modelling and response shaping (Davies and van der Gaag, 1992). It is about addressing communicative struggle by providing a supportive cue or ramp.

Reinforcement plays an important role in SLT. Hargie, Saunders and Dickson (1994) describe an investigation into the key communication skills used by the profession that was carried out by Saunders and Caves (1986). Videotapes of therapists conducting sessions with both children and adult clients were subjected to peer analysis. The behavioural category 'Using positive reinforcement' was one example of effective practice. Social rewards, including positive feedback or praise for a task attempt or an activity well done, serve to fortify the recipient and to encourage further endeavours.

Recasting, elicited imitation and modelling

Fey and Proctor-Williams in Bishop and Leonard (2001) consider the positive influence of recasting, elicited imitation and modelling on the performance of children with specific language impairment (SLI). A recast is designed to be a 'non-intrusive' procedure that is used in naturally occurring conversations. It immediately follows the utterance of the other person and shares the referential context. The original meaning, and major lexical items and referents, are preserved. The aim is to 'facilitate grammar development by creating an optimal environment for a child to actively compare target forms with structures generated by the existing grammar' (p. 179).

Elicited imitation is a direct request for an imitative response to a particular stimulus. It is usually tied into a contingent reinforcement schedule – as the stimulus is withdrawn, the individual acts more independently. The potential value of elicited imitation lies in its capacity to draw attention to particular communication forms whilst eliminating any competing stimuli, to structure opportunities for practice and promote exposure to target forms. It involves the repeated demonstration of the target form, which is observed/listened to by the person, who then attempts to produce it as instructed under similar conditions. Both modelling and elicited imitation involve differential feedback for informing the person about the quality of response. Typically, didactic teaching procedures are employed, although either procedure may utilize natural contexts and daily activities, e.g. milieu approaches. Fey and Proctor-Williams in Bishop and Leonard (2001) recommend an eclectic approach to optimize language development among children with SLI.

Reviewing what has taken place

During the course of therapeutic interaction, the act of summarizing is used to recycle content for the client (Button and Casey in Atkinson and Heritage, 1984). It provides the client/significant other and the therapist with the opportunity to review what has occurred in the session. It is used in the closure of a task or activity as well as in the formal procedure for concluding a session.

Maintaining the person and the context

Interaction with people with communication disabilities demands sensitivity to the human condition and the difficulties experienced by the individual. Individual needs, e.g. sensory or physical difficulties, are accommodated by therapist actions and the organization of the physical environment. Conditions that make the environment and interaction accessible and comfortable for the person are created, e.g. drawing the blinds to minimize glare from the window, placing equipment so that it is within arm's reach, checking glasses or hearing aids as required.

It is inevitable that human communication will involve the expression of affect. Furthermore, in situations where communicative struggle, loss of skills and changed expectations are likely, emotional difficulties may occur. Hargie, Saunders and Dickson (1994) identify three ways in which affect is communicated:

1) Explicit: The person conveys his/her internal state through verbal content, e.g. 'I am fed up today'.
2) Implicit: The person conveys internal feelings through implication of what is said. There is no direct statement or words that label the inner condition. The emotional message overlays the content, e.g. the parent of the child who has recently been diagnosed with learning disabilities conveys a low mood state by saying, 'I am so tired. I am off my food and can't stand all the noise of his screaming. I haven't a clue how I'll cope.'
3) Inferred: The verbal and non-verbal/paralinguistic behaviours of the person are signal bearers of internal state. The therapist infers what is going on for the person separately from the content of the message, e.g. the client's response of 'Things are going really well' may appear to be incompatible with the listless movements and flat affect of the person facing the therapist.

The experience and emotional response of the individual requires acknowledgement and sensitive responding by the therapist. Para- phrasing content and reflecting displays of affect are used to demonstrate acknowledgement of the person's condition and its relevance to communication.

Glossary of enactment processes

The reader is referred to the Appendix: Glossary of enactment processes. Seven categories of enactment process are described, which serve particular functions in the intervention process. In each case, a definition of the enactment process is provided with a rationale for its use. Concrete examples of overt technical skills that represent the enactment process are supplied, although the list is not exhaustive!

- *Engagement techniques* are used to support the attention of the individual and/or significant others in the therapy process, so that they can attend to the objective or focus of assessment and therapy activities.
- *Modification techniques* are applied to the therapist's use of communication skills in response to those of the client, so that competencies are revealed and a balanced interaction achieved.
- *Facilitation techniques* are invoked to provide timely and appropriate assistance or support to the individual, so that communicative access is improved and available skills are used.
- *Feedback techniques* are used to promote therapeutic change, so that individual contributions are affirmed, modified, positively encouraged and reviewed.
- *Personal maintenance techniques* are employed to establish the personal comfort of the individual by acknowledging and supporting individual needs and behaviours.
- *Context maintenance techniques* are used to preserve the adequacy and comfort of the therapeutic environment and the organization of materials so that optimal responding will ensue.
- *Transaction techniques* are used to ensure the timely release of information that is pertinent to the therapeutic process. This is so that the shared knowledge base on the individual's communication skills and other aspects of lifestyle is current and relevant. In a sense, the therapeutic process is shored up by transactional activities.

Gauging the need to intervene

Gauging the need to use an enactment process is informed by acute observation of a given situation and inner knowledge of how to effect change in this situation (Bray, Ross and Todd, 1999). Technical skills are used in a fast and fluid way that appears almost 'intuitive' to the naked eye. Indeed, some may identify 'clinical intuition' as an artefact of this process. Byng (1995: 4) elaborates on this:

There seems to be an 'automatic pilot' that a good therapist develops and then switches on which suggests how to present a task, how and when to modulate it, how to respond to a specific response by the person (with aphasia), and so on.

Selection and use of enactment processes

Three aspects of the interaction between client and therapist appear to be important to the online selection and use of enactment processes as illustrated in Figure 5:2: the *antecedent* conditions, the client's *contribution* and the *outcome*. Although identified separately, they are all inter-related.

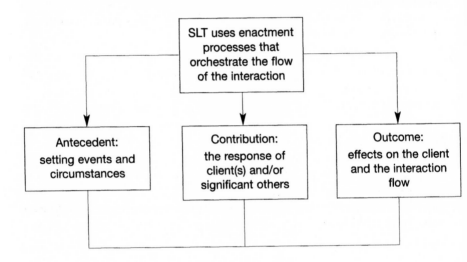

Figure 5.2 Online selection of enactment processes

There is no fixed starting point to the online selection of enactment processes. It may start with a contribution made by the client. Alternatively, it may be at the antecedent stage when the therapist presents a task or activity to the client, or at the stage after the client contributes, i.e. the outcome. Three linked questions guide the online appraisal of the therapeutic interaction. The first question focuses on the actual response(s) emitted by the individual. The second question relates to the antecedent conditions of the client's responding behaviour. The third question looks at the outcome. A form of 'online' processing occurs as the therapist goes through a hierarchy of information derived from various sources, including the current situation, so that the most appropriate technique is selected.

Question 1: the contribution of the individual
What are the features of the individual's contribution that prompt the use of one enactment process as opposed to another? The therapist observes,

listens and interprets individual contributions and behaviour that may reveal evidence of:

- Lack of engagement and poor attention, e.g. lethargic, despondent, bored, distracted, extremely passive, hyperactive.
- Difficulties with conventional interaction or use of particular ways of communicating, e.g. failure to understand what has been said, use of non-verbal signals, use of single words to express ideas, use of other modalities such as pictures, drawing or writing.
- Variable content and quality of responses, e.g. incomplete or delayed response, successive attempts that take the person closer/further away from target.
- Inadequacy of therapy context, e.g. the level of lighting is insufficient for lip reading.
- Sensory, physical or emotional needs that must be dealt with, e.g. the person's hearing aid is whistling due to an incomplete seal in the external auditory meatus or the person is showing signs of tiredness.
- Inadequate information and explanations, e.g. the person does not understand why therapy is focusing on a particular area.

Question 2: the antecedent conditions

What are the setting events or circumstances that prompt the therapist to invoke the use of one technique as opposed to another? The therapist evaluates the client's contribution against the setting events and circumstances in the situation:

- The antecedent stimulus, i.e. the communication demands presented to the person.
- The communication profile of the individual, i.e. what is already known and understood about the person's communication difficulties and their responses to therapeutic techniques.
- The current and immediate situation of the individual, i.e. what is known about the personal circumstances, including psychological state of the individual.
- The learning process, i.e. the planned process of prevention, change or maintenance as appropriate to the individual's needs.

Question 3: the outcome

What are the effects of the client's contribution: on the client and the interaction flow? The therapist scrutinizes the effects of the individual's contribution on the current situation and makes an evaluation of its relative worth. This includes the effects of any technical skills that have been used. This involves observation of the different aspects of the outcome, including:

- The client's general demeanour or overt show of satisfaction, e.g. was the response/contribution satisfactory to the individual?

- The clarity and accessibility of the client's response, e.g. was the therapist able to interpret the meaning accurately within the expected time frame?
- The continuation of the interaction, e.g. were the therapist and client able to move on from the specific interaction sequence?

Because the interaction process is dynamic and continuous, the outcome becomes the antecedent or setting events/circumstances of the next interaction sequence, and so on.

Selection of technique

By immediate and full appraisal of the interaction, the therapist makes a decision regarding:

1) the location for introducing an enactment process within the interaction sequence, e.g. antecedent condition, contribution or outcome;
2) what enactment process to introduce to the identified location, e.g. facilitation of contribution, attention maintenance, emotional support, etc. Included in this process is, of course, the decision *not* to intervene.

In this way, the therapist affects the antecedent, contribution and outcome of an interaction sequence, using enactment processes much as a conductor uses a baton to orchestrate a piece of music. The discipline is learned and therapeutic vigilance is maintained. Technical skills are used in response to the online appraisal that takes place. The client also brings his or her own expertise to the situation, which in turn influences the therapist's manoeuvres.

Process of intervention

There is a need to externalize the therapy process as characterized by the centre of influence, the role of therapist and the use of enactment processes. Exploration of the latter reveals therapists' use of technical skills. Definition of these skills is not meant to 'conflate theory and methodology' (Boyle, 1999: 133). Nor does it represent the whole story. It is an attempt to examine the interaction between therapist and client by articulating the underlying function of the enactment process. This is relevant to the development of therapeutic skills and in realizing the full potential of speech and language therapy services (Byng, 1995). The reader is referred to the second part of this book, where the glossary in the Appendix is used as a coding framework on transcribed excerpts from therapy sessions.

SECTION 2
PROCESSES OF INTERVENTION

Chapter 6
Therapeutic interaction with the individual

Intervention where the individual is a major centre of influence is concerned with internal processes that affect the way information is received, organized and interpreted. The interface between client and therapist is important to the mechanism for change, where individual competencies and functional use of skills are of primary interest. Technical skills are employed in the therapist's interaction with the client.

Although intervention activities may target the individual, it is not to the exclusion of any other centre of influence. An intervention may initially focus on the individual with the aim of revealing as much about the person as possible. Significant others may be involved at separate times or at a later date during the intervention period. The focus of intervention may move to broader centres of influence in an effort to secure a generalized effect. Moving from the centre of the individual in an outward direction through the communication partnership, environment and finally to society represents the broadening of the individual's social and political horizons (Bronfenbrenner, 1979). Alternatively, the intervention process may start within the environment, tackling more general communication issues before plotting a route back to the individual for some specific input.

The continuum of direct–indirect approaches

Direct intervention is a term that is found often in the intervention literature on speech and language therapy. It refers to therapy that focuses primarily on the interface between therapist and client(s). The term 'direct intervention' does not mean that more directive methods are used. Indeed, a variety of strategies may be employed, including non-directive ones. Nor does it mean that significant others are not involved. Bray, Ross and Todd (1999: 27) state that significant others may be present; however, 'The essential feature is that the client, or client(s), and clinician are physically together in the interaction.'

The interrelatedness of the different centres of influence places direct and indirect intervention on a continuum. For example, the therapy session that has client and significant other present during the session may feature some individual work with the client (individual communication) as well as joint work with the client and significant other (communication partnership). The direct therapy process shifts between individual and partnership communication.

A focus on the individual centre of influence does not imply a series of 'individual' therapy sessions. The context for the therapeutic interaction may vary from individual to group-based therapy. The main feature that they share is that interaction takes place between therapist and client.

Mechanism for change

The 'mechanism for change' is a term used by Byng and Black (1995). It is how we attribute any change in an individual's communication skills. Explanations are formed to assert the relationship between the intervention activities and any measurable differences. Usually, the design of the therapy activities considers how change will be brought about. This is partly dependent on the professional judgements of the therapist and how theoretical knowledge is used to make sense of the individual's presenting difficulties (Bray, Ross and Todd, 1999).

Individual factors of influence

In the early stages of the intervention cycle, it is not uncommon to centre on the person as a starting point. This means considering individual factors that may affect the overall intervention process. Scherer's (1993) 'Matching Person and Technology' model (MPT) cited by Lasker and Bedrosian (2001) provides a model for considering salient factors in the use of assistive communication technology. This has been adapted here to provide a practical framework for considering the factors of individual relevance – person, milieu and intervention (PMI):

- person – positive factors and any difficulties relating to the individual, including age, health, skills and abilities, emotional wellbeing, attitude, temperament, life-course experiences and intervention history, amongst others;
- milieu – the significant others with whom communication partnerships are formed and characteristics of the social environments used by the individual;
- intervention – critical features of the assessment and therapy approach such as the goals, themes, activities, materials and methods.

The person

As well as the positive factors and difficulties that are part of the person's presentation, there are also the values that an individual brings to the therapy process. These are all relevant to the design of the intervention and the individual's uptake of therapy opportunities. With reference to acquired language impairment, Sarno (1993: 326) states that:

A person's values play an important role in all stages of recovery, rehabilitation, and reintegration into the community. Impairments, disabilities, and handicaps mean different things to different people, and one's previously held concepts of them will greatly influence the new 'self' which the disabled person must develop, since the activities that contributed to the previous definition of that person are changed or no longer there.

Patterns of augmentative and alternative communication (AAC) use and acceptance may be informed, although not exclusively, by the individual's own values base. Lasker and Bedrosian (2001) observe that the attitudes held by the AAC user, together with those of the familiar communication partner, are integral to the acceptance of a new way of communicating. Both client and partner have the potential to influence uptake of the AAC device. Their individual experiences across the life course and their connections to particular social groups will affect how each responds to the current situation (Brumfitt, 1999).

Client degree of wellbeing or distress is another important variable in the intervention equation (Enderby, 1992; Enderby and John, 1999). The psychological and physical health of the individual and significant other(s) is central to therapeutic progression: a person who is depressed or is in a state of anguish may find it difficult to engage in the intervention process (see Chapter 3).

Individual uptake of the intervention is dependent on how and to what extent the main objectives are integrated into the individual's life (adapted from Lasker and Bedrosian, 2000). Optimal uptake suggests a willingness to use the strategies learned in therapy in everyday situations. The integration of an AAC device into an individual's lifestyle is dependent on the ease with which it is operated. If a person feels well practised and confident in the use of a system, it is more likely to become part of daily functioning (Lasker and Bedrosian, 2001).

The converse of acceptance is dissociation, abandonment or even outright rejection of the therapy recommendations. All therapies, because they are very much about the individual's needs, carry this risk. It is managed by early and ongoing negotiation with the client and/or significant others. The work of Connect – the Communication Disability Network – provides some very good examples of negotiation between client and therapist (Pound et al., 2000). People with aphasia and their significant others have been involved in planning the development of a satellite centre in Bristol, right from its inception. At the London centre of Connect, newcomers are invited to join a beginners group for a period of about ten weeks, where listening to the expressed needs of individuals is a priority.

The milieu

The support of significant others is crucial to the individual's acceptance of and commitment to the course of intervention. Motivation does not operate in isolation: the interest and attention of others feed the individual's inner drive. Even when it is the individual with whom the therapist interacts primarily, the contribution of the significant others who are in contact with the person on a daily basis should not be overlooked. Individual change does not occur in a vacuum.

Countless reports have been made of the contribution of significant others to the individual's therapeutic gains. Sacchett et al. (1999) highlight the importance of skilful interpretation by communication partners of the communicative drawing attempted by people with severe aphasia. The attitude of communication partners may affect the individual's acceptance and use of a communication device (Granlund et al. in Cockerill and Carroll-Few, 2001; Lasker and Bedrosian, 2001).

Cockerill and Fuller in Cockerill and Carroll-Few (2001: 82) propose a layered model for developing communicative competence within a supportive layered environment. At the heart of the model is the communicative competence of the child, defined according to the four areas of competence outlined by Light (1989): linguistic, operational, strategic and social. Key environmental factors that are inextricably linked to the individual's developing competence are identified in the outer layer and include funding for aids/training, attitudes to AAC, technological and training support, communication opportunities and policies, as well as collaborative team working.

Therapy approach
The therapy approach aims to be relevant and amenable to the individual situation. Amenability refers to the ease with which a therapy goal may be realized. It underlines the importance of the link between the individual's current communication skills and the selected target of therapy. Care is taken to avoid setting unrealistic goals that bear no relationship to the existing situation. For instance, Enderby and Emerson (1995), in their review of the speech and language therapy literature, report that stimulability is a critical factor in articulation therapy, i.e. the individual must be able to produce the target sound with relatively little effort.

Assumptions
Intervention activities that target change in the individual's communication system are underpinned by a number of basic assumptions. First, there is the notion that by practising the relevant tasks that have been selected for this purpose, change will be effected in the internal speech and language processing mechanisms. This implies some 'implicit relationship between the task and the deficit' (Byng in Code and Muller, 1995: 9). Another assumption is that the therapist's use of certain enactment processes (technical skills) facilitates the individual's ability to address tasks.

Generalization of therapy effects
Generalization of therapy effects is an important consideration in intervention that centres on the individual. Robson et al. (1998a) provide a

postscript to their therapy study of written communication with a person with jargon aphasia. Picture stimuli were used to help the client to access written word forms in the initial phase. Facilitation of functional use of the written vocabulary was tackled in a second phase through question and answer routines. The authors point out that individual gains made to picture stimuli did not extend to spontaneous use at other times. It seems that establishing a skill in the confines of the clinical setting is no guarantee of improvement elsewhere in the person's daily life. The authors suggest that the individually centred therapy applied to their subject served as a foundation on which a vocabulary was established for future therapies.

In order to move the effects of therapy into everyday life, focusing solely on the individual's communication skills is probably not enough. Its contribution lies in preparing the ground for any further investigations, and for identifying and addressing potential obstacles in the communication environment that may affect the individual's functional use of established skills.

Bringing about change

Bringing about change presupposes the development of competence in some way. At the individual centre of influence, change is roughly subdivided into improving the underlying system, addressing the individual's psychological state and exploring the functional use of skills. None of the approaches are mutually exclusive.

Addressing the underlying system

There are a number of therapy approaches to improve the way an individual both processes incoming data and performs communication acts. Some approaches seek to strengthen the individual's speech and language system in such a way that an existing problem is ameliorated or circumvented. Alternately, therapy may be targeted at the system underlying language and communication acquisition in an effort to boost development.

Strengthening the processing system
The therapy application of cognitive neuropsychology is 'directed at a specific language processing problem' (Edmundson and McIntosh in Code and Muller, 1995: 147). The selection and design of activities are influenced by the formed hypothesis about the nature of the speech or language difficulty (Howard and Hatfield, 1987). Therapy approaches may be specifically geared to re-route the individual's processing of information, thereby addressing an aspect of communication difficulty that is experienced. Frazier-Norbury and Chiat (2000) describe how a semantic intervention was used to promote word recognition in an eight-year-old

child who had problems with phonological processing. Therapy activities that aimed to overcome the child's phonological difficulties were deemed crucial to a fluent reading ability. Yampolsky and Waters (2002) combined the use of phonological information with semantic information to improve the reading of an individual with deep dyslexia.

Marshall, Chiat and Pring's (1997) published case study provides a detailed account of a specifically tailored therapy programme based on a diagnosed language processing deficit. Formulated hypotheses about the nature of the impairment were tested out using a range of assessment and therapy tasks. The aim was to improve the client's processing of verbs' thematic roles.

PB was a monolingual English speaker who had a cerebrovascular accident (CVA). Prior to his stroke, PB worked as a chiropodist. As a result of his stroke, PB was left with a persistent right hemiplegia, right visual field deficit and severe dysphasia. In the initial stages of recovery from his stroke, PB's communicative output was restricted to two phrases: 'Tuesday afternoon' and 'everything about it'. Approximately two years post-onset, his speech was assessed to be fluent with some word-finding problems, semantic and phonological errors and paragrammaticisms. PB received intensive speech and language therapy over an extended period of time that resulted in some gains to comprehension of nouns.

At the time of the case study, it had been six years since PB's stroke. Language therapy had ceased although he was attending a social group. Based on the findings of some preliminary assessments, a further course of therapy was offered to PB. It was hypothesized that his difficulties with verbs were 'primarily semantic, and that these particularly affected his processing of thematic information' (p. 860).

Furthermore, it was predicted that

> PB would have problems with mapping between syntax and semantics of verbs in both input and output, but that he would be able to understand and express other aspects of verb meaning relatively well, and would be able to judge and produce appropriate verb syntax (p. 860).

A series of subtests was devised to evaluate the strength of the hypothesis and predictions. It was suggested that PB's word-finding deficit with verbs originated in the semantic system. This led to the design of a therapy programme based on the hypothesis that access to thematic information would bring about improved verb comprehension and production.

Therapy was delivered in two-hourly sessions once a week over a six-week period. In the latter stages of therapy this was supplemented by homework. Activities were designed to test out the hypothesis in a hierarchy of gradually increasing demands. Colour coding was a critical feature of therapy tasks. It was used to facilitate both input and output on the comprehension and production tasks, e.g. differentiating the roles of the people in a sentence by always marking the recipient of the action in red, and to provide a sentence frame to support PB's production. The demands on PB were increased according to his success rate on the previous set of tasks. The final stage looked at story telling and involved more open production as PB was expected 'to comprehend, recall and effectively retell stories containing several three-argument events' (p. 872).

The gains made by PB included improved picture descriptions both in terms of the linguistic content and the communicative value to observers. There was evidence to suggest that this skill extended to the more open condition of story telling. Some limited generalization was also reported. The authors attribute this change to the possible restoring of 'information about perspective and the mapping between thematic and syntactic roles' (p. 875).

Marshall, Chiat and Pring's (1997) case study demonstrates therapy where the mechanism for change is centred on the individual. The specific design of the tasks was based on the defined clinical predictions. The hierarchical presentation of therapy items and the practice element of therapy procedures contributed to positive outcomes in PB's verb processing.

Strengthening speech and voice production

Improving speech production for the purposes of promoting accuracy, intelligibility and self-monitoring is a common theme in speech and language therapy sessions. Therapy activities involve a range of methods that help the individual to concentrate their efforts on speech production. They usually involve some of the following (Enderby and Emerson, 1995):

- explaining the nature of the particular problem with production so that the speaker is able to appreciate the rationale underpinning therapy activities;
- experimenting with different ways of producing the aspect of speech targeted in therapy;
- discrimination training for detecting the difference between aspects of speech production, and target and non-target responses;
- providing sensory feedback, e.g. auditory, visual, kinaesthetic and tactile, that emphasizes the distinctive features of target and non-target aspects of production;
- training in the use of specific strategies and system support, e.g. use of respiration to support an increase in volume, such that production of speech is improved.

Developing language and cognition through non-directive play

Many authors have written about the relationship between play and cognition. Reports of positive correlations between the play level and developmental stage of children with learning disabilities support this argument (Coupe O'Kane and Goldbart, 1998). Play is an important feature of some interventions, providing the milieu for the development of language and cognition.

Non-directive play is a therapy approach where the child leads the interaction, and therapist and or significant others shape their responses according to the child's observed behaviour. It is based on the work of Rogers (1951), who expounded on a person-centred philosophy. It is not about the acquisition of specific skills; rather it is designed:

> ... to work at a systems level ... thus underpinning future language and communication development. It aims to equip the child with experiences of language and communication strategies that are powerful and effective, so that children can make use of all the learning opportunities in their environment (Cogher, 1999: 7).

Non-directive play as an approach does not exclude any possible involvement of significant others. Based on developmental cognitive principles, it is about creating the conditions for the child to explore and develop at a pace (Bray, Ross and Todd, 1999; Cogher, 1999). The emphasis is on experiential learning in play contexts. The therapist or significant other provides the scaffolding that is conducive to language acquisition (Bruner, 1975), and s/he performs the role of observer and commentator providing a verbal account of the action in the child's play. The adult will frequently engage in 'play' alongside the child, imitating and reflecting his or her activities. Non-directive play seeks to match the child's level of ability based on the premise that children attend to those aspects of communication that are meaningful to them (Harris, 1992).

Addressing psychological state

Counselling is an integral part of the interpersonal skills used by therapists in developing and sustaining a therapeutic relationship with someone with a communication difficulty. Bray, Ross and Todd (1999: 94) identify 'genuineness, warmth and empathy' as core qualities of this relationship. It is about providing the individual with the opportunity for addressing the psychological effects of having a communication difficulty or to support change in the individual's life course, e.g. accommodating an altered way of communicating. Wintgens in Kersner and Wright (2001: 200) urges specific consideration of the emotional needs of children with communication difficulties and additional behaviour problems: 'Many such children are disenchanted with their experience of life: they may be underachieving and have often been socially excluded.'

DiLillo, Neimeyer and Manning (2002) describe a narrative approach used in the counselling offered to people who stutter. Grounded in personal construct theory, the aim is to deconstruct the 'stuttering-dominated personal narrative' so that an alternative narrative may be reconstructed 'that is more compatible with being a fluent speaker' (p. 19). This type of approach may have a role to play in the maintenance of therapeutic gains. The person's altered constructs make it easier to accommodate a different and more fluent way of speaking.

Counselling running alongside speech and language therapy

There are times when individual speech and language therapy is not sufficient to address the underlying issues of a particular communication difficulty. In the case of psychogenic voice disorder, there is evidence to suggest that some individuals would benefit from a two-handed approach that involves not only speech and language therapy, but also some form of psychological intervention (White, Deary and Wilson, 1997).

Marcia was a young woman in her early twenties who was referred to SLT with ventricular fold voice disorder. She had been raised by her mother who had kicked her out in her late teens. She subsequently lived in a squat in an inner city area and worked as an administrative assistant. Her voice problem developed at about the time she lost her job. The referral represented a second attempt to gain help for Marcia's voice disorder. She had previously received counselling and was keen for this to continue.

At her initial appointment, Marcia presented as somewhat unusual. She arrived wearing many layers of clothing: she wore three coats, multiple scarves wound round her neck and several pairs of gloves worn on top of each other. It was considered that this could have been due to a lack of heat in her accommodation; however, this was not the case and she continued to wear many layers even in the warmest weather and in centrally heated environments! Conversation with her revealed a nature that was inclined to magnify life experiences. She was convinced that she had cancer. Later on in the episode of intervention, Marcia was encouraged to take off her outer layers, which took a large part of the session. It was discovered that her arms were a mass of scratches.

Therapy was negotiated between therapist and client. Marcia was keen to receive counselling for her voice disorder and asked the SLT what she could do for her. The therapist countered this by defining clearly what she could contribute and what she could not. In short, she drew the boundaries for their working partnership: she could treat the symptoms, and counselling would indeed form part of that process, but a referral to a professional counselling service was also recommended. Marcia accepted this and a referral was made. Marcia was supported to articulate her own goals. The therapist responded by demarcating their various responsibilities in the partnership.

Marcia was seen once a week over a period of eight weeks. She achieved normal voice that generalized to all contexts. On her last session, she arrived wearing just one coat and one scarf. She had just enrolled in a college course and talked animatedly about going out with her friends. Her counselling from a professional service continued.

This case demonstrates the importance of a dual approach to intervention that addresses the overt symptoms of the voice disorder as well as the covert ones related to psychological state. The mechanism for change was dealt with at these two levels. Partnership practice between client and therapist proved enormously important in providing a holistic approach based on: observing and listening to the individual, supporting the person to express her own agenda; outlining the contribution of SLT as well as demarcating the boundaries; and defining the role of each person in the partnership.

Addressing functional use of language and communication skills

The term 'functional' refers to the effective use of language and communication skills in a range of contexts with people that matter and for a variety of reasons. Functional communication supports the individual to affect the actions of others and to influence their own experiences. By its very nature, functional communication cannot be restricted to the individual centre of influence. The contributions of partners and the broader communication environment are necessarily implicated, although intervention activities may concentrate on the individual in the first instance.

Key features of functional communication approaches
Self-instruction and problem-solving are key to the change process. Therapy aims to build awareness of covert processes so that they can be altered to affect the use of communicational skills in everyday life. Techniques used in this type of approach include:

- Systematic application of modelling procedures – reduce inappropriate responses and acquire new ones or extend repertoire.
- Skills rehearsal – scenes or communication tasks relating to the individual's life are set up for practising targeted skills.
- Role-play – real-life encounters are recreated in a miniature and artificial way.
- Assignments – used to locate therapy strategies in the context of the person's lifestyle.

Different purposes
The application of functional approaches to communication may have many purposes, including:

- Developing social use of language and behaviour:
  Social skills are described as a set of behaviours that can be learned through social experience. They are goal-directed, interrelated, vary according to the demands of the situation, and are under the control of the individual (Hargie, 1997). *Social skills training* is concerned with the development of self and other awareness (Kelly, 1996; Rinaldi, 1992). It is about 'shaping language in form and content towards normality and by incorporating the pragmatic and functional aspects of communication to help them become as natural a communicator as possible within the constraints of their handicap' (Rustin and Kuhr, 1989: 11).
  Conversational therapy allows individuals to experiment with their communication skills in a safe environment and to rehearse any strategies recommended to overcome or circumvent difficulties. This may

take the form of simulated conversations with the therapist or else participation in a conversation group.

- Alternative ways of communicating:
Therapy may introduce and develop alternative ways of communicating, particularly in circumstances where the usual mechanisms of communication are inadequate for normal speech and language production. This usually involves the client in the learning of a new way of producing voice or communicating messages. Such alternatives include the use of: an alternative method for producing speech, as in oesophageal communication; an external appliance or prosthesis for producing voice, such as the Blom-Singer valve; and an alternative means of communication that will replace or supplement a conventional communication system.

    Conversation training offers the new user of an AAC device the chance to review the relevance and utility of preprogrammed messages (Lasker and Bedrosian, 2001).

Therapeutic interaction

Regardless of what the intervention sets out to address, the interaction of therapist and client is central to the process. The question is: What makes this interaction *therapeutic* and how does it relate to the mechanism for change? What is it that makes the interaction between client and therapist qualitatively different to other types of interaction, for instance between friends and work colleagues, between teacher and child, or between health practitioner and patient?

Based on Byng (1995) and Byng and Black (1995), the therapeutic interaction is made up of:

Communication opportunities that are relevant to or tailored to the available skills of the client
A communication opportunity is defined as a clear chance for the other person to contribute to the interaction. Part of the role of the therapist is to engineer such opportunities based on what is known about the individual, i.e. the positive factors and difficulties. As such, the therapist attempts to control the demands that are placed on the individual's skill set. Opportunities may include certain tasks or exercises that have been selected to help the individual to build on strengths or else to address or circumvent any difficulties.

Observing and monitoring the contributions of the client
The therapist is alert to the responses of the client and uses this information to evaluate the demands of the communication opportunity, the

individual's communication skills, and his or her internal state of wellbeing. This may prompt the use of certain facilitation strategies that will shape the opportunity so that the client is able to use available skills.

Providing feedback on the client's contributions

The assumption is that much behaviour is guided by internal self-statements (Meichenbaum, 1977) and therefore it is important to change feedback. Schwartz et al. (1994) describe a problem-solving approach to sentence processing where the client was encouraged to check response attempts by looking at the answers on the reverse of the stimulus cards, i.e. the correct thematic roles were displayed, thereby enabling the client to make a judgement about the task attempt. In addition to verbal and non-verbal differential feedback that occurs online, a range of instruments are used in support of the feedback process, including:

- Video and audio playback for appraising individual performance – the process of identifying evidence of communicative success provides reinforcement for using the recommended strategies. Similarly, breakdown in conversation may be reviewed and the source of trouble located. There is the opportunity for both client and therapist to question why the trouble has occurred and to identify or devise solutions that will address it.
- Bio-feedback is the use of sophisticated means for providing detailed, timely and informative feedback to the individual about aspects of speech production. It involves the use of computer-aided devices that provide feedback in the forms of analogue or digital display. Feedback needs to occur simultaneously with production effort so that the client is able to assess the distance between a single production attempt and the target. A perceived narrowing of the gap between the two may encourage the client to pursue the target and to continue their efforts. It may also give critical detail about the attempt and therefore help the client to concentrate his or her energies on particular aspects of the target in any renewed effort. It helps to avoid a 'hit and miss' approach to practice, and encourages a process of target refinement (Enderby and Emerson, 1995).

Therapeutic skills in action

The next part of this chapter explores therapy techniques in action as therapist and client work together. Three short transcriptions are detailed here representing work with different client groups.

Coding of transcriptions

For the coding of transcriptions, the reader is referred to the Appendix: (Glossary of enactment processes), and Chapter 5. The use of technical skills has been indicated by annotating the transcription, found in the left-hand column, with the relevant code. The right-hand column provides labels for the technical skills identified in the transcript. Generally, each technical skill is mentioned only once in the column of enactment processes, unless it is used in a distinctive way, in which case the label is qualified using additional information from the transcribed interaction.

Transcription 1: review session with child in mainstream school

This is a transcription of a review session taking place in the learning support unit of a mainstream school. Review is once a month and is used as a basis for future teacher/learning support assistant (LSA) liaison work, to inform the types of activities carried out by teacher/LSA and the interaction going on in them. The therapist is keen for teacher/LSA to see the value of interaction, which supports the development of the speech/language skills, rather than concentrating too much on the type of activity.

Context details
* Activity – pelmanism card game as basis for work on: use of pronouns in sentence level picture descriptions; correct pronunciation of /sh/ and /the/.
* Therapist and child (ten-year-old boy) are seated around the corner of a table in the empty classroom.
* This transcription is taken from a session lasting about half an hour in all, and is about four minutes of therapy time.

Therapeutic interaction	*Enactment processes*
1. **T** ((shuffling picture cards)) [E.1] right now	E.1 Equipment organization
2. this is (.) can you read what it says on	
3. the envelope [C.5]	C.5 Checking understanding
4. **C** ((leaning forward)) ( )	
5. **T** it says <u>he</u> [C.2]	C.2 Modelling – target word
6. **C** he (.) I	
7. **T** she [C.2]	
8. **C** she	
9. **T** and [they] [C.2]	
10. **C** [they]	
11. **T** so we want to start all our sentences	
12. with he (.) she (.)	
13. or they [G.3 C.2]	G.3 Providing instructions
14. **C** ((nods))	

15.	**T**	(1.0) and you've got two things to think	
16.		about with she	
17.		(.) not only that it's a girl but you've got to	
18.		put your lips forward as well ^{C.4} ((fingers	C.4 Assisting contribution
19.		pointing to her lips) ^{C.2}	C.2 Modelling – target mouth shape
20.	**C**	she	
21.	**T**	that's very good ^{D.2}	D.2 Differential feedback – gives positive reinforcement for correct response
22.	**C**	she	
23.	**T**	((starts to lay cards out on the table	
24.		face down)) ^{E.1}	E.1 Equipment organization
25.	**C**	/tei/	
26.	**T**	((stops laying out the cards)) ah there	
27.		is that harder one we haven't	
28.		practised ^{D.3} (.) d'you want to get it	D.3 Evaluative feedback – prepare for demands of task
29.		right now ^{G.4}	G.4 Framing/negotiation – regarding execution of target sound
30.	**C**	((pushes lips out)) /ts'/ /ts'/	
31.	**T**	let me show you (.) it's like ^{C.2}	C.2 Modelling – demonstrates target sound
32.	**C**	/t'/ they	
33.	**T**	you're trying really hard [(.)]^{D.5}	D.5 Acknowledging contribution – for client's efforts
34.	**C**	[they]	
35.	**T**	can I stop you a second (.) just ((raises	
36.		finger briefly)) relax (.)^{C.4} right (.) now	C.4 Assisting contribution – by articulating demand
37.		just stick your tongue out slightly ^{C.3}	C.3 Production call – elicits target
38.		((sticks out tongue)) ^{C.2}	C.2 Modelling – demonstrates target response
39.	**C**	((sticks tongue out))	
40.	**T**	and go /the/ ^{C.2}	
41.	**C**	/the/	
42.	**T**	/the/ ^{D.4}	D.4 Summative feedback – by imitating client's correct attempt
43.	**C**	/the/	
44.	**T**	that's it (.) don't say they at all at the	
45.		moment (.)^{G.3}	G.3 Providing instructions – to support client's focus

46.   just go /*the*/ [C.2 C.3]

47. **C** /*the*/

48. **T** /the/ /the/ [C.2]

49. **C** /*the*/ ((velarized)) /*the*/ ((velarized))

50. **T** you know when you say like (.) the

51.   book [C.2] ((/*the buk*/)) [C.2]

52. **C** yeah

53. **T** say /*the*/ [C.3 C.2]

54. **C** /*the*/

55. **T** that's good ↓ [D.2] now say /*the*/ (.)

56.   book [C.2 C.3]

57. **C** the book

58. **T** that's excellent (.)[D.2] now it's the same

59.   sound as that (.) all right [D.2]

60. **C** they

61. **T** that's good (.)[D.2] and again [C.3]

62. **C** they ((tongue slightly protruding and

63.   curling up at the tip))

64. **T** you've <u>got</u> it (.)[D.2] well done (.)[D.2] do it

65.   again [C.3]

66. **C** they

67. **T** so now you're going to get she and he

68.   and they right [C.1] ((starts laying out

69.   cards)) [E.1] can you help me spread

70.   them out [G.4] ((T and C spread out the

71.   cards face down on the table)) [E.1] right

72.   is this how you've been playing it [B.4]

73. **C** yeah

74. **T** who's going first [G.4]

75. **C** (2.0) me ((turns over a card)) she's

76.   picking up flowers

C.2 Modelling – demonstrates target response

C.3 Production call

D.2 Differential feedback – gives positive reinforcement

C.1 Encouraging contribution
E.1 Equipment organization

G.4 Framing/negotiating – setting out activity with client

B.4 Checking understanding – of activity requirements

G.4 Framing/negotiating – setting out activity with client

77. **T** good (.) very nice and clear (.)$^{D.2}$ right | D.2 Differential feedback – gives positive reinforcement

78.   (.) turn another one over $^{C.3}$ | C.3 Production call – uses stimulus card

79. **C** ((turns over a card)) she is (.) putting

80.   water in her mug

81. **T** all right ((C turns cards back)) (.) ((T

82.   turns a card over)) she is washing $^{C.2}$ | C.2 Modelling – by having a turn at activity

83. **C** I just ( ) say he

84. **T** I wasn't sure with that (.) d'you think

85.   he $^{B.3}$ | B.3 Checking interpretation

86. **C** m:

87. **T** okay (.) he is washing his face (1.0) or

88.   d'you think she (.)$^{B.3}$ I'm in a muddle

89.   no

90. **C** oh just whatever what you want

91. **T** well what d'you think it is $^{C.3}$ | C.3 Production call – asks a question

92. **C** it's a he

93. **T** right (.) he is washing his face $^{D.2}$ | D.2 Differential feedback – affirms client's attempt

94.   ((turns over a card)) he is playing the

95.   piano $^{C.2}$ ((turns cards back)) | C.2 Modelling – takes turn in game to demonstrate

96. **C** ((turns over a card)) she is happy

97.   'cause she got a new cat

98. **T** mhm $^{C.1}$ | C.1 Encouraging contribution – by use of vocal acknowledgement

99. **C** ((turns over a card)) she ((/si:/)) is

100.   picking up flowers

101. **T** did you remember to out your lips

102.   forward $^{D.2}$ | D.2 Differential feedback – review of previous attempt

103. **C** whoops (.) <u>she</u> (.) is picking up flowers

104. **T** very good (.)$^{D.2}$ now (.) can I | D.2 Differential feedback – positive reinforcement

105.   remember where it was ((turns over a

106.   card)) she is picking flowers $^{C.2}$ ((turns

107.   a card over)) whoops (.) she is happy

108.   'cause she's got a new cat ((turns

109. cards back)) [C.2]	C.2 Modelling – takes turn in game to demonstrate target
110. **C** ((turns over a card)) <u>she</u> (.) is happy	
111. 'cause she is (.) picking up flowers	
112. **T** that's good [D.2]	
113. **C** ((turns over a card)) she is happy ( )	
114. she got a new cat	
115. **T** *very good* [D.2]	
116. **C** ((turns over a card)) she is (.) she's	
117. happy as she ( ) got a present	
118. **T** okay (.) what's she doing to the	
119. present [C.3]	C.3 Production call – asks a question
120. **C** she's unwrapping the present ((turns	
121. cards back))	
122. **T** good [D.2] ((turns over a card)) he is	
123. drying the cups [C.2] ((turns a card	
124. over)) he is writing [C.2]	
125. **C** ((turns over a card)) she is happy	
126. 'cause she's got a new cat ((turns over	
127. a card)) <u>she</u> is happy 'cause she's got	
128. a new cat ((keeps card pair))	
129. **T** good (.)[D.2] another go for you [C.3]	C.3 Production call – indicates client's go
130. **C** ((turns over a card)) he's wrapping up	
131. a present ((turns over a card)) /siː/ is	
132 dressing up	
133. **T** yeah (.) did you remember your good	
134. she [D.2]	D.2 Differential feedback – by getting client to review previous attempt
135. **C** /siːz/ dressing up	C.4 Assisting contribution – gives advice on production attempt
136. **T** bit more forward [C.4]	
137. **C** /sːiː/ is	
138. **T** make it get more /je/ in it (.)[C.4] <u>she</u> [C.2]	C.2 Modelling
139. **C** <u>she</u> is dressing up	
140. **T** very good [D.2]	D.2 Differential feedback – positive reinforcement

Evaluation of techniques in use

The interaction between therapist and client is focused on the production of /sh/ and /th/. Not surprisingly, facilitation mainly involves the use of *C.2 Production call* and *C.3 Modelling*. Feedback is provided through *D.2 Differential feedback* with plenty of positive reinforcement for client responses that are on target. The nature of the activity, i.e. pelmanism game, demands manipulation of the materials (*E.1 Equipment organization*). Some transactional skills that relate to the rules of the game and the production tasks are used, e.g. *G.3 Providing instructions*. By use of *G.4 Framing/negotiating* the therapist involves the client in setting up the materials. No specific modifications appear to have been made to the therapist's use of communication skills apart from one instance when she checks his understanding of the game (*B.4 Checking understanding*). This was a child who appeared to have good attention and therefore engagement techniques were not used.

Transcription 2: woman with aphasia and dyspraxia after stroke

The transcription is taken from a session in a hospital outpatient setting. The client was attending SLT once or twice weekly. The interaction is between the therapist and a woman who has had a stroke some months before. She has aphasia and dyspraxia.

Context details

The activity centres on dyspraxia drills with varying levels of support for word production:

1) written word;
2) therapist description and reminder of articulator positions;
3) linguistic definitions;
4) close or co-locative support.

- The therapist is supporting the aphasic client to become as reliant as possible on internal (i.e. self-initiated) mechanisms to support speech production, rather than remaining dependent on external mechanisms.
- The therapist and aphasic person are seated opposite each other at a table.

  This transcription is from a segment lasting about three and a half minutes.

Therapeutic interaction	*Enactment processes*
1. **T** I wanted to get onto some of these	A.1 Attention call – places object to attract attention
2. ((opens exercise book)) d'you want to	
3. choose a page ((places book down on	G.4 Framing/ negotiating
4. the table in front of C)) ᴬ·¹ are there	– deciding on the focus of activity
5. any you'd like to work on ᴳ·⁴	
6. **C** er (9.0) ((turns pages and scrutinizes	

7.   the exercise book)) ((points)) this

8.   **T**   that one [B.3]   B.3 Checking interpretation –

9.   **C**   yes   makes sure of client's
                                                  selection

10. **T**   okay (.) so (.) just to focus on it for a

11.   minute (2.0) just thinking about where

12.   you're going to start the word off (.)[C.4]   C.4 Assisting contribution

13.   and what it's gonna ((points to own   – helping client to prepare
                                                   for production task in stages
14.   mouth and chin)) [C.4] *feel like in the

15.   mouth* [C.4]

16.   *okay* (.) so it's right at the back [C.4]

17. **C**   yes

18. **T**   and you're going to have to start (with)

19.   your [mouth open each] time= [C.4]

20. **C**   [((pushing lips in and out))]

21. **T**   = in order to get the [beginning] [C.4]

22. **C**   [garden]

23. **T**   yeah (.) okay I'll take this ((removes

24.   book from the table top)) [E.1]   E.1 Equipment organization

25.   [away 'cause]=   – to alter demands of task

26. **C**   [grins and laughs]

27. **T**   = it's far too easy if you can read it ( )

28.   okay oh well ((looking at exercise

29.   book and reading out)) this week it's

30.   been nice and warm so you may

31.   well have been sitting out in the [C.3 C.4]   C.3 Production call – therapist

32. **C**   garden ((/*dirden*/))   starts sentence for client to
                                                     complete
33. **T**   in the [C.3] ((looks at C and holds her   C.4 Assisting contribution –
                                                         provides semantic cue
34.   own mouth open)) [C.2]   C.2 Modelling – demonstrates

35. **T**   garden   mouth shape

36. **T**   that's much better (.)[D.2] okay (.) *oh↓*   D.2 Differential feedback –

37.   ((reading out)) shooting with a [C.3]   gives positive reinforcement
                                                     C.3 Production call – therapist
38. **C**   gun   starts sentence for client to
                                                     complete

39. **T**	okay (1.0) erm when you're reading or	
40.	to *see* [C.4] things you might need [C.3]	C.4 Assisting contribution – provides semantic cue
41. **C**	(1.0) glasses	
42. **T**	perfect ( ) okay erm a field full of [C.3 C.4]	
43. **C**	(2.0)	
44. **T**	what the cows eat [C.3 C.4]	
45. **C**	(3.0) ((pushes her lips forward)) er	
46.	grass	
47. **T**	(1.0) that's brilliant (.) well done [D.2]	D.2 Differential feedback – gives positive reinforcement
48. **C**	((smiles and laughs))	
49. **T**	yeah ( ) okay erm if things (.) this is	
50.	where there's a couple of gs ((i.e.	
51.	letter G)) in the middle of the word [C.4]	C.4 Assisting contribution – helping client to prepare for production task
52.	okay so if things wind you up they	
53.	make you feel [C.3 C.4]	C.3 Production call – therapist starts sentence for client to complete
54. **C**	(4.0) ((shakes her head))	
55. **T**	the opposite of happy or contented [C.4]	C.4 Assisting contribution – providing a semantic cue
56. **C**	(2.0)	
57. **T**	(something) happens that makes you	
58.	want to hit out at somebody it's 'cause	
59.	you're feeling [C.3 C.4]	
60. **C**	(1.0) sad	
61. **T**	(1.0) ((cocks her head to one side)) [D.1]	D.1 Checking contribution – non-verbal questioning of client's response
62. **C**	no	
63. **T**	I was thinking of something a bit more	
64.	violent than that actually [C.3]	C.3 Assisting contribution – providing a semantic cue
65. **T**	(2.0) ((starts to lean forward))	
66. **T**	d'you want to see it ((shows the	
67.	exercise book)) [B.4] it's easier to it's	B.4 Checking interpretation – client's non-verbal behaviour in previous turn
68.	easier if you can (see it) [D.3]	D.3 Evaluative feedback – reading of target words as opposed to sentence completion task
69. **T**	oh↓ /waenwɪd/ ((smiles and laughs))	
70.	( )	

71. **T** think about

72. **T** ( ) just angry

73. **T** good (.) now can you cut out the just

74. **T** ((laughs))

75. **T** ((smiles))

76. **T** (4.0) o:h *just* ((laughs))

77. **T** ((smiles and laughs)) it makes you

78. feel [C.3]

79. **T** angry

C.3 Production call – therapist starts sentence for client to complete

80. **T** good (.)[D.2] yeah (.) okay (1.0) the

81. colour of grass (.) is [C.3]

82. **T** green

83. **T** perfect [D.2]

D.2 Differential feedback – gives positive reinforcement
C.3 Production call – therapist starts sentence for client to complete

Evaluation of techniques in use

Like the previous example, this is a session about speech production. The critical difference is that the client in this case has oral dyspraxia. Consequently, facilitation is invoked to support production, i.e. *C.4 Assisting contribution*. This usually takes the form of helping the client in the preparation phase by reminding her of the key features of the target sound or word. The other type of facilitation that is used is *C.3 Production call*, where the therapist offers a sentence structure for the client to complete. This is usually accompanied by a semantic cue (*C.4 Assisting contribution*). Positive reinforcement for successful responses is given (*D.2 Differential feedback*). Occasionally semantic cues are offered to the client, i.e. *C.4 Assisting contribution*, particularly at points of struggle or lack of response from the client. At the start of the activity, the therapist uses *G.4 Framing/negotiating*, where the client is given the chance to direct the focus of the next target sound/word.

Transcription 3: pre-school child with dysfluent speech

This is a transcription of a pre-school child with dysfluent speech being treated using the Lidcombe approach (Onslow, O'Brian and Harrison 1997). Therapy was delivered at once-weekly intervals. This session comes a few weeks into the child's therapy.

Context details

The transcription is from a clip of part of the session with therapist and child working at the table top, with speech being elicited by the therapist. Fluent ('smooth') speech is rewarded with tokens, which are accumulated by the child to be traded for stickers at the end of the session.

- The activity uses a story picture board and a series of 'stickers' to build a scene.
- The child's mother is in the room but not taking part in this particular interaction.
- The transcribed clip lasts about three and a half minutes (from a 30–40 minute session).
- The therapist is holding a book of stickers, while C is describing a scene on a large picture board on the table.

Therapeutic interaction	*Enactment processes*
1. **T** okay let's start now (.) we've got a	A.1 Attention call – focuses child on materials
2. street haven't we (1.0) [A.1] and what are	C.3 Production call – solicits response from child
3. all these along there ((pointing to the	
4. picture board)) [C.3]	
5. **C** houses	
6. **T** that's right and that was smooth	
7. ((dropping token into a cup on the	
8. table)) good talking [D.2] (.) and=	D.2 Differential feedback – provides positive reinforcement for smooth talking
9. **C** ((reaches over and takes the cup	
10. looking into it))	
11. **T** =we've got our first squirrel nut	
12. ((moves the cup to the left of C)) [B.2]	
14. d'you want to put them in there (.) so	B.2 Ascribing meaning – responds to non-verbal behaviour of client
15. you can see them growing (.) and what	
16. kind of [shop] is this [C.3]	

17. **C** [no] they can't grow

18. **T** well (.) the numbers are growing but

19.   you're right they can't grow (.) what've

20.   we got over here ((points to the

21.   picture board)) [c.3]

22. **C** er an ice cream shop

23. **T** that <u>is</u> an ice cream shop and that was

24.   smooth talking too ((puts token in the

25.   cup)) well done [D.2]

26. **C** well (.) well I can tell I've had the best

27.   ice cream I have

D.2 Differential feedback – positive reinforcement given

28. **T** have you

29. **C** I've had (1.0) er an ice cream with

30.   loads of sprinkles (.) <u>and</u> (.) chocolate

31.   stick and ice [cream]

32. **T** [(((makes sound of eating an ice

33.   cream))] making me hungry (.) was

34.   that the best ice cream ever [c.2]

35. **C** huh

C.2 Modelling – demonstrates 'smooth talking' as part of continuing interaction

36. **T** [wow]

37. **C** [ou:t] the ice cream van

38. **T** let's see if we can make this street

39.   really interesting [c.2]

40. **C** yeah

41. **T** would you like ((C stands up and

42.   reaches for the sticker book)) a dog or

43.   would you like a car ((raising index

44.   finger)) [G.4]

45. **C** um er a taxi ((still standing))

46. **T** a taxi okay (.) and that was smooth

47.   talking ((gives a sticker to C)) so I'll

G.4 Framing/negotiating – client is given chance to influence next stage in activity

WITHDRAWN FROM UNIVERSITIES AT MEDWAY LIBRARY

48.   give you a little nut ((drops token into

49.   the cup)) [D.2] okay (.) pop the taxi on

50. C ((sitting down puts the sticker onto

51.   the story board))

D.2 Differential feedback – provides positive reinforcement for smooth talking and token is placed in cup

52. T now d'you want another car or do you

53.   want a person

54.   this time [C.3]

C.3 Production call – therapist uses conversational turn to solicit response from client

55. C er an another taxi ((standing up and

56.   pointing at the sticker book))

57. T another taxi (.) well that's just the

58.   place where that goes but I can give

59.   you a car [C.2]

60. C yeah

C.2 Modelling – therapist uses turn to demonstrate 'smooth talking' in naturalistic exchange

61. T okay ((gives a sticker to C)) we'll put

62.   the car on the road [C.2]

63. C there th: there's another picture of a

64.   car ((sticking the picture to the story

65.   board))

66. T that's right (.) can you say (.) there's

67.   ((slightly prolonged)) another

68.   picture [C.2 C.3]

C.2 Modelling – therapist demonstrates 'smooth talking' based on client's previous turn where the talking was 'bumpy', together with ...
C.3 Production call – soliciting a response from the client

69. C there's another picture of a car ((trying

70.   to reach for a sticker))

71. T very smooth ((handing a token to C))

72.   d'you want to take that nut (.) because

73.   you made the bump go away that

74.   [time] didn't you [D.2]

D.2 Differential feedback – therapist gives positive recognition for improved second attempt

75. C [((drops token into the cup))]

76.   ((sits down))

77. T so you've got another nut [C.1]

C.1 Encouraging contribution – therapist reminds child of achievement so far

78. C I'm getting all yellows

79. **T** you'll get ... get some different colour

80. next time (.) okay I'm going to give

81. you this one (.) what's this ((hands

82. sticker to C)) [C.3]

83. **C** (1.0) um person

84. **T** what kind of person d'you [know] [C.3]   C.3 Production call – solicits
                                                      response from client

85. **C**   [police]man

86. **T** <u>very</u> smooth talking well done ((drops

87. token into the cup)) [D.2] where're you   D.2 Differential feedback –
                                                 provides positive reinforce-
88. going to put him [C.3]   ment for smooth talking and
                                                 token is placed in cup
89. **C** (1.0) er (3.0) ((looking at story board))

90. **T** where does he go [C.3]

91. **C** (1.0)

92. **T** he goes in the ((points to the story

93. board)) [C.3 C.4]   C.4 Assisting contribution –
                                                 indicates item on story board
94. **C** (2.0)
                                                 C.2 Modelling – therapist sup-
95. **T** park [C.2]   plies the target response

96. **C** park

97. **T** that's right (.) [D.2] and when you said   D.2 Differential feedback –
                                                     provides positive reinforce-
98. park was that smooth [D.2]   ment for smooth talking and
                                                     also prompts client self-
99. **C** er   evaluation

100. **T** was it smooth when you said park [D.2]

101. **C** ((nods))

102. **T** it was ((gives token to C)) [D.2]

103. **C** ((drops token into the cup))

104. **T** and something else that goes in the

105. park ((showing sticker to C)) is a [C.3]   C.3 Production call – therapist
                                                 starts sentence for child to
106. **C** ((taking sticker)) see saw   complete

107. **T** good talking again ((drops token into

108. the cup)) well done [D.2]

109. **C** ( ) ((putting sticker onto the story

110.   board))

111. T goes in the park (1.0) okay (.) <u>a:nd</u>

112.   this goes in the park as well I don't

113.   know d'you know what this is ((C

114.   stands up to look at the sticker book))

115.   this is a boy on ^{C.3}

116. C yeah I know

117. T on a ^{C.3}

118. C on roller skate ((takes the sticker))

119. T very smooth well done ((drops token

120.   into the cup)) ^{D.2}

121. C ( )

122. T I think he's actually on a skateboard

123.   (.) ^{C.2} but you said it smoothly so ^{D.2}   C.2 Modelling – therapist
                                                        supplies the target response

124. C he can go wee ((putting sticker onto

125.   story board))

126. T yeah down the path can't he (.) good

127.   you're doing very well (.) ^{D.2} let's see   D.2 Differential feedback –
                                                        provides positive reinforce-
128.   what else we can put in [a park shall   ment for 'smooth talking'

129.   we] ^{C.3}   C.3 Production call – therapist
                                                        solicits response from child

130. C [l:ooks like] he's running over his

131.   foot

132. T does it

133. C yeah (ah)

134. T ah this can go in the park look

135.   ((shows sticker to C)) ^{C.2} what've we   C.2 Modelling – therapist
                                                        demonstrates 'smooth talking'
136.   got there ^{C.3}   in own conversational turn
                                                        C.3 Production call – therapist
137. C football   solicits response from the child

138. T football and that was smooth talking

139.   well done ((drops token into the
                                                        D.2 Differential feedback –
140.   cup)) ^{D.2} do you like playing football   provides positive reinforce-
                                                        ment for smooth talking and
                                                        places token in cup

141. **C** ((nods))

142. **T** have you got a football at home

143 **C** er yeah

144. **T** have you

145. **C** ( ) ( ) have

146. **T** you have got a foot ball at home

147.　okay (1.0) ^{C.2} what's this ((showing a

148.　sticker)) ^{C.3}

149. **C** ((taking the sticker)) um a a lady (.)

150.　pushing a pram

151. **T** that's right (.) can you say (.) a

152.　lady ^{C.3 C.2}

153. **C** a lady /pu/ pushing um a pram

154. **T** that's right well done ^{D.2}

155. **C** er

156. **T** you said a lady <u>really</u> well that time ^{D.2 C.1}

157. **C** oh (I want) ((putting sticker on the

158.　board))

159. **T** you got it right ^{D.2 C.1}

160. **C** how can I put it on ( )

161. **T** you just put it on there like that

162. **C** ((puts sticker on the board))

163. **T** good boy ^{D.2}

C.2 Modelling – therapist demonstrates 'smooth talking' by recasting the client's turn

C.1 Encouraging contribution – therapist encourages the child in response to his struggle, alongside
D.2 Differential feedback – positive reinforcement

Evaluation of techniques in use

In keeping with the session's aims of achieving a more fluent way of speaking, therapist use of technical skills follows a pattern whereby a 'smooth talking' style is modelled within the therapist's conversation turns (*C.2 Modelling*); the child takes his conversational turn, which triggers specific feedback from the therapist, as she reinforces his 'smooth talking' by qualitative comment and placing a token in the cup. Use of *C.3 Production call* occurs quite naturally within conversation turns, variously involving sentence completion, verbal comments on activity, and direct questions. From line 124 to the close of the interaction, the client appears to experience some verbal struggle, to which the therapist responds by linking *C.1 Encouraging contribution* with *D.2 Differential feedback*. This also occurs at an earlier stage – lines 54 to 60. The therapist encourages the child by reminding him of his achievements so far in the session at the same time as providing positive reinforcement.

Focusing on the individual

Therapeutic interaction with the individual focuses on the individual's underlying system. How information is received, organized and interpreted for use is of primary interest. Enactment processes define the therapy process where therapist and client are the main correspondents, although not to the exclusion of any other centre of influence. The selection and use of techniques is determined by the perceived relevance to the client's communication difficulties and observed responses to therapy tasks/activities. The overarching purpose is about revealing individual competencies by strengthening the underlying system, addressing issues related to identity and emotional state, and promoting functional use of skills.

Chapter 7
Enhancing the communication partnership

Intervention that has a primary focus on the communication partnership is seen as a negotiated course of learning and change where client and significant other(s) are both contributors. The individual's network of social contacts is integral to the establishment of a positive momentum of change and maintenance. Any difficulties experienced by an individual in the communication process impact not only on the person who has impaired communication skills, but also on their interlocutors. Enderby and Emerson (1995) report that speech and language therapists are frequently concerned with helping significant others to appreciate and understand the nature of the client's difficulties, as well as to learn new ways of facilitating communication with the individual.

Client and significant other(s)

Bronfenbrenner's microsystem (1979), discussed in Chapter 1, includes the notion of communication partnerships along with the familiar communication environments in a person's life. Clearly there is a close relationship between the two, and intervening at a partnership level is likely to influence the environment and vice versa. The environment is specifically dealt with in Chapter 8. At a partnership level, the therapist works with the client and the key person(s) in their life in order to establish optimal collaboration (Kagan, 1998). Kagan (1995) stresses the need to work with significant others who are the natural communication partners of the client. It is about involving the people who are relevant to the client's lifestyle, e.g. parent, partner, teacher, keyworker or other health professional, so that therapeutic outcomes go beyond the boundaries of the client–therapist interface. Kagan and LeBlanc (2002: 155) state that 'It is equally important that significant others learn how to be effective communication partners.'

There is exploration of the ways in which communication takes place between two or more participants. New strategies and supportive techniques are invoked in order to establish interactions that demonstrate mutuality and balance. Some individual sessions may run in conjunction with partnership practice. Ware and Healey (1994: 10) reason the importance of involving significant others:

Learning is interpersonal. Any child (or learner) is able to do more with the assistance of a person more skilled than themselves than they are able to achieve alone. Initially the more skilled person in a teacher–learner pair may take responsibility for reaching the current goal; learning occurs as the less skilled person takes over that responsibility.

Interest in communication partnership

Interest in the role of the communication partnership is derived from a number of sources:

Study of pragmatics

Work in the field of pragmatics has highlighted the importance of communication in context. It refers to the individual's own unique ability to handle language for the purpose of communication (Mey, 1993). Coupe O'Kane and Goldbart (1998) describe it as the study of language in context. Exploration of the social context from the perspective of the individual is integral to our understanding of communication disability, because language use does not occur in a vacuum (Lund and Duchan, 1988).

Conversation analysis and social interaction approaches

Conversational analysis (CA) finds its roots in ethnomethodology, where social methods are employed flexibly to be responsive to the peculiarities of the interaction at any point in time (Lesser and Perkins, 1999). In a similar way to the study of pragmatics, CA is concerned with communication in real contexts. Its focus is not restricted to the individual's ability to handle language for communication purposes; rather it investigates communication as a naturally occurring social phenomenon between two or more people where the contributions of both speaker and listener are examined. It goes beyond the basics of information exchange and looks at how *sense of self* is revealed and relationships are constructed (Schiffrin in Frederick, 1988).

Assessment and therapy activities attend to the distinctive features of conversation and how language is used in real contexts (Alm and Newell in von Tetzchner and Jensen, 1996; Wilkinson, 1999). Lesser and Perkins (1999) state that the usefulness of this type of data lies in the information it provides about difficulties occurring in conversation and any corresponding strategies that are employed, as well as the effects that each has on the resulting interaction. CA is of interest to therapists because it 'has the potential to go beyond what is merely disordered or deviant in the conversations of the communicatively impaired partner ... analyses of conversation ... provide an opportunity to investigate how both parties work together to restore order and coherence in conversation' (Watson et al., 1999: 196).

Kagan (1995) states that the ability to converse is critical to revealing competence. The limitations brought about by communication disability whether developmental or acquired in nature, may have a deleterious effect on self-determination and relationships. The information arising from CA provides direction for the construction of partnership-based approaches and 'allows the therapist to develop interaction which is client-led and individually tailored to the unique interaction patterns that emerge from the linguistic impairments and strategies that have been developed by the person (with aphasia) and his or her key conversational partner' (Lesser and Perkins, 1999: 94).

Early interaction
Interest in early interaction between parent and infant stems from a general recognition of the importance of early life experiences in child development. Adults (in Western cultures) assume the responsibility for creating a conversational framework for interactions to take place (Grove, Bunning and Porter in Columbus, 2001). Goldbart (1996) reviews the mother's role in interpreting the infant's behaviour from a social constructivist viewpoint (see Grove, Bunning and Porter in Columbus, 2001). Very early on, the caregiver responds instinctively to the infant's expression of affect and it ascribes meaning to the behaviour accordingly. Over time, there is the mutual refinement of the infant's behaviours and the parents' responses: the infant is reactive to responses by caregivers and the caregiver becomes attuned to subtle differences in the infant's behaviours: 'mothers' interpretations of their children's behaviour change as infants develop goal-oriented behaviour and contingency awareness, leading to displays which are increasingly purposeful' (Grove, Bunning and Porter in Columbus, 2001: 94).

For some individuals this interactive process may be threatened by certain factors, which may be internal to the child (biological), e.g. the infant born with Down's syndrome, or external (environmental), e.g. low level of stimulation in the home environment due to a variety of reasons – parent has special needs, or low socio-economic status affecting nutrition, care, etc. Lack of caregiver sensitivity or alternatively reduced responding by the infant will have a reciprocal effect, thereby inhibiting the development of social interaction.

For the timely response to the needs of such children and their families, intervention is introduced at a very early stage in the child's life. It involves the identification of specific needs, and the institution of suitable approaches to promote development and address any complicating factors. It is based on the assumption that the earlier you start the better chance you have of preventing or minimizing problems later on. Mitchell and Brown (1991: xii) offer a definition of early intervention as 'systematic strategies aimed at promoting the optimal development of infants and toddlers with special needs and at enhancing the functioning of their families and caregivers' (Mitchell and Brown, 1991, p. xii).

Communication partnerships in education

The communication partnership between educational staff and children occupies a large chunk of time in the child's growing up. The teachers and learning support assistants (LSAs) are instrumental in helping the child to access the language of the classroom and in promoting the development of communication skills. The inclusive education agenda means that therapists need to work closely with educators who are in a position to provide the daily support that a child with communication difficulties requires. There is an absolute need for teachers and SLTs to work together (McCartney, 1999). The centrality of language to the child's development in the schooling years makes it essential that opportunities for developing speech and language skills are utilized to full effect (Wright and Kersner, 1998). Collaborative working practice between therapist and teacher demands a clear understanding of the 'interdependency between language and learning' (Wright and Kersner, 1998: 35). The sharing of knowledge and skills enables the teacher/LSA to perform the role of facilitating communication partner 'so that the children will be adequately equipped to follow instructions and receive information related to everyday events in the classroom and the school' (p. 35).

Communication partnership

A communication partnership is defined as the relationship between two people who contribute to the mutual exchange of ideas and meanings (Bartlett and Bunning, 1997). The knowledge, experience, attitude and cultural identity of the participants and their relationship to each other will affect the style of communication partnership. It involves the significant people in the individual's life, and any one person may experience a variety of communication partnerships during the cycle of a day and as their life course progresses, ranging from intimate and highly familiar (e.g. parent and child, husband and wife) to formal and distant (e.g. boss and employee, bank manager and customer).

Communication process

Communication is a complex process where mutuality and social co-ordination are features (Grove et al., 1999). Meanings and ideas are communicated through a range of different forms, including formal linguistic code, e.g. speech, writing, sign and symbol, and non-verbal behaviours, e.g. gesture, body language, eye gaze and vocalization, etc. The continuous process model of communication proposed by Fogel in Nadel and Camaioni (1993: 15) describes the 'continuous interplay of perception and action in a co-regulated social context' where the traditional roles of *sender* and *receiver* (see early model of communication based on information processing by Osgood, 1957) are difficult to decipher (Stamp and Knapp, 1990). Both participants are involved in coding and inference (Sperber and Wilson, 1995). Both speaker and listener are active contributors. This continuous activity implies that meanings emerge and change in the course of the interaction.

Interpersonal communication

The study of language development and communication-based interventions places a growing emphasis on the interactive nature of communication: communicative competence is not viewed in isolation as an intra-personal trait but is seen in context with the communication partner as a wider inter-personal phenomenon (Hargie, Saunders and Dickson, 1994). Relevance theory (Sperber and Wilson, 1995) suggests that the effort involved in the giving or receiving of information should be appropriate to both the communicative content and the context of the interaction, with neither participant having to do a disproportionate amount of work. The role of the listener is an active one. It encompasses the ability to *both* interpret the message *and* make inferences based on knowledge of the individual and information arising from the context (Grove et al., 1999).

Asymmetrical partnership

Kagan (1998: 817) views the conversation partnership as an 'equation' which is balanced by the skills and experiences of the participants and the availability of relevant resources. This 'equation' is susceptible to imbalance when differences exist between the skills and experiences the interactants can draw on.

Differences in available skills

Differences in available communication skills can result in difficulties for one or both of the partners (Bartlett and Bunning, 1997; Bradshaw, 1998; Bunning and Grove in Carnaby, 2002; Grove et al., 1999). Difficulties range in severity and type, e.g. problems with speech intelligibility, verbal comprehension, social use of language, fluency, etc. The domination of the person with intact communication and related lifestyle skills is an inherent risk in any interaction. The power base is likely to be settled with the more able person, leaving the communication-disabled person vulnerable to their suggestions and ideas. It is much easier to influence the actions of others when you have effective use of a complete communication skill set.

Unevenness/imbalance in communication skills that each person brings to a communication partnership may lead to a chain reaction where there is:

• A struggle to express ideas and feelings or to understand what is being communicated, which may lead to ...

- A breakdown in communication where there is failure to exchange ideas, which may lead to ...
- Disempowerment, where the communication-disabled person does not participate using available skills, which may lead to ...
- Feelings of low self-esteem and frustration, which may lead to ...
- Inappropriate ways of responding, withdrawal or problem behaviour, which results in ...
- Social isolation and exclusion.
  (Adapted from Bunning and Grove in Carnaby, 2002: 87)

Communication inflation and devaluation

Because communication is interactive, the discourse style of communication partners may promote the skills or alternatively cast doubt on the abilities of the individual (Simmons-Mackie and Kagan, 1999). There are two types of communication error. The first is the partner's failure to recognize the language and communication skills of the person. Opportunities for social participation, inclusion and personal development are limited, thereby masking the person's competence. The second communication error is attributing skills and competencies to the person that they do not possess. The way the communication partner contributes to an interaction demonstrates their judgement of the individual's competencies.

The potential for communicative vulnerability is demonstrated in Figure 7.1, which has been adapted from two contrasting models by O'Brien in Tyne (1981) and Bartlett and Bunning (1997). Two types of risk at the level of communication partnership are identified: the inflation or overestimation of the person's communication skills, and, the reverse of this, the devaluation or underestimation. These are described in two interlocking cycles.

Cycle of communication inflation

The advent of a communication disability, whether developmental or acquired, may induce normalizing beliefs in communication partner(s). There is an unswerving conviction that if you carry on as normal, things will right themselves. The risk is that real needs may be denied and expectations of the individual may be too high, leading to the provision of inaccessible opportunities for social interaction. The consequences for the individual are negative or diminished experiences with a corresponding increase in social isolation and weakening of self-esteem, e.g. the person is constantly put in a position of failure, etc.

Cycle of communication devaluation

The flip side of the coin is that disabling beliefs held about a person's skills and potential might lead to low expectations regarding their ability to contribute. Reduced opportunities for social interaction follow. The consequences for the individual are the same: negative or diminished experiences, which have a dampening effect on self-esteem, social partic

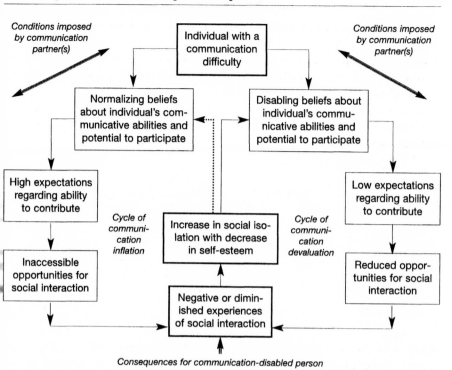

Consequences for communication-disabled person

·········· indicates that 'normalising beliefs' may continue in spite of an increase in social isolation and decrease in self-esteem of the communication-disabled person because of the fixed mind set of the communication partner(s). It does not feed into the *cycle of communication inflation* in the same way that disabling beliefs exacerbate the conditions in the *cycle of communication devaluation*. Movement from one cycle to the other is possible, e.g. communication inflation shifts to devaluation over the course of time.

Figure 7.1 Cycles of communication inflation and devaluation (Adapted from O'Brien in Tyne, 1981; Bartlett and Bunning, 1997)

ipation and the development and use of skills. A vicious cycle of devaluation may be set up, where disabling beliefs are 'confirmed' by the negative cycle, i.e. the consequential lack of social participation by the person who has a communication disability.

Facilitated communication

'Facilitated communication' (FC) (Biklen, 1990; Crossley and Remington-Gurney, 1992) demonstrates the risk brought about by unconscious inflation of a person's communication skills. In FC a linguistically intact facilitator gives physical assistance to a communication-disabled person to reduce the psycho-emotional and/or neurophysiological problems hypothesized to affect access (Grove, Bunning and Porter, in Columbus,2001). The technique involves physically supporting the individual to point at a communication board displaying letters, pictures or graphic signs letters or to operate an electronic communication device or computer (von Tetzchner, 1997).

Proponents of this method argue the importance of the role of touch in supporting people to put their ideas into visible form, e.g. spelt words, selected pictures, etc. (Crossley, 1997); however, validation studies suggest that the resulting communications originate from the facilitator rather than the individual (Wheeler et al., 1993; Datlow-Smith, Haas and Belcher, 1994). Prior and Cummins (1992) question the validity of the resulting communications, which often demonstrate a more sophisticated level of language than that produced independently by the person. The problem of communicative misrepresentation through FC has had far-reaching effects for both individual and facilitator. For some individuals and their families where abuse has been disclosed through FC, it has brought about enforced separation whilst allegations are checked out. For some facilitators extensive counselling has been needed when the problem of unconscious facilitator influence has been fully revealed (Grove, Bunning and Porter in Columbus, 2001).

Differences in primary mode of communication

Asymmetry in conversation has been observed in partnerships where one participant uses an alternative method of communication. Aided communicators are less likely to initiate interactions, introduce new topics or to use a broad range of communicative functions compared to normal speaking partners (Light, Collier and Parnes, 1985; von Tetzchner and Martinsen in von Tetzchner and Jensen, 1996). Muller and Soto (2002) noted significant differences in the conversation patterns of dyads made up of aided speakers (AS/AS) and those made up of aided speaker and natural speaker (AS/NS). Conversations between AS/AS achieved greater symmetry, evidenced by the balance in topic initiation and number of contributions, and the range of communicative and conversation maintenance functions. Conversely, repair featured more highly in conversations between AS/NS where less time was made available for AS participants to complete their turn, with NS partners more likely to engage in 'lengthy guessing sequences' (Muller and Soto, 2002: 86).

Muller and Soto (2002: 77) summarize the explanations for conversational asymmetries in AAC that have been put forward, although the reasons suggested are probably relevant to any communication partnership where inequalities or differences in communication skills exist:

- differences in individual characteristics, e.g. communication style, personality, disability, etc., may affect the person's contributions to an interaction (Kraat, 1987; Linell and Luckmann, 1991, cited in Muller and Soto, 2002);
- inequalities in status of participants, e.g. teacher–student relationship, parent–child, etc. (Linell and Luckmann, 1991; Muller and Soto, 2000b, cited in Muller and Soto, 2002);

- compensatory efforts on behalf of the natural speaker to address the constraints on time and communicative effort experienced by people who are dependent on alternative communication methods (Higginbotham and Wilkins, 1999, cited in Muller and Soto, 2002).

Role of communication partner

Being a good communication partner means treading a fine line between communication inflation and communication devaluation. If we inflate the competencies of the person, their self-image and real contributions may be compromised. Conversely, if we assume a low level of competence we may be guilty of contributing to a self-fulfilling prophecy, i.e. we do not believe the person can communicate, so we do not provide opportunities for them to communicate, therefore they do not communicate. Duchan (2001) observes that if we assume people *are* competent and provide them with appropriate opportunities to participate effectively, they are more likely to develop the relevant skills. Participation is an outcome of collaborative effort. This means negotiating, with the individual, what would constitute adequate support and accessible engagement opportunities.

The good communication partner is sensitive to the nuances of the other person's communication style. Conversational conventions may not necessarily apply. Flexible and creative use of communication skills to support the person who experiences difficulties is important. Alm and Newell in von Tetzchner and Jensen (1996) assert that successful communication between a natural communicator and one who uses aided communication is dependent on altering 'the conversational rule that participants take equal shares of the conversation' (p. 171).

Contributions of communication partner

The tendency is to assume that all expressive behaviour is representative of conscious inner intention and to ignore the mediating role of significant others. Arthur, Butterfield and McKinnon (1998) state that the contributions of the communication partner are just as important to the assessment process as the communication skills of the individual. Singular assessment of the person who experiences communication difficulties provides only half of the picture. It reveals something about the available skills of the person but neglects the supporting role of significant others and the reciprocity of interaction. The contributions of the one are affected by the contributions of the other. It is about how utterances are formed and presented, how meanings are accessed and inferred, how active listening and sequential responding occur.

Message formulator

Von Tetzchner and Martinsen (2000) discuss the attributes of the good conversation partner to users of alternative communication systems.

Knowledge about the characteristics and functions of a technical aid, plus awareness of the particular characteristics of communicating through alternative systems, is vital. Aided communication may require a 'message formulator'. This is a role usually assumed by the communication partner and involves a range of acts, including waiting for the message to be encoded, reading and articulating messages transmitted by the person, making interpretations 'online' even when the message is telegraphic in nature, etc.

Communicating through drawing

The role of communication partner has been considered in approaches that involve drawing as a means of communication. As a therapy technique, drawing has been variously used with people who have aphasia (Lyon, 1995; Weniger, 1995). The therapy programme described by Sacchett et al. (1999) focuses on the generative drawing of people with severe aphasia. Therapy activities involved both the individual as the primary communicator and the significant other as the main communication partner. The specific aims regarding the individual centred on the ability to 'think of an idea, call up its visual representation and translate this into drawing ... to promote "economic" drawing by improving subjects' ability to focus on the important aspects of the message to be conveyed and to draw only these' (p. 269).

The aim for the carers was to improve their skills of interpretation so that they became more efficient at extracting the meanings from their partners' 'drawn' contributions to the interaction. Initially, some of the carers tended to make random guesses at proffered drawings; however, as the course of therapy progressed, improvements in the elicitation and interpretation skills of carers were noted. The authors suggest that the improved communicative viability of the participants' drawings owed much to the training and participation of the carers.

The positive 'face' of communication

'Face' theory is described as the positive and unconditional value that is a basic human requirement of the person in a social encounter. It is the need of individuals to be appreciated by their communication partners (Brown and Levinson in Goody, 1978; Goffman, 1955). Leudar in Beveridge, Conti-Ramsden and Leudar (1989) suggests that an individual's value and self-respect may arise from and be maintained within interactions. For example, some speech situations are systematically biased with respect to the 'face' of the interactants, due to the nature of the activities involved and the participants' power differentials. Formal assessment makes explicit the distribution of power between therapist and client. It is the therapist who directs and the client who attempts responses. For some individuals, the process whereby their communication difficulties are exposed is a painful and face-losing one.

Process of repair

The phenomenon of intersubjectivity, whereby the participants demonstrate understanding of each other's contributions, is important to face (Wilkinson, 1999). Repair of trouble sources in conversation helps to bring intersubjectivity problems to the surface. The process of repair is described in the literature as interactionally delicate, because it presents a 'threat to face'. Schegloff, Jefferson and Sacks (1977) looked at the management of repair within ordinary conversations and identified four main types of repair that occur:

- Self-initiated, self-repair
- Other-initiated, self-repair
- Self-initiated, other-repair
- Other-initiated, other-repair.

In conversations between linguistically intact communicators there is usually a preference for self-initiation and self-repair. Repair management within the current speaker's turn (self-initiated, self-repair) brings a clear interactional advantage as it leaves the next turn free to carry on with the topic of discussion. A high incidence of other-repetition and 'other-initiated other-repair' has been found in interactions between learning disabled people and their carers (Sabsay and Kernan, 1983). This pattern is also seen between aided and natural speakers (Fishman, Timler and Yoder, 1985), people with aphasia and their linguistically intact partners (Wilkinson et al., 1998), and in adult–child interaction sequences (Tarplee, 1993: 96).

Good communication partners

The question of what makes for a 'good communication partner' is important to partnership-centred interventions. Simmons-Mackie and Kagan (1999) conducted a study which attempted to identify the conversational strategies of partners who had been rated as 'good' or 'poor' communicators. 'Good' conversation partners were found to accept responses as 'truthful' and 'sufficient' even when minimally informative. In contrast 'poor' partners projected doubt about the participant's competence and failed to acknowledge acceptable or adequate responses. They suggest that interaction is just as important as the exchange of information.

> The 'good' partners actually sacrificed transactional goals to some degree to help partners ... save face and foster positive engagement. Partners judged as 'poor' tended to focus significant effort on 'getting information' and attended less to building the social relationship. (Simmons-Mackie and Kagan, 1999: 818)

Pound et al. (2000) stress the facilitator role of the communication partner. Techniques are learned and used in communication situations in order to alleviate struggle and to boost the person's confident use of communication skills. The good communication partner creates the conditions for the individual to reveal their own competencies. Maneta, Marshall and Lindsay (2001) demonstrate the value of involving a partner in what they refer to as an 'indirect' approach to treating word sound deafness in a person with aphasia. An advice booklet was created, tailored to the new communication needs of an aphasic man and his wife. The idea was to recreate a balance in their communications and to reduce the incidence of trouble by training the wife in the use of facilitative strategies. The authors make the important point that:

> Indirect therapy, as practised in this study, is not a time saving option ... (it requires) ... careful preparatory assessment and the same number of hours as many other treatments. (Maneta, Marshall and Lindsay, 2001: 104)

Communicative competence is not a static state where the contributions of an individual are immune to those of the communication partner. Light (1989: 137) stresses the functionality of communication that underpins 'a relative and dynamic interpersonal construct'. How we respond to each other will affect how we are able to contribute. All of us can think of situations where we felt inhibited from showing our true ability, whether it was because of factors to do with the other person's behaviour or with the immediate context.

Partnership interventions

Partnership interventions focus on the active communication process and relationship between people with communication disabilities and their significant others. The therapist deals directly with both client and primary communication partner and they work collaboratively towards mutually agreed goals.

Partnership interventions include both assessment and therapy activities. When someone has a restricted ability to communicate, a more deliberate and focused input from significant others is required (McConkey, Purcell and Morris, 1999; Purcell, McConkey and Morris, 2000). This requires significant others to make conscious and consistent changes to the ways they offer support. Greater responsibility lies with the communication partner. If they are sensitive and responsive, the person may be able to demonstrate more skills. If they are not sure what to do, fail to recognize communicative signals, or dominate an interaction with their own words, the person's skills will remain hidden.

Appraisal of communication partnership

Appraisal of the communication partnership involves examination of the individual's communicative vulnerabilities and the corresponding barriers that may exist within the communication partner's repertoire. Once this has been done, appropriate communication supports may be invoked

Table 7.1 Illustration of linguistic vulnerabilities, potential barriers and supports

Vulnerable area	Communication barriers	Communication supports
Linguistic competence in communication. The individual may experience difficulty with language, including: • understanding the communications of others; • putting ideas and feelings into linguistic code for others to understand; • communicating ideas in a way that is intelligible to others; • organising language use in context; • remembering what has been said.	Potential barriers lie in a lack of adaptation to the individual's communication skills, influenced by the partner's: • overestimation of individual's abilities, e.g. using complex sentence structures with a person who has understanding for single words; • underestimation of individual's abilities, e.g. using single words with a person who has complex inner language but is unable to communicate in sentences due to a lack of motor control.	Supports to communication lie in the flexible use of a range of communication skills designed to make language accessible and appropriate to augment meanings as required, including: simplified use of language, eye gaze, facial expression, body language, gesture, sign, drawing, writing, photographs, symbols, objects of reference, use of touch and movement, extended use of pause between conversational turns.

Table 7.2 Illustration of operational vulnerabilities, potential barriers and supports

Vulnerable area	Communication barriers	Communication supports
Operational competence in communication. The individual may experience operational difficulties in communication for various reasons, including: • associated sensory impairments such that hearing/vision affect access to and participation in social events; • impaired muscle control for speech and execution of voluntary movements for communication, e.g. direct eye gaze, pointing, pressing switches, etc.; • problems affecting physical posture and motor control; • mismatch between available skills and demands of communication situation such that access is hampered.	Potential barriers lie in the partner's lack of sensitivity to sensory, motor and cognitive needs of the individual for a variety of reasons, including: • inadequate information about the individual's hearing and vision, e.g. providing mainly verbal opportunities to someone who is deaf; • strongly held beliefs by significant others not necessarily based on real evidence, e.g. 'S/he can hear when s/he wants to!', leading to denial of individual's needs; • lack of suitable or adequately functioning assistive devices, such as communication or hearing aid, leading to high level of dependence on others.	Supports to communication lie in: • helping the individual to use and maintain any recommended aids to hearing, vision and communication as recommended, e.g. make available individual's communication aid, book or other supports; • using appropriate tactics to support access to communication, e.g. allow more time for responding, physical and visual support when required.

Table 7.3 Illustration of social vulnerabilities, barriers and supports

Vulnerable area	Communication barriers	Communication supports
Social competence in communication. The individual may experience social difficulties in communication for various reasons, including: • limited or inappropriate use of social skills such as turn-taking, use of eye gaze, gesture, body language, social use of language; • lack of experience of social interaction or limited opportunities, e.g. meeting new people, going out to different places and social venues, developing a range of relationships including friendships and intimacy with a chosen partner; • individual's emotional state or level of arousal, affecting contributions.	Potential barriers lie in limited, inappropriate or inflexible opportunities for social interaction such that participation is constrained, influenced by: • the existence of rigid routines that preclude the use of a range of social skills, e.g. decisions are made on a daily basis without the involvement of the individual; • the relationship between the communication partner and individual, and the communication style used, e.g. limited degree of interpersonal advocacy, disempowering communication style.	A deliberate approach to communication by significant others aims to facilitate the social participation of the individual: • within the communication partnership, prompting the use of social skills, e.g. indicating the person's communication turn, inserting waiting time; • within the communication environment, establishing social routines to promote successful exchanges, e.g. greeting at start of day.

Table 7.4 Illustration of strategic vulnerabilities, barriers and supports

Vulnerable area	Communication barriers	Communication supports
Strategic competence in communication. The individual may experience strategic difficulties in communication for various reasons, including: • lack of flexibility in use of communication skills, e.g. unable to speak louder when required (or quieter), unable to use more generic gesture when faced with a non-signing communication partner, etc.; • lack of confidence to use communication skills in situations outside those which are immediate and familiar.	Potential barriers lie in the scope of the individual's communication network, which is affected by: • restricted social horizon or opportunities for meeting people outside the familiar and immediate partnership; • narrow approach to communication with the individual, e.g. one that excludes the use of alternative and augmentative communication approaches.	Supports lie in negotiating the opening up of communication with the individual: • in a variety of situations that extend beyond the familiar communication partnerships, e.g. classroom, workplace, supermarket, social club, pub, further education college. • with a range of communication partners with different knowledge, skills and experiences of the individual, e.g. volunteer workers, neighbours.

to ameliorate or circumvent any difficulties experienced in the communication partnership. Light's (1989) definition of communicative competence provides a useful framework for looking at the various aspects of the communication partnership in Tables 7.1–7.4. Four areas of competence are considered:

- Linguistic competence: mastery of linguistic code.
- Operational competence: the ability to transmit message and methods for accessing communication opportunities.
- Social competence: involves knowledge, judgement and skill in the social rules of communication.
- Strategic competence: compensatory strategies to deal with limitations of their communication.

Direction of therapy

Intervening with the partnership gives the opportunity to examine individual contributions to the communication process and for solving any difficulties. Open discussion between therapist, client and significant other(s) may help to reveal individual perspectives and relevant issues. The therapist draws on knowledge of the particular aspect of communication and functioning; the client and significant other(s) draw on their separate experiences.

Intervening with the partnership may have a promotional or adaptive/compensatory aim, or a combination of the two.

Promotional

The aim is to advance certain aspects of an individual's communication skills and functioning where there are concerns about natural progression or recovery. There is a concentration of effort on the advancement of conventional communication skills, i.e. speech, language and communication. Techniques may be employed to support progression. This may involve consciousness-raising of communication partners so that they become more active with regard to promoting the skills development and use of the person concerned. Daily therapy activities may be advised for the parent and child to engage in. For example, this may require the parent of a pre-school child with language delay to accentuate active listening in a range of play activities. A child's early fluency difficulties may be positively supported by parental reinforcement of fluent behaviours.

Adaptive or compensatory

The aim is to minimize or cancel out the effects of any known impairment by the conscious use of recommended techniques and/or devices. The primary client and his/her communication partners work collaboratively with the SLT to adjust to partnership conditions that are different from the normal circumstances. For many linguistically intact communication partners this means suspending their usual set of communication skills and employing a modified skill set where specific techniques might be introduced. For example, the parent of the young child with learning disabilities may employ the use of signing in order to match the child's needs. A keyworker may introduce sensory stimulation to the interaction opportunities offered to adults with profound and multiple learning disabilities. Massage may form one component of the interaction between a mother and her infant with Down's syndrome. Drawing and use of a communication book may be used in the conversations between aphasic and non-aphasic partners. Both teachers and parents collaborate with the cerebral palsied child whose primary mode of communication is via a computer-aided device, learning new ways of 'listening' to the child and adopting a different rate of conversational turn-taking.

Role of communication partners

The role of the communication partner will vary according to the theoretical principles driving the approach, the over-arching purpose and the goals that have been identified. Intervention approaches roughly fall into two categories: 'naturalistic' and 'direct' (McCormick and Schiefelbusch, 1990). 'Naturalistic' interventions may be described as organic in that they focus on the interplay between a changing individual and a dynamic environment. Based on a social constructivist view of language and cognitive development, the responsiveness of significant others in the child or adult's life is of primary interest (Coupe O'Kane and Goldbart, 1998). 'Direct' approaches embrace a behaviourist structure whereby the behaviour of the individual is shaped by the organization of contingencies.

Early interaction skills

Interest in early interaction skills is shared by a range of communication partnerships, e.g. between parent and child, support staff and adult with learning disabilities, and partner and older person with dementia. There are a number of approaches that target the familiar partnerships in the person's life. Significant others require a high level of commitment and a desire to effect change. There is the development of therapy activities that can be integrated into daily living from the outset. Implementation is promoted in naturally occurring contexts. The impairment is not viewed as a static impediment; rather it is 'based on the premise that development results from a continual interplay between a changing organism and a changing environment, so that both the individual and their settings experience change' (Gompertz in Fawcus, 1997: 70).

Early parent–child interaction
Intervention that is targeted early on in the child's development has two main purposes (Launonen in von Tetzchner and Jensen, 1996):

- primary prevention, which seeks to avert any disability threatening conditions;
- secondary prevention, where early identification of the child's needs highlight the risks to development and there is a corresponding move to minimize the effects of any disability that might follow.

The Hanen early language parent programme was developed by Manolson (1983). It is concerned with building a positive communication partnership between parent and child. Parents are encouraged to consider the consequences of being a poor interaction partner to the child, and this helps them to understand how they make a difference. The programme employs the use of 'easy to remember' acronyms so that accessibility and implementation are optimized. For instance it describes the responsive partner in relation to its '3A's way to encourage communication':

- Allow our child to lead
- Adapt to 'share the moment'
- Add language and experience.

Levels of communication development are identified as a guide to parents. At level 1 the child responds primarily on a reflex basis. The parent is encouraged to notice the child's reactions to events in the environment and to follow identified interests. Level 2 is where the child begins to explore the immediate environment and starts to imitate actions and sounds. Level 3 is described as when conventional sounds and gestures start to emerge. Level 4 is where word use is evident.

The Swedish Early Language Intervention Programme was developed by Johansson (1994) to promote the language development of children with Down's syndrome. It recommends an early beginning to therapy, when the infant is only a few weeks old or whenever the parents wish to start. Continuity and repetition are key features of implementation, with parent and baby going through the same activity every day for a number of consecutive days. Much of the emphasis in the early stages of the programme is on preparing the parent to be a sensitive respondent to the infant's signals. This means being alert to subtle changes in ongoing behaviour and other small body actions. Activities are recommended that are amenable to daily life, with objectives that are clearly defined for the parents (Thomas, 1990). For example, structured tactile stimulation in the form of body massage is carried out several times a day at opportune moments, e.g. at nappy changing times or after a bath, to promote social contact and relationship building. Babble play and conversational turn-taking are also encouraged.

Early introduction to signing
The introduction of signing to the early interaction context provides a bridge for partnerships where the child has particular cognitive and communication needs. Use of visual communication support is considered invaluable as an alternative means of communication for some children (Le

Provost in Buckley et al., 1993). It facilitates development of eye contact, visual attention and selective listening (Abrahamsen, Romski and Sevcik, 1989; Hurd, 1995; Le Provost in Buckley et al., 1993) and spontaneous verbal communication (Buckley et al., 1993). The provision of a more accessible communication mode may help to reduce personal frustrations at not being able to communicate, which in turn may prevent the development of further behaviour problems. Valuable insights may be offered to parents about the way the child perceives the word, thereby enabling the monitoring and correction of errors (Gompertz in Fawcus, 1997).

Interacting with children and adults with severe to profound learning disabilities

A number of programmes focus on the development of basic interaction with children and adults who have severe to profound learning disabilities. Consideration is given to the development of social routines and spontaneous exchanges.

Intensive interaction is an approach based on the early development of communication between parent and child (Nind and Hewett, 1994; 1998; 2001). It has been developed primarily for use 'with pre-verbal students who were experiencing extreme difficulty in learning and in relating to others and who were demonstrating ritualistic and challenging behaviours' (Nind and Hewett, 1994: 8).

Intensive interaction focuses on the development of a sensitive response network to expressive acts made by the learner. The content of interactive sequences varies and is spontaneous and responsive rather than pre-planned. Essentially, the communication partner is encouraged to 'tune in' to the behavioural repertoire of the individual.

Individualized sensory environment (ISE) seeks to extend the interactive behaviours of people with severe–profound and multiple learning disabilities by introducing sensory stimulation, e.g. tactile and vestibular sensations, to the interaction process (Bunning, 1996; 1997). The therapist works with the familiar communication partnerships in a person's life. Sessions resemble interactive workshops where the therapist, client and significant other(s) explore different ways of establishing, maintaining and extending human interaction. The therapist demonstrates appropriate models of interaction for the significant others and provides feedback on the interactions taking place.

Developing a communication partnership with a woman who relies on mainly non-verbal communication

Flora is a 27-year-old woman who has severe learning disabilities. She communicates in a mainly non-verbal way, e.g. eye gaze, hand-arm gesture and vocalization. She has a few echolalic-type utterances that she uses, such as 'Hello Bill!', 'Look!', etc.

The therapist is working with Flora and her keyworker. The principal aim is to develop their communication partnership by:

- revealing Flora's communicative competence in an interaction;
- demonstrating the role of the communication partner in ascribing meaning to communication behaviours;
- helping the keyworker to identify the possible meanings of Flora's non-conventional communication behaviours and to facilitate her self-expression;
- establishing the principles for a 'good communication partner' with Flora, thereby addressing communication barriers at this level.

Context
- the therapist, Flora and the keyworker are working in a small room in the day centre.
- the therapist is interacting with Flora using a range of items that provide sensory feedback – the example here is a soft brush.
- the keyworker is observing in situ.
- the session is being videoed for mutual appraisal between therapist and keyworker after the session.

Therapeutic interaction	*Enactment processes*
1. **T** ((reaches behind her back and brings	E.1 Equipment organization – presenting sensory item to client
2. forward a large soft 'blusher' brush)) [E.1 A.1]	
3. Look/ [A.1 B.1] ((uses brush on own hand [C.2]	A.1 Attention call – emphatic presentation of item and verbal call 'look'
4. and then holds it up in front of Flora	
5. looking at her)) [A.1]	B.1 Adapting communication – therapist uses minimal verbal code throughout the interaction to reveal client's communicative competence
6. **C** ((reaches for and grabs the brush	
7. head)) Look/	
8. **T** ((takes brush)) [E.1 C.3]	E.1 Equipment organization – withdraws item
9. **C** ((outstretches hand towards **T**))	C.3 Production call – act of removal creates new opportunity for client to respond
10. **T** ((brushes C's outstretched hand)) [B.2 D.2]	
11. **C** mhmm	B.2 Ascribing meaning – client's non-verbal behaviour is read to mean 'more' or 'again'
12. **T** ((stops brushing and places brush	
13. behind back – out of view of C)) [C.3]	
14. **C** Oh	
15. **T** Flora ((looks at C)) [A.1]	
16. **C** ((looks at **T** and moves arm towards **T**))	
17. **T** ((brushes C's forearm)) [D.2] Gone ↓[B.1]	

18.   ((places brush behind back and looks

19.   at C)) [E.1] [C.3]

20. C   ((pats T's knee and reaches for the

21.   brush))

22. T   ((brings brush forward and brushes

23.   C's forearm)) [D.2] ((removes brush to   D.2 Differential feedback –
                                                        sensory stimulation is applied
24.   behind back)) gone↓ [C.3]   as positive reinforcement

25. C   ah ((moves forward and touches T's

26.   hair briefly)) /ker: / ((sits back))

27. T   gone ↓ ((looks at C)) [C.3]

28. C   ((touches index finger of right hand

29.   with index of left hand))

30. T   more? ↑[B.2]

31. C   ((touches index finger of right hand

32.   with index of left hand))

33. T   ((brushes C's hand [B.2] [D.2] and then   B.2 Ascribing meaning –
                                                        client's non-verbal behaviour is
34.   withdraws behind back)) [C.3]   read to mean 'more' or 'again'
                                                        D.2 Differential feedback –
35. C   ((pats T's hand)) hello Bill   sensory stimulation is applied
                                                        as positive reinforcement
36. T   ((brushes C's hand)) [B.2] [D.2] gone ↓

37.   ((withdraws brush behind back)) [E.1] [C.3]   C.3 Production call – act of
                                                        removal creates new
38. C   ((pats T's knee then touches index   opportunity for client to
                                                        respond
39.   finger of right hand with index of left

40.   hand))

41. T   ((brushes C's hand and forearm [D.2]

42.   – withdraws brush behind back)) [C.3]

43. C   ((pats T's knee)) hello Bill

44. T   gone ↓[C.3]   C.3. Production call – reminds
                                                        the client that the item is no
45. C   ((reaches towards item on floor))   longer there

46. T   ((follows C's direction and picks

47.   up fan)) [B.2]

Evaluation of enactment processes

The interaction is characterized by therapist use of minimal verbal coding, which serves to check potential verbal domination whilst revealing Flora's communicative competence (*B.1 Adapting communication*). Each 'conversational turn' is characterized by the therapist attracting the client's attention (*A.1 Attention call*). This is frequently accompanied by the presentation of an item which serves to further enhance the attention call (*E.1 Equipment organization*). The application of the sensory stimulation provides positive reinforcement for the client's contributions (*D.2 Differential feedback*) and the withdrawal of the item serves to create a further opportunity for the client to respond (*C.3 Production call*). In order to preserve the flow of the interaction and to build the client's functional communication repertoire, the therapist ascribes meaning (*B.2*) to the non-verbal and echolalic phrases used by the client.

Once the different communication tactics had been identified by the therapist and keyworker, it was decided to work on them within social routines that involved the use of sensory stimuli. Sessions resembled interactive workshops where Flora, her keyworker and therapist were participants. Use of a minimal verbal code was practised, prefaced always by an attention call, such as 'Flora look' or 'Flora here'. Feedback was provided in the form of sensitive responding to Flora's contributions, following her lead whenever possible and providing the chosen form of sensory stimulation. In this way, Flora and her communication partner were able to develop social interaction that carried forward to other times outside the workshop-style sessions.

Interpreting communication

'See What I Mean' (SWIM) is a set of guidelines that has been developed for use by significant others of people with profound and multiple learning disabilities (Grove et al., 1999). Communication is viewed as an interactive partnership of mutuality and social co-ordination. The attribution of meaning is acknowledged as an essential constituent of the communication process with such individuals because of a reliance on non-conventional forms, such as eye gaze, body language, vocalization, etc. Partners frequently have to 'second guess' the meaning of behaviour, running the risk of 'getting it wrong'. A series of steps have been devised to guide communication partners in checking their interpretations of their clients' behaviours. They are encouraged to gather and use available information about the person and the context, and to try out an interpretation of the underlying meaning. The resulting communication is negotiated between the individual and the communication partner.

Conversation skills

Some of the consequences of having a communication disability are addressed by focusing on the interactants and their contributions to the construction of meaning and social engagement (Pound et al., 2000). Perkins (1995) suggests that by focusing intervention on naturally occurring social exchanges, the clinician is able to move away from 'prescriptive judgements of appropriacy ... or correctness'. Studies have shown that 'deviation from what is normal does not necessarily equate with failure or communicative ineffectiveness' (Perkins, 1995: 373).

Conversation analysis (CA) defines social interaction as a dynamic process to which the participants contribute. It is not some rule-based state (Lesser and Perkins, 1999). As a method of investigation, it seeks to uncover processes whereby participants achieve shared understanding in the sequential organization of talk. In order to build up the partnership-based approach, the contributions of the interactants are scrutinized.

> 'Evidence is sought inductively from the sequential unfolding of the interaction. Participants reveal directly, by their responses, their analysis of the preceding speaker's turn' (Lesser and Perkins, 1999: 91).

Conversation coaching

Conversation coaching is used with aphasic adults and their spouses (Holland, 1991). Intervention looks at pre-morbid interaction patterns and concentrates on selecting and developing verbal and non-verbal strategies to improve communicative interactions between the couple (Hopper, Holland and Rewega, 2002). Unlike supported conversation for adults with aphasia (SCA: see Chapter 8), it does not focus on generic communication strategies; rather it considers the idiosyncrasies that are part of a familiar communication partnership. Conversation and communicative exchanges in natural contexts are emphasized, e.g. relaying telephone messages, talking about what to have for dinner, or discussing family issues. Citing Kagan and Gailey in Holland and Forbes (1993), Hopper, Holland and Rewega (2002: 757) state that 'A person with poor communication skills but a skilled communication partner can do well in conversations, whereas one with excellent skills and an unskilled communication partner may do poorly.'

Communication and challenging behaviour

Challenging behaviour (CB) is a feature in the lives of many people with severe learning disabilities. It is defined as behaviour that presents serious risk to the physical safety of the individual or others around them, or prevents the individual from taking part in everyday life in the community (Emerson, 1995). The social constructive nature of CB, i.e. that it is related to both individual and environmental characteristics, is generally acknowledged. It is 'the outcome of complex interactions amongst a range of interaction factors – organic, psychiatric, environmental, ecological, historical' (Emerson, McGill and Mansell, 1994: 6).

Published research reveals an inverse relationship between communication skills and incidence of CB (Bott, Farmer and Rohde, 1997; Bunning, 1998; Chamberlain, Chung and Jenner, 1993; Desrochers, Hile and Williams-Moseley 1997). Where communication skills are more severely restricted, there is a stronger likelihood of CB. The relationship between communication and challenging behaviour is a reciprocal one: abnormal behaviour patterns may challenge the communication process and failure to communicate effectively may be a catalyst in the establishment of problem behaviour. The likely consequence of this is fragility in social situations and a reliance on the skills of communication partners to make themselves understood (Grove et al., 1999). There may also be a risk in the way significant others respond to the demands of clients who challenge. Staff may function to avoid prolonged contact with challenging behaviour that they find aversive, thereby exacerbating the negative effects of isolation (Emerson, 1995; Hastings and Remington, 1994).

Albert, a man with severe learning disabilities and challenging behaviour

The case of Albert and his communication partners illustrates how the development of unique and varied ways of communicating with the client can have a positive effect on presenting difficulties. The positive momentum in Albert's team of support staff influenced the types of interactions with the client. This helped to build a warm and mutually satisfying communication partnership between Albert and the significant people in his life.

Albert was a 52-year-old male with severe learning disabilities. He had lived in a community house with four other residents for nine years. Prior to this he lived in a long-stay institution for over 15 years. A referral was made to SLT because staff wanted an evaluation of the way they interacted with Albert. They were concerned that the 'in-house' communication style they had developed with Albert appeared to 'fly in the face' of age-appropriate communication and as such might be in conflict with the values of the service, i.e. treating adults as adults. This had led to feelings of insecurity amongst staff.

Albert was on five different types of medication, one of which was to control his epilepsy. One of the side effects of his cocktail of medicine appeared to be an unquenchable thirst. He had no apparent hearing or vision problems and good motor skills. Albert had a history of severe challenging behaviour characterized by aggression to self and others, anal stimulation and faecal smearing, stereotypic behaviours and ritualistic routines.

Assessment activities involved semi-structured interview with two of the staff team who knew Albert very well, and videoing Albert interacting with his primary communication partners at different times and in different situations. The aims were to examine the nature of Albert's interactions with familiar partners in everyday environments; to identify structures and patterns that illustrate how the interaction is constructed; and to identify conversational strategies of partners who are rated as 'good' communicators. Transcripts were made of a sample of the interactions.

Interactions between Albert and familiar staff member

The interactions took place in the living room, between Albert and a familiar member of staff. Three interaction segments are presented here, each occurring at different times on different days. The same member of staff features in each one. On each occasion, Albert was sitting in his favourite armchair with the staff member sitting on the edge of a sofa beside him.

The transcription conventions are to be found in the preface. In this context 'S' refers to significant other, and 'C' refers to client (Albert). For enactment processes refer to the glossary in the Appendix at the back of the book.

Interaction (i)	*Techniques used by partner*
1. C ((waves left hand in front of face))	
2. S ((moves close and waves hand)) [D.5]	D.5 Acknowledging contribution – S observes and imitates non-verbal behaviour
3. C ((turns and looks at S)) I cry	
4. S You're too lovely and handsome to	
5. cry↑ [C.2]	C.2 Modelling – S expands on C's familiar utterance
6. C ((turns away and waves left hand))	
7. S ((moves close to C and whispers)) [A.1]	A.1 Attention call – S whispers in C's ear which breaks up repetitive hand waving
8. C ((laughs, turns to S and laughs))	
8. S Oh yes! [D.5]	D.5 Acknowledging contribution – uses words and intonation from familiar verbal routines
9. C ((turns away and waves left hand))	
10. S Anyway big boys/ ... [C.3]	C.3 Production call – S calls on C's usual response to familiar verbal routines
11. C ... don't cry	

Interaction (ii)	*Techniques used by partner*
1. S ... it matches your lovely blue eyes	
2. C [((looks and smiles))]	
3. S [Oh yes!/] [D.5]	D.5 Acknowledging contribution – uses words and intonation from familiar verbal routines
4. C ((looks away))	

5.   S   And you have got lovely blue eyes

6.   Let's see let's see your lovely blue

7.   eyes [C.3]   C.3 Production call – S uses un-
                                             conditional valuing in familiar verbal
8.   C   Oh yes /((turns round, looks at S   routines to stimulate C's usual
                                             response
9.   and smiles))

Interaction (iii)	*Techniques used by partner*

1.   C   ((stamps feet on floor and waves

2.   left hand in front of face))

3.   S   ((taps arm of chair and sits

4.   back)) [E.3]   E.3 Behaviour acknowledgement/
                                             support – S indicates that she has
5.   C   ((stamping stops))   noticed the start of C's feet stamping
                                             and withdraws
6.   S   Is that river dance? [C.3]
                                             C.3 Production call – S solicits
7.   C   ((waves hand)) Oh yes!   familiar verbal routine with same
                                             intonation pattern
8.   S   It was very fast. Oh yes! Oh yes
                                             D.5 Acknowledging contribution –
9.   my lovely [D.5]   as per familiar routine

10. C   ((gets his biscuit from plate to

11.   his left, breaks biscuit, turns to S

12.   and eats one half)) Oh yes

13. S   Oh yes/ [D.5]

A summary of the techniques used by Albert's communication partner is
to be found in A.6 of the individual profile (p. 186).

Stage 1: Appraisal of individual profile

The individual profile draws on information from the keyworker interviews and the naturally occurring interactions between Albert and his
communication partner.

**A: Positive factors – e.g. What can this person do communicatively,
or what resources can they draw on?**

A.1 Albert uses a highly individualized and functional vocabulary, which is
     understood by the staff team, e.g. 'jams' = pyjamas or bedtime, 'best'
     = getting dressed, 'I cry' = I'm not happy OR I want attention, etc.

A.2 Albert uses a range of non-verbal behaviours, e.g. eye gaze, body language, vocalization, intonation, etc. to communicate his ideas and feelings.

A.3 A number of strong social routines have been established that are familiar to both Albert and his interactants with use of intonation that invites participation in the verbal ritual, e.g. 'Oh yes'/'Oh no' sequences, etc.

A.4 Staff express a warm regard for Albert denoting a positive relationship.

A.5 Communication partners use a 'playful' communication style with Albert that denotes positive 'face' and is characterized by:
- soft, quiet voice;
- repetitions of familiar words and phrases;
- a range of non-verbal behaviours including touch, vocal and facial gesture, hand play;
- positive value vocabulary and phrases, e.g. 'You're too handsome', 'Oh you're lovely'.

A.6 Staff employ the use of certain techniques in their interactions with Albert, including:
- *A.1 Attention call* – varying proximity/orientation and using non-threatening communication style to attract attention, e.g. whisper in ear;
- *C.2 Modelling* – recasting phrases from familiar verbal routines;
- *C.3 Production call* – using familiar utterances that provide unconditional value to Albert;
- *D.5 Acknowledging contribution* – using words and intonation from familiar verbal routines, and imitates actions;
- *F.3 Behaviour acknowledgement/support* – showing evidence of notice of C's feet stamping routine by non-verbal gesture and withdrawing social contact.

B: Difficulties – e.g. What does this person have difficulty doing, or what are the complications and barriers to overcome?

B.1 Albert emits a number of stereotypic behaviours including: hand waving/flapping, feet stamping, rocking, twirling and throwing his handkerchief, slapping own face, etc.

B.2 Albert engages in a number of rituals frequently during the course of a day, usually in the bathroom, e.g. one ritual includes turning the taps on and off, stamping his feet and drinking water repeatedly.

B.3 Albert may be aggressive to others, particularly when either they are unfamiliar to him or his personal space is invaded, e.g. during rituals.

B.4 It is difficult for new members of staff/novel interaction partners to 'tune in' to Albert's interaction style.

B.5 Albert finds it difficult to deal with variation in daily events, preferring a certain amount of predictability and routine.

B.6 Staff do a shift pattern of working, which means that staff who are less familiar with Albert may be on duty at any one time.

B.7 There is no SLT available to Albert and the current contact is on a consultancy basis.

Stage 2: Activity planning

Content

Step 1: Goals of intervention	The main goal is to establish a consistent approach to social interaction between Albert and all potential communication partners. Support Albert's growing identity and self-determination by use of positive face in interactions. Address barriers in daily life that inhibit participation, e.g. lack of familiarity of some newer members of staff.
Step 2: Focus of approach	Identification, use and development of the 'in-house' interaction style in spontaneous interactions and in domestic routines with reference to those members of staff considered to be 'good' communication partners.

Building on positive factors – A.1, A.2, A.3, A.4, A.5, A.6

Addressing difficulties – B.3, B.4, B.5, B.6

Process

Step 3: Centre of influence	The communication partnership is the primary centre of influence. The planned trajectory is outwards to Albert's communication environment.
Step 4: Role of SLT	Therapist assumes role of 'video' profiler of interaction – listening and exploring staff ideas, analysing interactions and organizing them on video, inserting commentary to affirm positive characteristics of 'in-house' interaction style.
Step 5: Enactment processes	Video profiling – capture the positive characteristics of interactions with Albert. What are the interaction techniques used by the familiar communication partners? Convert these into an accessible commentary for the video. Record the domestic/

communication routines for dissemination to
all staff members. Therapist advises senior
member of staff on profiling interaction
features of domestic routines.

Building on positive factors – A.3, A.4, A.5

Addressing difficulties – B.3, B.4, B.5, B.6, B.7

Context

Step 6: Implementation arrangements	Consultancy approach whereby initial exploration and identification of interaction characteristics takes place in direct contact with staff members and Albert, moving to indirect once the video profile is produced.
Step 7: Physical setting	Exploration of interactions takes place in Albert's home in collaboration with staff and Albert. Construction of video profile takes place in technical suite off site.
Step 8: Individual maintenance	Observe Albert's ritualistic routines, avoiding direct intervention and crowding of personal space.

Building on positive factors – A.3, A.4, A.5

Addressing difficulties – B.1, B.2, B.3, B.7

In summary, Albert's intervention was centred on the communication
partnership and environment. As a piece of consultancy work it was delivered through brief direct contact with the familiar partnerships in Albert's
life, and indirectly through a video profile. The intervention process was
focused on the real and spontaneous interactions that took place. It was
concerned with revealing the competencies that occurred in the dynamic
partnership between Albert and his interactants, supporting the consistent use of the 'in-house' interaction style across the staff team, and
externalizing the interaction scripts of domestic routines. A video was
produced to demonstrate the positive interaction style in Albert's communication partnerships at home so that both existing staff and new
recruits could learn from it.

Partnership as centre of influence

The direction of therapy and the mechanism for change in partnership interventions are supported not only by the individual who has a communication disability, but also by the people with whom interaction takes place on a regular basis. The person who experiences communication difficulties, and the communication partner(s), work together to explore and develop new and more effective ways of constructing meaning, expressing and asserting identity, facilitating a communication relationship that is acceptable to both, and addressing any barriers to a mutually beneficial communication partnership.

Chapter 8
Restructuring the social environment

Intervention that is focused on change in the environment is concerned with the broader social network of the individual and the ethos of the setting in question. The social environment is described as the settings or milieu in which people engage with each other for a variety of reasons. It provides the critical foundations upon which positive change is built. Without a fertile communication environment, individual and partnership-based interventions fall into a vacuum. The environment or culture 'can have a major influence on both the method and the success of speech and language therapy intervention' (van der Gaag and Dormandy, 1993: 109).

The term 'social environment' covers the many different settings and contexts that a person enters during the course of daily life. It involves the people with whom they live, work and play. It is about the activities that they participate in, the jobs that they undertake and the social engagements that occur as part of it. It is about the physical setting, the understood function of a place and the level of ambient stimulation. Dockrell and Messer (1999) comment that there may be subtle differences in any of these 'microsystems' (after Bronfenbrenner, 1979). They recommend that special attention should be given to the establishment of links between the different systems that a person inhabits, e.g. between school and home, between day centre and residential home, between therapy group and home, etc. This is what Bronfenbrenner (1979) refers to as the 'mesosystem'.

Source of interest in environment

Communication is a constant variable in the main settings where learning, work and leisure take place. Because communication does not occur in isolation, the implementation and evaluation of interventions must necessarily take account of the wider contexts (Dockrell and Messer, 1999). The success of an intervention is dependent on environmental support for the individual's learning, and use of language and participation in social interaction (Martinsen and von Tetzchner in von Tetzchner and Jensen, 1996). Interest in the infrastructure of the communication environment stems from a variety of sources:

Interactionist approach

An interactionist view of language acquisition and intervention considers the role of the communication environment. The child's experiences and the reinforcing and differential feedback that occurs in the context of everyday interactions are associated with the development and use of language and communication skills (Dockrell and Messer, 1999; McLean and Snyder-McLean, 1978). Van der Gaag (1989) shares the view that there are factors within the environment that alternatively support or restrict the communicative competence of adults with a learning disability. McCall and Moodie (1998) identify a specific training need amongst people who support AAC users, particularly for communication partners of high technology AAC users. This finds resonance in Lourenco et al. in von Tetzchner and Jensen (1996):

> The limited efficiency of the communication behaviours at home and in broader environments has made it necessary to increase the awareness of people in the environment about communication opportunities, in order for more generally understood alternative ways of communication to be established. (von Tetzchner and Jensen, 1996: 310)

Social and educational influences

Social and educational policy influences the way interventions are designed and delivered. Service providers are given a direction for service developments based on a review of existing practices and a vision for the future.

• Educational directives:
Two major policy documents highlight the importance of collaboration between SLTs and teachers. The Government's consultation paper on special educational needs (DfEE, 1997) 'links better collaboration with raising of educational potential' (Miller, 1999: 141). The report of the working group on SLT provision to children with special educational needs in England states that schools, local education authorities (LEAs) and the National Health Service (NHS) are required to make a commitment to supporting children with communication difficulties (Law et al., 1998). It follows that partnership practice between educational settings and local SLT services is a necessity if the needs of children in educational settings are to be addressed. Corresponding service developments and practice models have been reported in various texts and clinical practice journals (McCartney, 1999; Miller, 1999; Rinaldi, 2000; Roux, 1996; Wright and Kersner, 1998).

• Social model:
The World Health Organization recognition of the complex relationships between biological and environmental factors (WHO: ICF, 2002) has prompted developments in the field of SLT (Threats, 2000). Assessment

and therapy activities consider not only the individual, but also the immediate personal and social environment. This is evidenced in services for adults with learning disabilities in the UK where an emphasis has been placed on environmental modification by the training of significant others. Over the past two decades there has been an increase in the commercial availability of assessment and intervention packages in the area of learning disabilities particularly, which include a focus on environment (Communication Assessment of Speech Profile: van der Gaag, 1988; Intecom: Jones, 1990; Personal Communication Plan: Hitchings and Spence, 1991).

The environmental view extends to the formal and informal structures of services, the attitudes and ideologies that are held by people, and the overarching approaches and systems established in the culture. Kagan and LeBlanc (2002) state that the recent trend in the development of therapy approaches based on a model of empowerment and social participation (for example Byng, Pound and Parr in Papathanasiou, 2000; Jordan and Kaiser, 1996; Pound et al., 2000) prompts a closer look at the social context of communication.

The interface between the individual and the context is essential to the success of interventions. Pound et al. (2000) recommend the exploration of communication in everyday environments as relevant to the aphasic person's use of total communication strategies beyond the clinical setting. For Dockrell and Messer (1999: 140), 'Intervention in isolation from real-life situations and functions can be seen to be counterproductive.'

Communication environment

The communication environment is made up of:
- The underlying values of the setting and the relationship between individuals, the separate roles that they perform and their social standing in the environment: the relative power or influence that each person has within that setting.
- The significant people who are present in an environment and with whom individuals with communication disabilities may come into contact and have cause to communicate: individual knowledge, experience, attitudes, communication style, skill mix and sensitivity to the presenting needs of others.
- The conditions of the setting: the degree of formality, which may be affected by its main function, e.g. business, leisure, etc., and general ethos of the environment.
- The communication acts that take place within the environment: the reasons for communicating and the range of forms that act as signal bearers of meaning, e.g. soliciting information verbally, supplying information in document form.

- The activities and communication opportunities that are available to people who are present and use that environment: the range and type of demands that are placed on individuals participating in the social milieu and how connections are made between the different communicators.

Purpose of intervening in the environment

Ecological interventions aim to address the social consequences of communication impairment. There is the identification of barriers that make individual use of available communication skills difficult. Corresponding communication opportunities and supports are devised to ameliorate or to overcome any complicating factors. There is the notion of 'directing ... attention away from the impairment' and creating an environment that is amenable to the individual's needs (Parr and Byng, 2002: 847).

Manipulation of the social environment is about establishing an appropriate infrastructure to support accessible and responsive communication. Cullen (1988) points out that success of an intervention is essentially related to the behaviour of significant others. Before effecting change in an individual's behaviour it may be necessary to change the behaviour of the significant people in that person's life. Powell in Kersner and Wright (2001) states that staff use of AAC in the environment supports an increase in usage by children and adults with learning disabilities. Kagan (1998) talks about expanding the communicative and social horizons of people with communication difficulties and creating a sense of empowerment.

Hamilton and Snell (1993) identify four principles for addressing the needs of individuals with severe disabilities through the communication environment. First, that communication should be tackled in the natural contexts that occur on a daily basis. Second, that many opportunities should be created and offered for the individual to use his or her available skills. Third, that the significant others should be sensitive and responsive to the communication attempts of the individual. Fourth, that some effort should be made to ensure that the communication options put before an individual are relevant to the assessed capabilities.

Rationale

Bjorck-Akesson, Granlund and Olsson in von Tetzchner and Jensen (1996) report on the rationale of an in-service training programme. Based on empowerment theory, its main aim is to promote carer awareness of communication issues with adults with profound and multiple learning disabilities. Adaptation of the five key principles that underpin the programme provide a suitable rationale for interventions where the centre of influence is the communication environment:

- Communication is interpersonal and dynamic: it involves not only the individual but also the range of people in the environment.

- There are mutual influences present: the degree of impairment does not tell the whole story about an individual's communication – environmental factors may alternately support or inhibit the extent to which skills are used.
- Environmentally based interventions must be appropriate and amenable to the actual environment used by individuals and to the individuals themselves.
- The methods employed to bring about change to the communication environment need to focus on the process whereby significant others are able to apply newly acquired knowledge and skills to real-life situations, to receive feedback about the application of skills and to problem-solve relevant issues as they arise in communication contexts.

Communication ecology

A communication environment may be conducive to inclusive communication and support the individual to reveal competencies. Alternatively, it may restrict participation. People who experience communication difficulties are at risk of social isolation because of differences in competence and generally fewer communication opportunities being available (people with developmental disabilities: Bradshaw in Abudarham and Hurd, 2002; people with aphasia: Parr et al., 1997; schoolchildren with special educational needs: Shevlin and O'Moore, 2000). Finkelstein and French in Swain et al. (1993: 28) observe that the presence of physical or social barriers may lead to 'the loss or limitation of opportunities', which in turn brings about inequalities in normal life.

Enabling vs. disabling environments

The people with aphasia interviewed by Parr et al. (1997) identified numerous barriers to communication, including:

- environmental factors, which included invasive ambient noise levels, inaccessibly fast rates of conversation and elliptical turn-taking;
- structural resource barriers, which included opportunity restrictions and poor or limited support;
- attitudinal barriers, which included the ignorance and lack of comprehension of others, leading to insensitive responses;
- informational barriers, which included poor access and many unanswered questions.

The communication environment that supports participation and inclusion of people regardless of existing competencies pays due consideration to:

- access to events, activities and situations, whether physical, communicative or emotional, e.g. to learning and leisure opportunities;

- free expression of knowledge, skills and understanding;
- the breadth of knowledge, understanding and specialist skills held by significant others and those who act as communication partners in some capacity;
- the shared experience of all as paramount to participation (Corker in Swain et al., 1993).

Implications of a 'poor' communication environment compared to a 'positive' one

Martha was a 73-year-old woman with advanced stage Alzheimer's disease. Up until the time of her admission to the care system, she lived with her husband in the family home. In the circumstances of her husband's ill health and after a brief period of respite care, Martha was moved into a residential home for continuing care. She lived in a small unit with five other residents, four of whom had general dementias. After a period of less than three weeks, it became clear to Martha's family that there were problems in the placement that were affecting Martha's general state of health and psychological wellbeing. The communication environment was poorly resourced and there was a general lack of staff engagement with residents. Observations included:

- Lack of engagement: staff members were not a visible presence in the environment, very often leaving residents to their own devices. Communication was most frequently initiated by staff when some form of physical care or intervention was required by a resident, such as washing or helping to the toilet, or else when the day's menus had to be submitted and food dished out. There was limited social engagement on topics outside immediate physical care.
- Lack of opportunity to express self: although choice was present in the daily menus that were circulated, it was not an integral part of everyday events. For instance, one member of staff was observed to manipulate the controls of the television in the sitting room without consulting the three elderly residents who were also present. It was discovered that two of the ladies had a preference for classical music, which they only heard on family visits.
- Limited understanding of resident behaviour: certain members of staff showed a lack of respect for Martha and her fellow residents. Their choice of vocabulary revealed a prejudicial attitude to Martha because of the care challenges raised by her Alzheimer's disease. Her resistant behaviour at times of personal care was described as 'aggressive' and 'disruptive'. There was little attempt to understand the behaviour in any other terms, e.g. 'Martha is an intensely private person who becomes extremely anxious during personal care supplied by another person.' Martha's family were made to feel that Martha was a problem.
- Lack of empathy for individual circumstances: Martha spent much of the day searching for her husband or anticipating his return from work.

She repeatedly questioned staff as to his whereabouts and attempted to use the fire exit to look for his car in the car park. There was a general lack of acknowledgement and understanding displayed by the staff in relation to Martha's expressions of anxiety. After 50 years of marriage, she was entitled to be anxious about her husband's whereabouts. The main response of the staff at the home was to call in the local GP so that Martha could be sedated through the use of medication. There was no corresponding staff engagement with Martha, acknowledging her right to her anxiety. When she searched for her husband's car via the fire exit, the response was simply to get her away from the exit whilst not engaging with the possible reasons for her action.

The poor environment and inadequate care had a major effect on Martha and her family. Martha declined rapidly during her stay at the home. She became depressed and lethargic. At a time of change and emotional stress, she was robbed of her sense of self and the means for dealing with the challenges of lifestyle change. Her human dignity and privacy were compromised. Her already limited life skills were further reduced, affected by the prescribed sedation and the disempowering home environment. She was denied the basic human right to express her anguish and concern regarding her husband's illness and his consequential absence from her life. It was obvious to visiting members of the family that certain staff members resented Martha's presence in the home and their negative attitude transmitted itself to her family.

A formal complaint against the home was commenced and Martha was duly moved to a new home. In contrast, this home provides a good-quality communication environment. Its professed values of 'care with dignity' permeate life in the home. Staff members are accessible at all times and mix freely with the residents. Communication has a strong interactional base and is not dependent on the transfer of information. Efforts are made to group people at mealtimes and in the sitting room, thereby encouraging social interaction. The choice of vocabulary used by staff members and their knowledge and understanding of the personal backgrounds of the residents reveal a positive attitude. Three months on, Martha has settled well in her new home and has recovered from the deterioration that occurred in the last home:

- She initiates social communication with staff members, some of her fellow residents and visitors.
- She expresses shared humour and enjoyment by laughter, makes quips and presents a relaxed social demeanour with members of the family.
- She comments on the clothes and jewellery that people wear, flowers and soft furnishings around the home.

Martha is not taking any medication. She continues to ask where her husband is; the difference is that now, there are people with whom she can talk!

Values underpinning a positive environment

Values are not standards that articulate the decisions and actions that are integral to professional practice, e.g. RCSLT *Communicating Quality 2* (1996). Rather they are statements that attempt to capture the vision and philosophy of a service. Byng, Cairns and Duchan (2002: 94) observe that 'Values emerge in the way that healthcare staff behave towards each other and towards patients and in the attitudes they evince.'

Davis and Watson (2001: 684) state that 'personal and cultural values need to be addressed' if difference is to be minimized. This finds resonance in Byng, Cairns and Duchan's (2002: 90) comments on Worrall (2000), where the importance of human values is emphasized: 'Far from being marginal, the issues that underlie how we engage with people in the process of providing a therapy service to them should be fundamental to our practice.'

Value base of provider

Byng, Cairns and Duchan (2002) question the effectiveness of interventions and the optimal uptake of resources if values operating within a service give rise to negative feelings amongst service users. They suggest that the value base of the service provider is 'a significant variable affecting outcome' (p. 95) and 'value-based judgements (are) at each level of clinical practice' (p. 98). Each decision that is taken in the process of constructing intervention is linked to a framework of personal and professional standards that shape the direction of practice. For instance, a clinical decision to train significant others is informed by a belief that change in the communication environment is necessary to improving the communicative effectiveness of the individual.

Kagan and LeBlanc (2002) report on the values base of the Aphasia Institute in Toronto, Canada. As part of its mandate it embraces the notion of *communicative access* as key to life participation. They stress the need for interventions to take into consideration both individual and environmental factors. This is reiterated by Pound et al. (2000), who advocate a range of therapy approaches designed to address both issues that are internal to the person as well as external barriers in the environment.

Impact of values

A dehumanizing experience can lead to a lack of engagement by service users. They are less likely to commit personal energies to a situation where identity and human dignity are compromised. When an individual is made to feel appreciated as a *human being* rather than simply as a number, the intervention is likely to have a more positive impact. The negative experiences of service users with aphasia have been recounted (Parr et al., 1997). Systematic devaluation of people with learning disabilities was seen in the institutional care provision of the 1900s up until the inception of new community-based services in the latter part of the last century (O'Brien in Tyne, 1981). More recently, a report of the experiences of children with special educational needs within mainstream schools reveals that 'integration and inclusion ... is far from complete' (Davis and Watson, 2001: 671).

Values influence the way a service is provided. The London Centre of Connect, the communication disability network, provides a therapeutic environment that reflects their ethos of ensuring that people with aphasia and their significant others 'are able to live healthily with communication disability' (Byng, Cairns and Duchan, 2002: 98). Many community services for people with learning disabilities were originally fashioned according to the principles of *social role valorization* (SRV), where value is given to the many different social roles that an individual may have (Wolfensberger, 1992: 32): 'the enablement, establishment, enhancement, maintenance, and/or defence of valued social roles for people – particularly for those at value risk – by using, as much as possible, culturally valued means'.

Inclusive communication

Inclusive communication is the cornerstone of the positive communication environment. Von Tetzchner et al. in von Tetzchner and Jensen (1996) point out that communication is at the heart of the relationship between an individual and society. Adapted from Kenworthy and Whittaker (2000), inclusive communication is about the person having an equal place in situations where human engagement happens. The social standing and participation of an individual is dependent, in part, on the dominant communication form of the culture. Users of alternative or non-conventional ways of communicating, e.g. signing or computer-aided device, are in a minority. Use of such communication forms is rarely seen in naturally occurring situations other than in those planned routines that are part of the person's immediate environment, e.g. within the familiar and informed communication partnership, etc.

Inclusion in education

Inclusion is a term that is commonly used in relation to educational provision for children with special needs. Inclusion demands attention to the infrastructure of service provision. Alterations are made to cater for diversity of pupil need. Rinaldi (2000) suggests that the language-based approach in education provides a method for restructuring the curricular provision within the framework of the National Curriculum. Grove (1998) offers a creative solution to the English curriculum, by using drama and story telling as enactive routes to quite complex texts (Grove and Peacey, 1999).

Gascoigne in Kersner and Wright (2001) summarizes the 'inclusion agenda': 'The ultimate goal is to achieve a fully inclusive society where the handicapping effects of disabilities and impairments are reduced by changes made to the fabric of society' (p. 64).

In the context of education, inclusion refers to learning in the *least restrictive environment* (Millar, 2001). That is, educational and social opportunities are made available to the child that might otherwise be denied in a more specialist, segregated setting. Additionally, there is the advantage of experiencing real community life *with* a disability so that facilitating strategies may be developed as required in 'preparation for later life in wider society' (Gascoigne in Kersner and Wright, 2001: 65) – at least that is the theory!

Only rhetoric?

Davis and Watson (2001) argue that the 'rhetoric of inclusion' is often articulated but little attention is paid to the *process* whereby integration becomes a reality for the children concerned. They found that the teachers in their study had strategies for dealing with the individual but lacked ideas for dealing with the broader group culture. The focus of change is usually on the child with special needs whilst the infrastructure of the social environment is neglected. Cuckle and Wilson (2002) suggest that the development of social relationships and friendships for children with Down's syndrome in mainstream schools requires a deliberate approach by the organization. True inclusion is not simply the physical integration of individuals, e.g. a child with special needs placed in a mainstream class; rather it requires openness from all at the heart of the organization (Lindsay and Dockrell, 2002).

Social inclusion

Social inclusion is one of the guiding principles of the government white paper *Valuing People: a new strategy for learning disability for the 21st century* (DoH, 2001b). The definition of inclusion can equally apply to almost any group of individuals who find themselves in a socially compromised position because of a disability: 'Enabling people with [learning] disabilities to do those ordinary things, make use of mainstream services and be fully included in the local community.'

Charness and Holley (2001: 69) suggest that the ideal environment for people with dementia is one that 'maintains control, choice and personal autonomy over the circumstances of one's final days'. Based on Bronfenbrenner's (1977) ecological system, Calkins (2001: S77) provides an 'integrated model of place' to delineate the multiple dimensions in a dementia care setting. It is a series of nested areas of influence within the four interlinked dimensions of: the physical environment, the social context, the organizational context and people with dementia. The same model provides a useful summary of the key factors in the communication environment as illustrated in Figure 8.1.

A receptive environment

When applied to communication, the term *inclusive* suggests acceptance of and support for diverse ways of communicating and engaging socially.

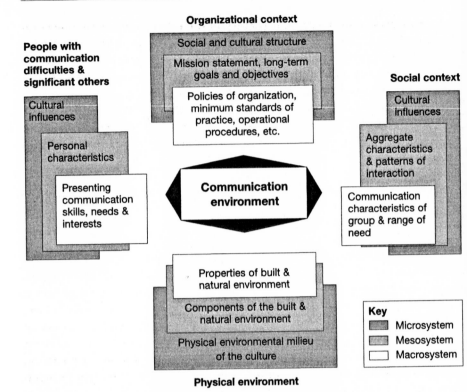

Figure 8.1 Integrated model of the communication environment (Adapted from Calkins' 'integrated model of place', 2001)

Table 8.1 Examples of variables across the dimensions and levels of the communication environment

	Microsystem	Mesosystem	Macrosystem
Organizational context	Staffing ratios and training on communication-related issues.	Value base of organization that underpins practice.	Current social/educational/health policy that directs the way forward.
Social context	Prevailing and immediate communication needs of group: use of AAC, etc.	Means, reasons and opportunities for communicating.	Group identity and social infrastructure.
Physical environment	Physical properties: furnishings, lighting, ambient noise level, etc.	Composition of natural and built space, functions of space and access to space.	Construction standards; space registration requirements.
People with communication difficulties and significant others	Immediate competencies, skills, needs and interests.	Values held by individuals, personality, sense of self.	Cultural influences; religious affiliations.

This requires that equal value is placed on the different ways people communicate in any given setting. Ware (1996: 1) uses the term 'responsive environment' and defines it as one in which 'people get responses to their actions, get the opportunity to give responses to the actions of others, and have the opportunity to take the lead in interaction'.

In short, the contributions of the individual are valued by others, as demonstrated by their reactions and the types of opportunities on offer. A receptive environment is one that does not judge difference as a reason to exclude; rather it seeks to learn from the new situation and to make changes to the environment-based on the learned experience. For example, the London Centre of Connect acknowledges the importance of graphic forms of communication for people with aphasia: notepads and pencils are placed in wall-mounted boxes at strategic points throughout the building.

The standing of the individual is addressed by the provision of communication opportunities for everyone, regardless of available competencies and skills (von Tetzchner et al., 1996). An exclusive communication environment is one that observes the conventional communication of the majority, or attributes communicative control to those in positions of power, e.g. to the paid staff even though the users are in the majority. Alternative or adaptive ways of communicating become subordinate in the culture of the dominant communication style. This is evident in meetings where professionals and client come together to discuss topics of mutual interest, e.g. case conferences, medical consultations and progress reviews.

Review meetings for adults with learning disabilities

Person-centred planning is the principal forum for reviewing a learning-disabled client's service and for identifying personal goals for the future (DoH: *Valuing People*, 2001b). In the past, a system called *individual programme planning* (IPP) fulfilled a similar function. Meetings were arranged for the client, significant others and interested parties to review relevant aspects of a person's life, e.g. communication, domestic skills, living arrangements, educational opportunities, leisure activities, therapy needs, etc. Appropriate goals were selected, action plans devised and responsibilities for implementation assigned. The trend was to encourage the presence of the individual whom the meeting was about. The idea was that participation of the focal person was essential to the good procedural conduct of the meetings; however, in reality little was done to address the issue of inclusive communication. The main forms of communication were verbal, with notes of meetings and agendas in type print. Since there is a high level of communication difficulties and literacy problems in this population (Rondal and Edwards, 1997), as well as hearing impairments (Yeates, 1989; 1991; 1995), the majority of clients were left out in the cold.

Communication across the modalities

Inclusive communication embraces the notion of Total Communication (TC), which involves the flexible use of communication across the modalities (Bradshaw, 2000; Jones, 2000; Lawson and Fawcus in Byng, Swinburn and Pound, 1999; Pound et al., 2000). Communication is viewed as having multiple representations that move beyond conventional linguistic code (e.g. the spoken and written word), and include the use of facial, vocal and body gesture, writing, drawing and objects, pictures and environmental points of reference, and specific communication devices.

Balancing act

Establishing the rights of people with communication difficulties within the communication environment whilst also progressing individual competencies is a balancing act. The way in which society ascribes value to difference is part of the inclusion equation. Campbell (2002: 472) states that society needs to find ways of making people with disabilities 'powerful enough to influence the future'.

Tensions may arise between discrete services in the health and educational sectors. Sometimes the ethos of the SLT service may be at odds with the prevailing medical or educational paradigm (Byng, Cairns and Duchan, 2002). For instance, the practice biases of the main setting, e.g. a dominant medical model that influences practice in an acute hospital site, may provide an uncomfortable backdrop for the SLT service where priorities relate to a social model of intervention, e.g. intervention that is focused on empowering the individual and looks to manipulate barriers to communication in the environment.

Interventions in the communication environment

Intervening in the communication environment raises the question of what needs to happen so that people with communication disabilities can break into the communication environment. Charness and Holley (2001: 65–73) recommend what they call a 'human factors approach'. It provides a more global focus by considering the interaction between 'human capabilities and environmental demands'. The relationship between these two is a dynamic one; environmental demands need to correspond to changes in capabilities.

Kagan and LeBlanc (2002: 163) identify four key principles that are considered critical to SLTs aiming to motivate for infrastructure change. First, they recommend the securing of a strategic partner for sharing and developing aspiration. Second, they urge perseverance, as significant change is not won overnight. Third, they suggest that drawing on real-life examples in the targeted environment or organization is more likely to bring about the desired outcomes. Finally, the current 'client-centred' model of care may be used effectively 'to address the real-life concern' of individual service users.

Interventions that are organization-based must necessarily look at the practice of significant others within the focal environment. Consideration is given to reliability – individual compliance with the agreed standards and the consistency with which intervention is carried out.

Planning for change

Bringing about change in the communication environment requires meticulous planning. It is about recognizing the need and mobilizing the commitment for change. The first step is to explore the present state of the host organization and its culture. In order to build a vision for the future, that vision needs to be seeded. Building up a positive working relationship with the key players in the environment is critical to moving forward and developing an intervention strategy and identifying the methods for restructuring the social environment.

Service provision in other settings

SLT provision within settings that are organized and staffed on the basis of their overall purpose, e.g. educational, medical, social or residential, requires ongoing negotiation and collaboration (Jordan and Kaiser, 1996; Kersner and Wright, 2001; McCartney, 1999; van der Gaag and Dormandy, 1993). The amount of contact that SLTs have with the significant others in the host environment may affect the uptake of intervention and its ultimate effectiveness. Wren et al. (2001) comment that when intervention with children takes place off site from their main environment (e.g. school), sporadic or infrequent contact between SLTs and teachers in mainstream educational settings results, making it 'more difficult to integrate therapy into educational activities' (p. 107).

Training significant others

The development of appropriate training initiatives for people who work in the health and social sectors is an expressed commitment of the British government (DoH, 2000a; 2000b). Communication is central to the provision of health, social care and education. In view of this, SLTs are called on to share their knowledge and skills with others in a variety of contexts (Bryan et al., 2002; MacMillan, Bunning and Pring, 2000; Patterson in Kersner and Wright, 2001). Law et al. (2002) report that as many as 94 per cent of health trusts are involved in training LEA staff. In recent years a number of training initiatives on communication-related topics have been carried out with staff teams and significant others in a range of contexts:

- Jones (1990) produced 'Intecom' in an attempt to formalize a joint planning procedure for the SLT and keyworkers of people with learning disabilities. It involves raising carer awareness of communication issues, so that difficulties may be detected and suitable facilitation strategies invoked.

- Bryan et al. (2002) report the effects of a training programme delivered to care staff working with older people. The programme is called Communicate and was developed in 1994–95 by the voluntary organization Action for Dysphasic Adults (ADA), renamed 'Speakability'. The aim of the programme is to encourage carers to reflect on their own communication skills in relation to the people they support. The programme is structured as a practical skills workshop, and participants are actively encouraged to relate their learning to the workplace.
- Pound et al. (2000) describe a programme developed by Connect. Volunteers learn how to be 'good' conversation partners to people with aphasia as part of Connect's outreach programme at its London base.
- MacMillan, Bunning and Pring (2000) recount a deaf awareness training programme designed and delivered to support staff working with people who had a dual diagnosis of learning disabilities and hearing impairment. The training involved a great deal of problem-solving. Participants were helped to select and apply hearing tactics to ameliorate a problem situation.
- Wright, Wood and Stackhouse (2000) have published a training package that addresses communication in the early years: *Language and Literacy Joining Together. An Early Years Training Package*. It aims to bring together early years practitioners and parents with the accent on collaborative working practice and facilitating the links between speech, language and literacy. The training is made up of four sessions that are supported by video, tutor's manual and handouts.

Interventions that target the communication environment frequently focus on changing the communication behaviour of significant others. This involves the provision of some form of training with the combined aims of promoting awareness and knowledge of communication issues, teaching specific skills and techniques, and developing problem-solving on practical issues. *Communicating Quality 2* identifies the training of colleagues and significant others as central to SLT practice in many client service groups (RCSLT, 1996).

One-off training sessions

Traditional staff training models have an emphasis on the acquisition of knowledge. There is a general reliance on handouts, talks and lectures that usually take place away from the workplace. Jackson (1988) criticizes modular training courses as providing a superficial learning experience. Blackstone (1991) emphasizes the need for research in this area and identifies a list of ten ways to facilitate adult learning and to modify attitudes and behaviours. Amongst the strategies proposed are: keeping topics highly relevant and encouraging the active learning of participants. She suggests that there might be limited advantages to the provision of one-off training sessions whilst acknowledging that stresses on service, both in terms of finance and staffing resources, may make this more likely.

Transferring learning from the classroom

The transfer of newly acquired skills and the application of learning to the real-life context present some challenges. McLeod, Houston and Seyfort (1995) investigated the effectiveness of a two-and-a-half-hour teaching session to naive and experienced carers of non-speaking adults with severe disabilities. Five principles of communication were taught: eye contact, being at the same physical level, waiting, responding, and structuring the environment to encourage communication. Importantly, they found little difference between the knowledge and skills of the two groups at baseline, thereby concluding that experience alone did not 'teach' people good practice. Participants were found to have increased knowledge of communication strategies and to be more open to the use of communication facilitation techniques. Although the shifts in staff knowledge and attitude are welcomed, there is no reported evidence of changes to staff practices in the communication environment. Furthermore, some participants expressed their apprehensions regarding the amenability of the working environment for the use of the new strategies. Clearly, the issue of skills transference from 'classroom' to 'natural environment' needs to be addressed.

Managerial commitment to the training of staff is needed if new practice is to be established in anything like a consistent and reliable way (van der Gaag and Dormandy, 1993). Preparation should involve exploring the 'best fit' with the targeted environment. Time is spent identifying the roles and responsibilities of significant others in order to ensure the amenability of training plans and the practical application of new skills.

Training from the 'bottom up'

Changing staff behaviour demands a different approach. Mittler (1984) states that in order for staff training to be effective it should be on the job, practical and related to the teaching of a whole range of personal and community living skills. This is supported by Cullen (1988), who recommends a practical 'bottom-up' approach to training. This enables the content to be tailored in a way that is broadly relevant to current issues within the service. There are some key features that are considered to be essential to communication training (McLeod, Houston and Seyfort, 1995; Nind, 1996; Pennington and McConachie, 1999):

- Because staff learn by seeing and doing, an *active learning* approach is preferable.
- The content of the training must be *relevant to the workplace* or communication environment because it is the context that supports new or changing practice.
- It needs to be *person-centred*: staff need to tune into an individual's idiosyncrasies before they generalize their learning out to other individuals;

- Training should *promote teamwork* so that an individual's communication needs are not centred on the skills of just one person.
- Training needs to be made *available to all staff and significant others* in order to maximize the effects on the communication environment.

Changing practice in situ
Changing the communication style of staff is a complex proposition. The use of techniques that provide feedback on staff practice is recommended (McConkey, Purcell and Morris, 1999; Purcell, McConkey and Morris, 2000; van der Gaag and Dormandy, 1993). Staff are encouraged to reflect on and alter their practice by use of video playback, guided observation to identify effective strategies, verbal feedback on implementation of techniques, keeping records of clients' progress over time, open discussion about individual goals, etc.

Learning process
Consideration of the ways in which people acquire new knowledge and skills is relevant to the design of training courses. Kolb (1984) defines four learning styles that an individual may engage with in the process of learning: concrete experience, reflective observation, abstract conceptualization and active experimentation. There are variations in the way people learn: one person may have a bias for abstract conceptualization (i.e. 'theorist') whilst another favours practical experience (i.e. 'pragmatist') (Honey and Mumford, 1992). Naturally, it is impossible to predict the learning style range of a particular cohort and, therefore, the planned training package should incorporate a variety of learning opportunities that feed into the different learning styles, to ensure that there is something for everyone in the course content.

Expanding the social network

Intervening with the communication environment is not always about altering the behaviour of those already present. Training and introducing new communication partners may help to expand the individual's social network.

Supported conversation for adults with aphasia
Interest in the training of linguistically 'intact conversation partners has arisen based on the principle that competence can be revealed via conversation and with reference to the published work of conversational analysts (for example, Schiffrin, 1988). Supported Conversation for Adults with Aphasia (SCA) is an approach that has been developed by Kagan and Gailey in Holland and Forbes (1993) and Kagan (1998). Similar to conversational coaching (CC: Holland, 1998 – see Chapter 7), it focuses on communication within real-life social contexts (Simmons-Mackie, 1998). Training in the use of generic skills is emphasized but does not preclude the develop-

ment of techniques at the familiar dyadic level. SCA consists of three main components:

1) Training potential communication partners.
2) Using appropriate resource materials.
3) Providing appropriate communication opportunities (Simmons-Mackie, 1998).

A central aim of this area of work is to reduce the isolation experienced by people with communication disabilities by making skilled communication partners available to the individual. The targets of the training are not the individuals with aphasia but the potential communication partners. By enskilling communication partners to reveal the competence of the aphasic person, both the communication of the aphasic person and partnership interactions will improve (Simmons-Mackie, 1998).

It is through the contact with trained partners and the experience of effective communication that re-engagement with community life occurs. Pound et al. (2000: 108) aptly refer to the communication partnership as 'a vehicle for reintegration'. This includes taking up with people and activities that were previously enjoyed, as well as pursuing new contacts and ventures (Pound et al., 2000). The social and communication horizons of the person change as the experience of partnership training boosts confidence and use of communication skills.

Training communication partners
In many cases, volunteers are recruited to establish a network of skilled communication partners that are available to people with aphasia (Kagan and Gailey in Holland and Forbes, 1993; Pound et al., 2000). The volunteers perform the role of conversation partners and are given training to meet the needs of people with aphasia. An important distinction is made between transaction and interaction. An over-focus on information exchange, i.e. transaction, may compromise the quality of social engagement and the relationship between the communication partners (Simmons-Mackie and Damico in Lemme, 1995). The idea is to show others how to be a supportive partner through providing communication supports so that individuals of variable communication abilities are able to access everyday social opportunities.

Pound et al. (2000) describe a conversation partners training scheme based on a programme developed by Lyon et al. (1997). Based at Connect, it is carried out in collaboration with a local SLT service provider. First-year SLT students and volunteers are recruited to the scheme, the former possessing a given interest in working with people with communication difficulties. Training is carried out in two group sessions, which cover the nature of aphasia: 'its communicative and social consequences outlined, and basic communication techniques are introduced ... also elaborate the anticipated benefits of the Conversation Partners scheme' (Pound et al., 2000: 121).

Volunteers are encouraged to videotape their first encounters with an aphasic partner for joint review with the scheme facilitators so that communication strategies may be introduced to meet observed needs. Additionally, monthly meetings of all concerned provide a valuable forum for mutual support, progress monitoring and problem-solving. Adapted from Kagan and Gailey in Holland and Forbes (1993), Pound et al. (2000: 107) identify a range of conversation techniques designed to establish a facilitative social environment. Techniques to facilitate comprehension include the use of 'natural gesture and drawing in communication ... allow(ing) extra time for the processing of information ... signal topic change through the use of Total Communication'.

Worrall and Yiu (2000) describe the effects of a structured approach to involving volunteers in carrying out a functional communication programme with aphasic adults in their own homes. The programme was called 'Speaking Out' and comprised ten scripted modules covering themes such as: 'What is aphasia? Communication breakdown, Communication repair, Starting a conversation, Managing finances, Using the telephone, Leisure – going out, Leisure – at home, Daily planning, Surprises and gift giving' (p. 918).

The lived experience was central to the training scheme. Each of the identified themes (listed above) was introduced to the partnership by use of a trigger. This usually took the form of a casual observation made by the volunteer that was related to the theme. Exploration of its relevance to the aphasic person's lifestyle then followed. Relevant information was then accessed and suitable strategies identified to inform an action plan that could be executed.

Promoting appropriate interaction patterns
Basil and Soro-Camats in von Tetzchner and Jensen (1996) recount the intervention carried out with a school-aged girl with multiple impairments. Although the intervention concentrated largely on key partnerships in the child's life, creating an appropriate language environment was integral to its success. The two main contexts of the child's life were the home and the school. Intervening with the environment involved video-recording interaction patterns in both contexts, supported by a series of intervention sessions in both settings, plus some joint meetings. Strategic advice was given and there was the opportunity for problem-solving. The enhancement of the child's main learning and social environments supported her communication skills development.

Environmental support

Environmental support is a term that is used to describe the establishment of external cues to help deficiencies in the memory of older adults

(Craik, 1986, cited by Charness and Holley, 2001). For example, an album of family photographs and written labels may prompt an individual to talk about particular family members.

Communication access

The development of accessible information is essential to the inclusive communication environment. People with communication disabilities represent a large constituency of service users who are frequently excluded and marginalized in the planning and provision of health, educational and social services. Problems with literacy skills, difficulties with understanding and use of language, and associated sensory and motor impairments compound the difficulties experienced by individuals on a daily basis.

The Communication Access Resource Centre (Communication-ARC) is located in the Compass Centre for Clinical Education and Therapy at City University London. It is an initiative set up to explore and develop accessible ways of presenting information. The Communication-ARC undertakes a range of information projects, including:

- health promotion materials, e.g. leaflets, posters;
- information leaflets and operational procedures, e.g. residential or day service booklet, complaints procedures, clinical audit;
- resources for therapy activities, e.g. group newspaper, organization of outings and projects;
- record keeping, e.g. minutes of person-centred planning meetings;
- participation in assessment and intervention procedures, e.g. self-assessment formats, intervention plans.

A three-stage methodology is carried out:

1) *Communication in focus*: In the first instance, an assessment of communication access need is carried out. This involves assessing the communication environment and the materials already in use and identifying any barriers to communication access.

2) *Communication by design*: The second phase deals with the specific development of materials to address the communication access problem. Consideration is given to the language, symbolic reference, organization and display. Relevant environmental images, e.g. relevant photographs, are collated as required. Accompanying guidelines on how to use these materials in context are also drafted at this stage.

3) *Communication in context*: This involves piloting the access material with service users and their carers, with training support in their use. Trials are carried out with a range of service users, which are videoed for evaluation purposes. Based on the results and the feedback solicited from service users and staff, the access materials are modified for further piloting until they are considered truly 'accessible'.

Improving communication access to information about a respite care facility

A respite and emergency care facility for adults with learning disabilities requested the development of an accessible leaflet about its service for potential users. The facility had recently achieved a charter mark and was committed to improving the quality of its service.

Communication in focus – An information leaflet was already in use, aimed at carers and social workers. Some staff were trained in specific communication approaches, e.g. Makaton, etc. Examination of the communication environment showed the use of photographs and symbols to convey meaning, e.g. noticeboards displaying activity options, daily menu, etc. Detailed analysis of the content of the carer's leaflet revealed a heavy reliance on text and the use of complex sentence structures. Service users found the leaflet difficult to manipulate and follow. The design was in concertina style with organization of information in columns left to right on both sides. Interview of service users and staff indicated a need to alter the perspective of the leaflet from 'carer's respite' to 'service user's holiday'.

Communication by design – A new version of the leaflet was designed using a service user perspective. Concrete vocabulary was used and sentence structures were characterized by brevity, repetition and rhythm. Text was kept at a minimum with digital imagery and line drawings featuring heavily. A colour-matching index was used in an A4 booklet design. Guidelines for significant others helping clients to use the leaflet were produced.

Communication in context – Several pilot trials of the new materials were carried out with service users. The materials were also offered to the staff team and residents' committee for scrutiny. The accessible leaflet was printed for distribution to the borough's learning disability services. Evaluation of the leaflet revealed:

• improved ability to use the materials;
• increase in language concepts generated, with increased reference to own experience;
• evidence of social exchange with carer(s)/peers, e.g. turn-taking, alternating eye gaze, etc.;
• evidence of multi-functional use of access materials, e.g. accessing service, preparing for stay at respite home, making choices during stay, recalling aspects of stay afterwards.

Perhaps the most noteworthy piece of evidence is the manager's report on the first client to initiate respite care for herself. Ellen was a young woman with Down's syndrome who had previously resisted the idea of a respite stay. Upon looking at the new leaflet that had been strategically placed in the reception area of her day centre, she marched into the manager's office and demanded that he arrange for her to stay at the place. This set the ball rolling, which led ultimately to Ellen having her 'holiday'. She is now a regular visitor at the facility and her family is also happy with the arrangement.

Communication resources

The social environment can be rendered more accessible by the open availability of communication prostheses that will diminish the effects of the communication impairment and support individual participation. Observation of a conversation group taking place at the London Centre of Connect revealed the presence of a number of resources that the clients were able to access quite spontaneously, as supports for their contributions to the conversation, e.g. maps to help recount the location of a recent holiday, paper and pencil for writing or drawing, and up-to-date magazines for discussion of current affairs.

Communication passports are used with a number of different client groups as a means of facilitating interaction between communication-disabled people and those with whom they come into contact. Passports are 'a positive way of supporting people with sensory and communication disabilities who cannot speak for themselves by collecting together important information about them and making this accessible to others with whom they may interact' (Millar and Caldwell, 1997: 1).

The idea for presenting information about an individual's communication was conceived by the CALL Centre (Communication Aids for Language and Learning) at Edinburgh University in 1992. Millar and Caldwell (1997) comment that the process of making a passport in itself helps to raise awareness of communication issues amongst significant others. Various local initiatives have been reported recently in services for people with learning disabilities (Brown, 2002; Lord, 2002). Lord (2002) describes an SLT project to set up communication passports for people with a learning disability. A communication passport is defined as 'a written, videoed or object-based record of how a person communicates and some of the things they might like to communicate about' (Parkside SLT Service, cited by Lord, 2002). The governing aim of the work was to promote social interaction between client and significant others by providing basic information to get a conversation started. Initial work was conducted collaboratively with care staff who were instrumental in collating images and information for individual passports. This was accompanied by a training package to promote successful use of the communication passports and to enskill staff in creating them. Lord (2002) comments that the passports provided a means for staff to discover more about client's communication skills.

A related idea is that of memory wallets for people with Alzheimer's type dementia (Bourgeois, 1992). Bourgeois describes these as scrapbooks that contain autobiographical information in the form of photographs and text, which function in much the same way as the passport idea. The idea is to establish a shared core knowledge that both individual and carer can access to promote interaction and relationship building.

Measuring effectiveness

How to measure change and prove the effectiveness of ecologically centred interventions is a challenging proposition. The philosophical and organizational features of the focal environment will affect the way evaluation is carried out, e.g. SLT intervention carried out in an educational establishment. McCartney and van der Gaag (1996) stress the importance of recognizing key differences between healthcare and educational contexts because 'they have a strong influence on how the relative effectiveness of practice is perceived' (p. 317).

Different perspectives
Judging the outcomes of an intervention must be seen from a number of different perspectives, e.g. the views of people with communication difficulties, significant others, non-participant observations, etc. Measures should attempt to look at changes in the social environment and the corresponding effects on individuals. Penn (1998) recommends a multidimensional approach for judging the effectiveness of SCA. Pound et al. (2000) recommend the use of qualitative methodologies alongside more traditional quantitative methods. In particular, they stress the importance of 'listening to service users rather than using therapist-determined perceptions of what these issues might be' (p. 257).

Auditing training
Evaluating interventions that are aimed at the communication environment is a complex business. There is a need to derive indices for many components that make up the social environment:

- the social ease experienced by participants;
- the quantity and quality of interaction opportunities that are made available and experienced;
- the availability and promptness of social contingencies within the natural environment;
- the knowledge and understanding of participants about relevant communication themes;
- the ability of participants to problem-solve and to select appropriate strategies;
- the engagement levels of individuals;
- the perception and judgement of those who use the environment and therefore have a vested interest in it.

Despite the prominence of staff training in learning disability services and the increase in commercially available training packages over the past two decades, there has been little published about the positive outcomes (Daniels and Sandow, 1987). Where attempts have been made to evaluate the effectiveness of a training programme, the focus has been on the knowledge and skills of the trained significant others (McCleod, Houston and Seyfort, 1995; MacMillan, Bunning and Pring, 2000) and underlying attitudes (Bryan et al., 2002) rather than actual benefits to users of the environment.

Environment as centre of influence

Interventions that centre on the communication environment are concerned with the social infrastructure that affects the individual's everyday functioning. A setting cannot provide support for people with communication disabilities if it is devoid of skilled communication partners, is insensitive to the needs of individuals, lacks contingent stimulation and contains inaccessible communication opportunities. In order to avoid the negative consequences of a poor environment and to address multiple needs within a defined setting, e.g. in a nursing home or a day centre, interventions seek to bring about change for individuals. This is done by reordering the environment in respect of the underlying values, the attitudes and behaviours of the people in supportive roles, the opportunities and resources available to individuals, and addressing any barriers that compromise participation.

Chapter 9
A place in society through advocacy

This chapter is concerned with the ways in which people who have communication disabilities find a place in society. Consideration moves from more immediate communication needs to citizenship and the human rights agenda. Two streams of activity support this: legislation and social policy to promote integration and to underwrite human entitlements; and advocacy as a process of empowerment, autonomy and inclusion (Atkinson, 1999). The two are not separate: the pursuit of choice and self-determination through advocacy is closely linked to the power base of society.

Legislation and social policy to promote rights

Legislation is one way in which the rights of vulnerable individuals may be defended and upheld. It can be seen as a mechanism for engineering the passage of change (Dalrymple and Burke, 1995); however, a political framework of rights and entitlements needs to move beyond simple rhetoric. It is dependent on consistent funding, the adequacy and accessibility of resources and a real commitment to hear what is being said. Young and Quibell (2000) point out that individuals will be placed at a disadvantage, regardless of legislation, if required to communicate with professionals and significant others using conventional linguistic code that they do not understand. In short, without the necessary modifications and resources in the communication environment, the individual will experience social exclusion.

Right to education

All people share the right to receive an education. There is the opportunity to acquire knowledge and develop skills in an environment shared by children from diverse backgrounds and with differing educational needs. Norwich (1996) offers a descriptive framework for 'educational needs':

- Individual needs arise from characteristics that are different from all others.

- Exceptional needs arise from characteristics shared by some individuals, e.g. visual impairment, musical ability.
- Common needs arise from characteristics that are shared by all, e.g. emotional need.

As Norwich states, 'Two children may share a special need but may have different individual needs, and their special need does not define fully their individual needs ... A child's special needs does not preclude common needs which are shared with other children' (p. 103).

Code of practice

The main intention of the Code of Practice (DfEE, 1994) was to support pupils with special educational needs and to ensure their fair treatment by schools and local education authorities (LEAs). A child is defined as having special educational needs if he or she has a learning difficulty, which needs special teaching. The Code of Practice places a duty on schools to plan strategically so that the needs of the individual child are seen as a priority (Gascoigne in Kersner and Wright, 2001; Lingard, 2001). The revised Code of Practice (DfEE, 2001) provides a simplification of the process whereby the school-based stages are reduced from three stages to two: school support and school support plus, respectively. The involvement of the child and their parents is encouraged and therefore advocacy in education takes on new importance.

Life in the community

Community care legislation over the past couple of decades has meant increasing control for service users. People are more actively involved in the planning of their own services and in appraising lifestyle choices.

NHS and Community Care (Caring for People) Act (DoH, 1990)

The aim of the new system of community care, introduced by the NHS and Community Care Act, was to enable people 'to live as independently as possible in their own homes or in 'homely' settings in the community'. It was about maximizing the achievement of full potential by providing the right amount of care and support (DoH, 1989). A duty was placed on social services to carry out an assessment of need so that individual packages of care could be developed; however, poor accessibility of care plans restricted the degree to which service users could be actively involved in the process. Barriers included the complexity of language used in the care plan, and the imprecise methods that were employed to involve individuals.

Community Care (Direct Payments) Act (DoH, 1996)

This act introduced statutory intervention into the care relationship. It potentially established a foundation for further rights-based developments in community care. The aim was to pay cash to people with disabilities rather than provide them with services, so that they could have some control over the purchase of resources. Holman with Bewley (1999) observe that greater personal choice and control over the services individuals would otherwise receive from the local authority leads to a superior quality of service; however, uptake and assertion of this right presupposes that individuals are already equipped to make such choices The reality is that for many people with disabilities, particularly where there is a cognitive disability, taking control of lifestyle is a very great challenge indeed.

Right to health and social care

All people share the right of access to public health and social services although inequalities within the health and social care systems may be present.

The NHS Plan – creating a 21st-century health service (DoH, 2000); NHS Reform and Health Care Professions Act (DoH, 2002)

The public agenda of the NHS centres on the relationship between user and providers of healthcare. The reforms outlined by the government establish new roles and rights for people using the NHS, including patient representation at all levels. Concern over the inclusion of people with communication disabilities on the developing 'user involvement' agenda is timely (Byng, Cairns and Duchan, 2002; Law et al., 2002) Partnership practice demands an organization that is committed to user participation as demonstrated by the values that inform professional practice, the local policies that direct service developments, the methods and procedures that are employed, and the settings in which care is provided.

The National Service Framework for Older People (NSF) (DoH, 2001a)

The National Service Framework for Older People is concerned with the quality of relevant health and social services. It seeks to preserve the dignity of individuals in the latter stages of life, whilst also promoting service accessibility. Communication issues are integral to the person-centred agenda.

Equal treatment and opportunities

There have been a number of pieces of legislation that share the common theme of supporting the rights of individuals, and abolishing discriminatory practice.

Disability Discrimination Act (DDA: DfEE, 1995)

Passed in 1995, the DDA sought to introduce new measures aimed at ending the discrimination that many people with disabilities face. The Act concerned with access and opportunities for people with disabilities specifically in the areas of employment, access to goods, services and facilities, sales and letting of property, transport and education. The legislation lays down a framework to encourage and hasten change in the prevailing culture; however, a change in attitudes cannot be forced. Casserley in Cooper (2000) cites a number of cases where discriminatory practice-led to tribunal.

Initially, a major flaw in the DDA was the lack of an enforcement body (Casserley in Cooper, 2000). The Disability Rights Task Force was formed by the government in December 1997 to consider the best ways of securing 'enforceable civil rights for disabled people within the context of our wider society and to make recommendations on the role and functions of a disability rights commission' (Disability Rights Task Force: December, 1999). In April 2000 the Disability Rights Commission was formally established to provide an effective mechanism to oversee and enforce the rights of people with disabilities.

Special Educational Needs and Disability Act (DfES, 2001)

The passing of this Act brought education within the scope of the DDA. New responsibilities have been allocated to local authorities to ensure that students with disabilities are not placed at any 'substantial disadvantage' in relation to their non-disabled peers. This means that institutions are required to take steps and make suitable adjustments to prevent any such disadvantage from arising, e.g. providing auxiliary aids and services such as a sign language interpreter.

Human Rights Act (DfEE, 1998)

The Human Rights Act (1998) came into force in October 2000. It allies itself to the European Convention of Human Rights, with which all public authorities and UK legislation must act compatibly. Where breaches occur, the Act provides the opportunity to make a legal challenge through the courts (Swain, French and Cameron, 2003).

Valuing people – a new strategy for learning disability for the 21st century (DoH, 2001b)

Collaboration between all agencies is considered germane to the achievement of social inclusion for people with learning disabilities. This white paper sets out the government's proposals for: 'improving the lives of people with learning disabilities and their families and carers, based on recognition of their rights as citizens, social inclusion in local communities, choice in their daily lives and real opportunities to be independent' (p. 10).

Encouragement is given to the establishment of a range of advocacy schemes on a local basis so that people can select the one that best meets their needs. Communication is central to its four major principles of independence, choice, civil rights and inclusion (Jones, 2001). There is an expectation on local service providers to develop workable communication policies, particularly in relation to person-centred planning (DoH, 2001b). This means the development of practical strategies to optimize inclusion and participation (Brown, 2002).

Contributions of legislation

What are the contributions of legislation to the wellbeing of people with disabilities? It has the potential for bringing more cohesion to social policy on disability (Waddington, 2000). The provision of a national framework influences the development of local initiatives that share a common goal, thereby minimizing inequalities across the country.

Tensions may exist between the legal and public arenas of equal opportunities. The government's proposals for 'Reform of the Mental Health Act 1983' (DoH, 1999) is one such example. There appeared to be a greater concern for public safety compared to the rights of individuals concerning the issue of compulsory treatment in the community.

It is impossible to legislate for a change in the attitudes of people in society. Furthermore, the law's impact will be constrained by the structural inequalities that exist within society. If people who have disabilities are always placed at a socio-economic disadvantage to their non-disabled peers, the concept of 'equal treatment' becomes unworkable. Ramcharan et al. (1997: 247) contend that 'where equality of opportunity ends, the right to entitlement to resources must begin'.

The right to be included

The right to be included at every level in society is shared by all human beings regardless of individual characteristics. Ramcharan et al. (1997: 253) state that

> Oppression, inequality and exclusion are not inborn characteristics of individuals, nor predetermined experiences, nor a function of individual impairment. They are socially produced phenomena to which socially contrived solutions can be applied.

Status and identification are important factors in accessing the public world (Beckett and Wrighton, 2000). Who we are, our perceived value to others and how we are identified at every level of society affect the quality of our lives. Gray and Jackson (2002: 7) comment on society's tendency to devalue people from marginalized groups and to neglect their 'right to a voice'. The presence of difference, such as experiencing difficulty with everyday communication, makes it difficult for some individuals to find a place in a society that caters for the majority.

'Border-crossing' is a term used by Ramcharan et al. (1997). It is used to refer to the idea of people breaking out of the roles and contexts that have been traditionally determined for them by society, and moving into mainstream society. In short, it is about fighting for the right to be included.

No society can enjoy full development without proper inclusion of all its members. The contribution of disabled people through their achievements, talents and experience is of immeasurable benefit to us all. (Disability Rights Task Force, 1999: 11)

Influencing the actions of others

Communication is the means whereby the needs, hopes and aspirations of individuals are conveyed to others. The experience of interacting with others influences self-esteem (Harter, 1999). The way in which others respond to the individual, and the feedback that is received, both positive and negative, contribute to a perception of self. Additionally, the ability to influence the actions of others, no matter how menial, is crucial to the development of self-worth. Scott and Larcher in Gray and Jackson (2002: 171) state that 'Having a communication difficulty is likely to mean that the person has even fewer opportunities to voice their opinions, to make choices and to be assertive than a person with similar cognitive abilities but without this additional problem.'

People who experience difficulty in communicating are at risk of not being heard by those in positions of power, for many reasons, including:

- compromised or limited communication skills that make influencing others effortful and difficult;
- being placed within a 'carer–being cared for' relationship that nurtures dependence and compromises individual autonomy;
- personal reluctance to challenge those in a position of power because of a fear of failure;
- a lack of confidence in own abilities, which restricts the placement of value on individual wishes and options;
- the individual experience of communication difficulties leading to various emotional reactions in order to protect or sustain self, such as exhibiting extreme passivity and apathy, appearing defensive or aggressive to others, etc.

A question of control

Autonomy in everyday life is about 'exerting influence and having control' (Barron, 2001: 431). Barron explains that having an impairment frequently means being dependent on the assistance of others on a daily basis. An individual's autonomy is expressed variously according to the context, the roles of others and the nature of existing relationships. For example, 'Parental control over their disabled children's decision-making serves as an obstacle to autonomy for the latter' (Barron, 2001: 441).

Sometimes it is difficult for people to realize their basic entitlements as human beings because of the barriers that exist in society (Ramcharan et al., 1997). Environmental and societal factors inhibit the individual right to voice ideas, viewpoints, concerns and desires and to challenge the ideas, judgements and decisions of others. For example, Garner and Sandow (1995) observe that there is limited opportunity for children to assert their views within educational law.

Impaired self-esteem

Children and adults with language difficulties are thought to be at greater risk of low self-esteem (Lindsay et al., 2002; Scott and Larcher in Gray and Jackson, 2002). The communicative struggles experienced by some may cause others to make negative judgements about the rest of their abilities. Such feedback from others is likely to affect the individual's self-perception (Scott and Larcher in Gray and Jackson, 2002).

> Also, a (child) [person] with language difficulties is likely to have more difficulty in social interactions, resulting in reduced ability to engage in those which either demonstrate competences per se, or allow negotiation of perceptions. (Lindsay et al., 2002: 128)

Harris-Cooksley and Catt in Garner and Sandow (1995) recount the experiences of children with special needs in mainstream education. Based on an interview with the class teacher and field observation notes, they found that the two pupils with statements of educational need in the class experienced difficulty in making friends. The teacher attributed this to their frequently disruptive behaviour in lessons and a lack of social skills.

Advocacy vs. communicating

The advocacy process is distinct from communication because of the different roles assumed by individuals. The role of the advocate is quite distinct from the role of the communication partner. The relationship between client and communication partner is based on familiarity and mutual appraisal of each other's contributions, so there is equal access to conversational floor. It denotes a certain reliance on the communication partner's ability to adapt to the individual's way of communicating. An empowering communication style used by significant others may be described as a type of interpersonal advocacy, whereby the individual has a 'voice' in everyday interactions. Advocacy, on the other hand, 'because of the potential conflicts between needs, wants and rights, and the inevitable presence of challenge, may be a less comfortable and "natural" human relationship' (Gray and Jackson, 2002: 9).

What is advocacy?

Goodley (2000: 3) views advocacy, in particular self-advocacy, as a 'counter movement to state paternalism', designed to oppose openly discriminatory practice. Goble (2002) argues that it is a political activity rather than a therapeutic one. He makes a distinction between *advocacy* with a small 'a' and *Advocacy* with a capital 'A'. The former is 'conducted within the limits and constraints of service systems' (p. 73). It forms part of the role of professionals who provide services. Advocacy with a capital 'A' is 'social and political, rather than systemic in nature' (p. 73). Regardless of scope and effect, both are concerned with opening the channels of communication so that individuals who are at risk of *not* being heard, *are* heard. There is the creation of opportunities for challenging the status quo and the active support of a cause or a course of action that helps to promote the self-worth of individuals (Mosely, 1994).

> 'Advocacy is the representation of the views, feelings and interests of one person or group of people by another individual or organisation' (Garner and Sandow, 1995: 1).

Types of advocacy

The attainment of human, civil and legal rights is at the heart of the advocacy process (Miller and Keys, 1996). Two types of advocacy are commonly identified: self-advocacy and citizen advocacy. The former has strong links to the disability movement and the social model of disability; the latter finds resonance in normalization theory, later termed social role valorization (SRV) (Walmsley, 2002). Another formulation of advocacy is to be found in the National Health Service (NHS) Plan (DoH, 2001c; d), termed the Patient Advocacy and Liaison Service (PALS).

Advocacy characteristics

Regardless of the type of advocacy employed, i.e. citizen advocacy or self-advocacy, there are basic principles and values upon which it is founded (Clement in Gray and Jackson, 2002). Kendrick in Gray and Jackson (2002: 40–48) views integrity as a prized characteristic of all types of advocacy. A lack of integrity would mean a process where the needs of individuals were vulnerable and likely to be misconstrued or ignored at the expense of the advocate's personal agenda. Adapted from Kendrick, there are a number of principles that underpin the advocacy process:

- *An intrinsic understanding of human worth* means that individuals should know how people can be expected to be treated. This is critical if practices are to be challenged and views defended.
- *The will and ability to face aspects of poor practice* require individuals to search beneath the surface of people in the community and service organizations. Coupled with this is the quest for truth. Care is taken to avoid exaggerating or distorting the facts of a matter.
- *Perseverance* is an important quality in the advocacy process. The battle is not easily won when challenges are made to existing practice or societal ways. Determination and staying power are needed in situations that demand problem-solving steps over time.
- *Reconciliation, restitution and improvement* are the projected out-

comes of advocacy. Each is dependent on a negotiated process of resolution. Although some types of conflict are unavoidable, 'doing battle' is not an integral part of the process.

- *Accountability* is about maintaining the best interests of those the advocate claims to represent. It means the honest construction of the agenda to be addressed so that personal influences are inhibited. Part of accountability is understanding the difference between the role of advocate and the people being represented. As Kendrick in Gray and Jackson (2002: 44) states:

> It is almost inevitable that advocacy groups or individual advocates will find themselves in situations where the interests of other parties than those being advocated for come into conflict with those being advocated for.

Baillie, Strachan and Gordon in Gray and Jackson (2002: 100) add a further characteristic that is considered crucial to the execution of the independent advocate's duties, particularly when dealing with professionals who are unclear about the legal basis for the decisions they have made regarding the client: 'a working knowledge of the key areas of law which may affect the particular client group'.

Citizen advocacy

Citizen advocacy refers to the representation of people at risk of devaluation, by those who are not. Thus non-disabled people practise the principles of advocacy by placing their 'skills, networks and prowess at the disposal of a devalued person' (Walmsley in Gray and Jackson, 2002: 33). In this way, attempts are made to influence the prevailing attitudes in society. Citizen advocacy is needed because of inadequacies in service organizations (Clement in Gray and Jackson, 2002). It is about establishing 'the links between the devalued person and the community through long-term relationships based on mutual choice and personal commitment' (Dowson in Ramcharan et al., 1997: 112).

Independent advocate

For unbiased representation of users' views, an advocate recruited from outside the host organization is required (Garner and Sandow, 1995). The independent advocate should have no formal or familial connections with the person(s) being represented. This determines the necessary impartiality so that actions are only influenced by the person. Clement in Gray and Jackson (2002) argues that the values base of the citizen advocate is critical to the ability to truly represent another. There should be an underlying belief in the advocacy process and the rights of all human beings.

Building a partnership

The building of a partnership between citizen advocate and service user is at the heart of the advocacy process. It involves the careful inspection of environmental factors and past experiences of the person concerned.

Only with knowledge of the individual, and familiarity with their lifestyle, is the advocate equipped not only to act as friend to the individual concerned, but also to represent their interests vigorously and to defend or exercise their rights.

Self-advocacy

Self-advocacy is about people who are marginalized in society giving voice to their own needs, as opposed to being represented by others. It refers to both the individual and group process. Solidarity is brought about by similar experiences and therefore people come together because of a shared interest (Walmsley in Gray and Jackson, 2002). There is the notion of 'revolt against disablement in a variety of ways, in a number of contexts' (Goodley, 2000: 3). Walmsley and Downer in Ramcharan et al. (1997: 36) state that 'Self-advocacy is about establishing an identity for yourself.' Walmsley in Gray and Jackson (2002) argues that locating self-advocacy within the disabled person's movement is useful because of its social model of disability, which 'opens the way for a defiant reassertion of pride in the disabled body or mind' (p. 31).

Promoting self-advocacy

The individual's ability to advocate for him/herself within a service will depend on a complex interaction of a number of factors (adapted from Gersch and Gersch in Garner and Sandow, 1995):

Service ethos and values base: The ethos of the service and the values that underpin it provide the setting conditions for self-advocacy (Byng, Cairns and Duchan, 2002). This includes the attitudes of the people who are in positions of influence and power, e.g. professionals and significant others (Ramcharan et al., 1997).

Operational policy: Mosely (1994) recommends that services develop a suitable operational policy that looks at service accessibility, amenability and responsiveness to the ideas expressed individually, collectively or by advocate representation. This should include avoiding disempowering practice that does not take into consideration the self-esteem of other colleagues and the service users.

The means of representation: The means for self-expression is crucial to the advocacy process, and this is tied intrinsically to the significant others in the person's life. Material resources and communication partner support must be available to the individual so that representation happens in whatever forum it needs to happen. Advocates who support and represent people with communication difficulties in the advocacy process need to develop expertise in the use of augmentative communication strategies and to access specialist help as appropriate (Scott and Larcher in Gray and Jackson, 2002).

Access to information: Having access to information is an important part of service operation (Grant in Ramcharan et al., 1997). For individuals with communication disabilities, this means presenting the relevant facts in an accessible format with support as needed and adequate time available for processing. Self-evaluation is very important, such that ongoing practice is monitored and positive action maintained.

The right of redress: People need to understand why a complaints procedure may be of interest to them, and supported to access and use it.

Individual characteristics: The life experience, skills and abilities of individuals will affect their contributions to the advocacy process. Having the ability to use the information provided, being able to process the relevant content, to express viewpoints and to exercise choices some way or other is crucial to the empowerment process (Grant in Ramcharan et al., 1997).

Characteristics of peers: The attitudes and behaviour of peers with whom particular experiences are shared may influence the individual. Identifying with another encourages reflection on the position occupied by oneself.

Real opportunities: The opportunities that occur on a daily basis to challenge the status quo and to assert individual rights are critical to the development of self-advocacy skills, expressing choices, making decisions and asserting self.

Learning in a multi-agency framework: Advocacy does not fall under the auspices of any one profession. It involves a process that crosses professional boundaries and may include the expertise of more than one agency according to the needs of the individual.

User empowerment

Although not advocacy, user empowerment is concerned with providing the opportunity for individuals to influence services in a variety of ways. User empowerment is frequently used in conjunction with user consultation. It is a recurring theme in public health and social services where there is a commitment to professionals handing over power to the service users (DoH, 2001c; d). It requires that the service provider recognize that users lack power (Garner and Sandow, 1995). Addressing the power base in service provision is based on two main principles:

1) The quality of services is dependent on their relevance and sensitivity to the needs and preferences of those who use them.
2) Achievement of this ideal requires service user participation in decisions affecting the design, management and review of services (Grant in Ramcharan et al., 1997).

'Empowerment' or 'taking power'?

Dowson in Ramcharan et al. (1997) makes a distinction between *empowerment* and *taking power*. *Empowerment* denotes the imbuement of power, casting the service user in the role of passive recipient and the professional as active delegator of power. Conditions may be attached to the act of empowerment and there is nothing to say that this 'power' can't be taken back again! *Taking power* captures the notion of 'action by the disempowered on their own initiative to wrest power from the powerful' (p. 105). This latter definition is more indicative of a process whereby individual agendas surface and are impressed on those who need to hear.

Consultation process

The process of consultation should provide opportunities for tackling the marginalization risk to those individuals who are disadvantaged in some way. It should also aim to ensure that the expertise of all the main players is utilized in the pursuit of a shared goal, i.e. good quality services. Grant in Ramcharan et al. (1997: 122) writes that 'Being based on the strengthening of interpersonal ties and natural networks, consultation allows change to be pressed for over time, and is a realistic option which can link "what is" with "what should be".'

Influencing an organization is a complex process, which involves appraising the options, determining the issues, dealing with searching questions, and problem-solving, such as 'What would help people like yourself in this situation?' Grant in Ramcharan et al. (1997: 129) identifies the gaps in the user consultation process: 'There is an urgent need therefore to consolidate knowledge and understanding of techniques and technologies for helping people to express their needs and views.'

Barriers to the exercise of control

Power is a relative concept that varies according to the lifestyle and circumstances of the individual. The kinds of power offered to and used by a person, e.g. voting rights, earning power, personal and social independence, may not be relevant to the individual's lifestyle (Garner and Sandow, 1995).

Stalker in Clark (2001: 50) questions how far people can realize their ambitions within 'the care, welfare and protection model'. The issue of unequal status may hamper the advocacy process. Generally, the staff employed within services occupy a higher status than those who use their services (Dowson in Ramcharan et al., 1997). Furthermore, there may be a conflict between service user and service provider agendas. The personal views, experiences and judgements of those recruited to represent those who are unable to speak up for themselves may interfere with an honest and relevant advocacy process. Goble (2002) provides an example of the staff member who holds strong religious views that provoke a negative judgement on the sexual orientation and behaviour of the service user.

Griffiths (1994) comments that there are some complex issues to deal with when working with the parents of children with disabilities. The process of coming to terms with the growing independence of a child may challenge some parents. There may be a heightened awareness of associated risks. Parents may fear handing over power and control or be ill-prepared to confront risk-taking. It may be difficult to perceive the changing status of the child growing into adulthood and to accept the need for individual privacy and confidentiality.

Tensions between the development of behavioural approaches with children and adults with learning disabilities may appear to be at odds with the process of self-advocacy, which demands a more facilitatory style (Garner and Sandow, 1995). This is overcome to a certain extent by involving the person in the setting of individual goals and the selection of reinforcement; however, as Garner and Sandow (1995: 26) suggest, the decision of whether to manipulate the overt behaviour of the individual by use of reinforcement schedules requires the practitioner to decide 'if the end justifies the means'. In short, does the introduction of rules for inhibiting problem behaviour and promoting desirable behaviour present an ethical compromise to the individual's right to self-expression? This question serves to remind the professional of the human right to self-determination when making some difficult clinical decisions.

Process of advocacy

Mosely (1994) describes a process whereby the individual is able to convey important messages so that positive changes to life are effected. Ludlow and Herr in Ludlow, Turnbull and Luckasson (1988) proposed a conceptual framework for advocacy work that encompasses three main response themes:

1) Preparation of the individual and provision of appropriate opportunities for individuals to represent their own interests.
2) Efforts made by major stakeholders in relation to the needs of the individual, such that their rights are protected and their views asserted.
3) Organized efforts in the pursuit of influencing society and the makers of policies.

Miller and Keys (1996) recognize the empowerment potential of all human beings, because empowerment and advocacy refer to the *process* and not to an arbitrary set of standards representing the outcome. It therefore follows that empowerment be construed flexibly and in relation to the skills and abilities of the individual with a communication disability. The process is about the development of self-knowledge and the acquisition of certain skills to do with self-efficacy, awareness and influence (Mosely, 1994).

Setting conditions

Choice-making by people with disabilities demands the setting of conditions that are conducive to the individual's exercise of autonomy (Twine, 1994). This cannot be legislated for and in order to achieve empowerment of the person, certain antecedent conditions must be in place. Ramcharan, McGrath and Grant in Ramcharan et al. (1997: 55) identify the 'ability to conceptualise choice and then pursue it' as critical to the process. This features as the foundation level in their *Basic model identifying needs* (original source: Ramcharan, 1995: 234). It is about individual recognition of wants, needs, rights and entitlement. The second level involves their articulation as well as identifying 'infringements of one's rights'. The third level focuses on having 'these articulations heard in an appropriate place'. The final level is 'To have your wants, needs or entitlements met, or to have redress for infringement to your rights.' Where an individual is unable to achieve these levels for one reason or another, representation by someone else is considered. That someone else is then placed in a position to speak and act on behalf of the individual. Ramcharan, McGrath and Grant in Ramcharan et al. (1997: 56) state that this is more a case of 'substitute decision-making than advocacy'.

The survival interests of the service agency may cause the active dampening of service users' self-expression and challenges, because of a desire to restrain any bad publicity (Goble, 2002, citing Brandon et al., 1995). There may be a conflict between professional interest and meeting the needs of individuals. Goble (2002: 74) refers to the 'widespread promotion and adoption of "normalisation" principles and ideals in the 1980s' in services for people with learning disabilities. He points out the pervasive influence on the way services were structured and delivered, without necessarily achieving the best deal for the people themselves. For instance, sometimes the notion of 'age appropriateness' was extended to communication regardless of the available skills and abilities of the individual (see Figure 7.1, Cycle of communication inflation and devaluation).

Advocacy approaches

The objective of any approach to advocacy is about consulting to involve or consulting to empower (Grant in Ramcharan et al., 1997). There are a number of different approaches that support the promotion of the individual's rights as a citizen. Working with people with communication disabilities demands original responses to obvious barriers to self-expression. As such, the approaches identified here do not represent an exhaustive list; rather they point the direction to some creative ways of addressing communication difficulties in the advocacy process.

Use of biography and narrative

Narrative inquiry is concerned with the lived experience. It involves accessing the person's story, sifting through the realities that are told and presenting them in a coherent way (Goodley, 2000). Life stories allow the reader to gain insights into the individual's life course and to sample the perspective of the narrator. Achievements and failures, joys and frustrations are revealed. The expertise of the person with a disability is realized through their role as 'story teller'.

Atkinson, Jackson and Walmsley (1997) recommend the use of personal narrative and biography in order to validate claims of marginalization. Atkinson (1998) identifies four functions served by the telling of life stories: bringing us into greater accord with ourselves, with others, with the mystery of life, and with the universe around us. The analysis of narrative accounts is said to strengthen stories (Goodley, 2000). Through historical accounts and lived experiences the personal agenda is connected with the broader political one. The user's agenda is impressed on those who provide services at many different levels (Pound, Parr and Duchan, 2001; Pound et al., 2000; Rees, 1991). If the experiences of the past are understood, the culture of the present and future may be influenced (Young and Quibell, 2000). Peters in Barton (1996: 224) puts forward a convincing argument for the power of life stories in combating potential obstacles to an inclusive society:

> If we teach [young] people with disabilities how to become border crossers at a personal level, the cultural symbols and metaphors prevalent in today's society will begin to disintegrate.

Life story research

Atkinson, Jackson and Walmsley (1997) highlight the contribution of life story research to development of identity. It provides a sense of history that is meaningful to the individual. The act of story telling is about 'bearing witness' to the past – 'to the social and political oppression of oneself and others' (Atkinson in Gray and Jackson, 2002: 131). The person performs the role of historian and ensures that the 'expert' view is heard. Personal histories become 'intertwined with the history of the self-advocacy movement' (Atkinson in Gray and Jackson, 2002: 122). The person whose individual story remains untold is vulnerable to the suggestions of others; however, the telling of a personal history from the perspective of the person who experienced it means that no external validation is needed. Citing Birren and Deutchman (1991), Atkinson in Gray and Jackson (2002) observes that 'Life story research treats people as "expert witnesses" in the matter of their own lives' (p. 122).

Life maps

Goodley (1996) acknowledges the many difficulties in undertaking life history research, particularly with individuals who find it difficult to recall and articulate their experiences. He recommends the construction of a life plan. Also called a life map (Gray and Ridden, 1999), it provides a visual representation of an individual's experiences across the life course, from birth to the present. Harris-Cooksley and Catt in Garner and Sandow (1995) used 'lifemaps' with statemented and unstatemented pupils in a mainstream class. The aim was to encourage pupils to build positive social relationships by providing opportunities to share information about themselves and to discover what they had in common. The process of life mapping is seen as a potentially liberating one (Gray and Ridden, 1999), where the individual has the opportunity not only to review the life course up to the present, but also to speculate on the future and even to make strategic moves based on an evaluation of the past.

Personal portfolios

Pound et al. (2000) describe the use of personal portfolios with people with aphasia at the London Centre of Connect. A portfolio contains information about the person's life that relates to the past, what is happening now, and any future goals, plans, hopes and aspirations. The format of the portfolio is entirely flexible and should correspond to the wishes and preferences of the author. They stress that portfolio work is crucial to the rebuilding of self-esteem and sense of identity. It also supports the decision-making process in therapy by revealing truths about the individual. The therapeutic value of portfolio work lies in 'the process of recalling, gathering, collating, selecting, explaining and representing autobiographical events and milestones' (p. 204).

The functions served by a portfolio are numerous (adapted from Pound et al., 2000):

- The personal portfolio provides the means for reflecting on *life course continuity*. Events and relationships occurring through the passage of time are identified and explored. Past experiences are reviewed in the same way as current ones. There is also the opportunity to look forward to and anticipate circumstances in the future.
- The collation of a personal portfolio in itself *asserts the realities* that are relevant and mean something to the author. It helps to build the person's sense of self and to establish self-knowledge. In a way, it presents the expertise that comes from the 'lived experience' in accessible format to share with others as desired.
- It provides the means for telling others about oneself and therefore helps to build *self-esteem* in the context of human relationships.

Role-play, discussion and committees of inquiry

Sweeney in Garner and Sandow (1995: 73) recommends that the best approach to advocacy and self-advocacy is through using a range of communication methods for exploring 'real-life challenges and opportunities'. He states that role-play and other related drama activities provide 'a powerful medium' for encouraging individuals 'to develop their inquiry skills and powers of communication'.

Two principles are considered to be crucial to the use of drama in advocacy and self-advocacy (Sweeney in Garner and Sandow, 1995): first, experimentation with non-verbal forms of communication so that individuals learn to 'voice' their innermost thoughts through physical activities; second, the trying out of other roles in situations helps to develop the individual's

> powers of self-expression by giving voice to the thoughts, feelings and experiences of others. In pretending to speak as another person, or as oneself in other circumstances, individuals can explore and experiment with approaches to self-expression and self-assertion. (Sweeney in Garner and Sandow, 1995: 69)

Out-of-role discussion happens in what Sweeney in Garner and Sandow (1995) refers to as 'forum theatre'. The audience and the people enacting roles have the opportunity to appraise the focal situation and to make changes as they see fit. One way is when the members of a role-play audience are able to pause the action flow to reflect on the thoughts and feelings triggered by what they have seen. There is encouragement and the opportunity to re-route the course of an interaction or to suggest alternative ways of dealing with the situation. Participants are able to experiment with new ways of asserting themselves and to evaluate the outcomes with personal risk kept at a minimum. Still images in picture books, posters, paintings, sculptures and toys can also be used to stimulate topic interest and discussion (Sweeney in Garner and Sandow 1995).

'Committees of inquiry' are sometimes formed. This is when individuals are encouraged to see different perspectives within the same story Alternatively the role-play itself may be used to present evidence from a number of angles. Subsequently, participants of the role-play are interviewed; opinions are challenged before making alterations to the course of a role-play. The process is akin to problem-solving by committee.

Advocacy groups

There are many different types of group where advocacy is either a central theme or is related to the main activity. It is sometimes useful to view the advocacy process as a multi-dimensional entity where the different types of advocacy-related activity are interconnected, e.g. social skills and assertiveness training, self-help, self-advocacy, personal portfolio, etc.

Self-help groups

The development of self-help groups is to be found across the range of client service groups, including: people with aphasia and their partner (Jordan and Kaiser, 1996; Pound et al., 2000); parents and children with special needs (Gibbs Levitz and Schwartz in Nadel and Rosenthal, 1995); carers of people with dementia living at home (Lévesque et al., 2002); people who stammer (Smith, 2002); and adults with learning disabilities (Winchurst, Stenfert Kroese and Adams, 1992). The groups have some variation in focus and in the membership criteria but generally the members share a core life experience. This is what unites the purpose of the group and sustains the 'self-help' momentum of meetings. There is the desire to take responsibility in the pursuit of meeting personal needs (Smith, 2002). Such a group provides individuals with the opportunity to 'enjoy the security of a group of people who also have endured the prejudices and unaccommodating practices of the non-disabled world' (Pound et al., 2000: 222).

Pound et al. (2000) describe some of the challenges that often feature in the running of self-help groups, such as tensions that may arise between different personality types, maintaining the equilibrium of the group and dealing with the domineering group member. They also provide a series of guiding questions to help the therapist to work out her or his relationship and responsibilities to the self-help group. The very nature of a *self-help* group means that the volition for change and movement in the group should emanate from the participants themselves and not be forced by someone else.

Self-advocacy groups

There are many different types of advocacy group or advocacy-related activities that have been written about in relation to the various client groups. Speech and language therapists may find themselves either directly involved with or otherwise associated with such initiatives. Harris (2001) outlines his experiences of a course called 'Self-advocacy for people who stammer' run at the City Literary Institute in London, where self-examination of communication difference and identity were encouraged. Openness of self-expression and assertiveness were key themes addressed by the course: 'The self-advocacy course gave me a valuable opportunity to question all the negative emotional baggage and to review my identity as a person who stammers' (p. 12).

Harding, Cheasman and Logan (2002) provide a more detailed account of the course aims and content. The current course advertised by the City Literary Institute in London is entitled: 'Be yourself – what it means to stammer'. It is a ten-week course of two hours a week. Participants are encouraged to explore identity issues through preparing a personal portfolio, using any media, e.g. essay, drawings, collage, poetry, photographs and even music.

Pound et al. (2000: 223) provide a chronological account of the development and progress of a self-advocacy group for people with aphasia. The group ran over a fixed period of ten weeks and set out to explore 'issues of confidence, lifestyle and speaking out'. *Living with disability* was central to group discussions and individual participants identified personal goals in relation to self-advocacy. The speech and language therapist assumed the role of co-facilitator in partnership with a person who brought teaching and group work skills to the group as well as their expertise of living with aphasia. The group facilitators assumed a non-directive approach and carried specific responsibility for recording group discussions. Evaluation of the group revealed an increase in self-esteem and participation in life, personally valued changes in communication skills and use of resources, and positive effects on social interaction and relationships with others, such as newly found assertion.

'People First' is a self-advocacy organization run by and for adults with learning disabilities that was founded in the UK in the 1970s. Since then many local groups have been set up, sharing some common goals and concerns, including:

• helping and supporting people to speak up for themselves;
• campaigning for improved rights;
• speaking up on policy issues;
• educating the general public on relevant matters;
• training and supporting advisers to self-advocates.

Change through the advocacy process
What is the mechanism for change in advocacy activities such as those discussed above? Pound et al. (2000) attribute a number of changes specifically to the group content and process, including the opportunities for review of one's life course through discussion, portfolio and biography work, making personal contributions to the debate on social issues and needs, and experiencing control of the group's agenda.

Citizen advocacy

For some individuals who are unable, for whatever reason, to represent themselves, citizen advocacy may be an option, although Hunter and Tyne (2001: 553) advise that it is not the *singular* solution to ensuring against the marginalization and devaluation of some individuals; rather, it offers 'one strategy for mitigating the vulnerability and dislocation in the social networks of some individuals'.

The idea behind citizen advocacy is to contribute an independent view of the individual quality of life and the service structures in support. It enables errors in service provision to be detected and opportunities for positive action to be identified; however, the process of citizen advocacy and the involvement of independent advocates is not without problems. Tensions may arise between the separate agendas of the independent agency and the service provider. Hunter and Tyne (2002) report on three citizen advocacy schemes. They reveal some of the many areas of struggle thought by advocates to constrain their efforts. These include conflicting staff loyalty, to client or to work colleagues and provider organization, and issues of power and control when authority is challenged by the outsider, i.e. the advocate.

Developing citizen advocacy

What constitutes an effective and fair citizen advocacy scheme? Hunter and Tyne (2000) resist efforts to regularize advocacy and to accredit such schemes under one bureaucratic umbrella, arguing that it does not suit the diverse and irregular nature of community. Furthermore, they state that professionalizing and standardizing independent schemes are directly opposed to the original sentiments of citizen advocacy, which are about open-ended relationships between advocates and service users, i.e. 'long-term, freely given, independent relationships which offer the possibility of belonging in a network of community connections' (p. 559).

An example of a citizen advocacy organization is Partners in Advocacy. It is an independent organization that provides both citizen advocacy and support for self-advocacy for children and adults with learning disabilities in Scotland. It originated from The Advocacy Service set up by Barnardo's in 1987, which became independent at a later date in order to avoid conflict of interests between the larger organization and the advocacy service. Partners in Advocacy is concerned with:

- safeguarding the interests of people with learning disabilities, and recognizing their talents;
- empowering such individuals so that they can influence decisions and assume control in their own lives;
- identifying and supporting the uptake of opportunities so that friendship networks are increased and social horizons broadened.

Safeguarding interests

Despite the long-term nature of citizen advocacy, it is commonly used in a crisis situation to safeguard the interests of individuals. This is when a third person is brought into a situation where an individual is deemed to be at risk of having their real needs and desires side-stepped by others in a position of greater power. In cases where the individual experiences difficulties in expressing their own needs and interests, the exercise of personal rights is at risk.

Porter et al. (2001) tell the story of one service user's involvement with an independent advocate. The story of 'Peter' illustrates some of the problems that arise when an advocate has to interpret the needs and wishes of the person who has severely restricted communication skills. Peter was a young man with severe learning disabilities and cerebral palsy. He communicated through eye gaze and had limited understanding of spoken language. He needed a gastrostomy because of recurrent chest infections due to aspiration. The speech and language therapist and keyworkers spent time discussing the operation with him, using photographs and video film to explore his difficulties with eating and drinking. It was the view of the professionals that the operation was in his best interests. A citizen advocate interviewed Peter for over an hour, with no witnesses, and produced a written transcript as a record of his views, stating that he did not want the operation.

Of course, Peter's story is fraught with problems, not least of which is how to separate out the professional view of what is in the individual's 'best interests' with what Peter truly wants. In this case, the role of the independent advocate is enormously important, both as a communication partner and a representative for the client. The story highlights the need for a process of openness and honesty so that the potential influence of personal agendas is minimized.

Interpersonal advocacy

Interpersonal advocacy refers to equal dispersion of communicative power within an interaction such that the views and judgements of the focal person, in this case the person who has communication disability, are revealed. Scott and Larcher in Gray and Jackson (2002) advise that the development of a relevant and equitable communication partnership does not happen overnight. The subtleties of an individual's communication style and the setting factors that are conducive to optimal communication may be far from obvious. In this way, citizen advocacy at crisis points in an individual's life is problematic for those who are unable to articulate their own interests and needs, as illustrated by the case of 'Peter' cited above.

'See what I mean' (SWIM: Grove et al., 2000)

The relevance of SWIM to the communication partnership is highlighted in Chapter 7. It is mentioned here also, due to its potential contribution to the advocacy process, particularly where the inference of meaning is complicated by the limited and sometimes unconventional ways that some individuals communicate. Although focused on the needs of people with profound and multiple learning disabilities, the guidelines produced by Grove et al. (2000) have something to offer the process of interpersonal advocacy across the client groups. As a starting point, SWIM views uncertainty and ambiguity as part of everyday communication and seeks to build on the intuitive skills that are in use naturally. It assumes that difficulties are inevitable when communicating with people who have speech and language impairments. Far from being glossed over, these difficulties should be made explicit. Guidelines are provided for the collection of observation-based evidence to support the decision-making process. In short, the person who is in a position to advocate for the client is encouraged to check out his or her own interpretation of an individual's communication behaviours. Individual perceptions of what the person might want and need are shared and compared with the perceptions of others. Evidence from the client's behaviour is gathered to support the different interpretations so that the most likely meaning may be identified.

Talking Mats

Another approach that lends itself to advocacy process is 'Talking Mats'. Murphy (1998) developed this low-tech communication resource so that people using some form of alternative communication system were able to express their internal judgements and feelings. Since its original conception it has been used with a number of different client groups: people with motor neurone disease (Murphy, 1999); people with aphasia (Murphy, 2000); and people with learning disabilities (Murphy and Cameron, 2002a). Murphy and Cameron (2002b: 8) describe Talking Mats as 'an interactive resource that uses three sets of picture symbols – topics, options and visual scale'.

Talking Mats uses a mat upon which the client places symbols. On the back of each picture symbol is the hook side of a piece of Velcro. The use of a video camera is recommended, to record the views expressed by the individual and to monitor the veracity of the process. A still photographic image provides a permanent record of each completed Talking Mat for feedback to the individual and their significant others.

Murphy and Cameron (2002b) observe that Talking Mats may support many different activities, including joint goal planning, planning communication passports (Millar, 1997), self-perception of intervention outcomes, developing relationships with others, and planning activities. They provide a number of examples of Mats that have been completed by individual service users. The views expressed range from a personal evaluation of activity preferences to feelings about different forms of transport and life-course aspirations, e.g. choice of occupation after leaving college, etc. Any one topic explored within Mats may be looked at in more detail. These are called *sub mats* (Murphy and Cameron, 2002b: 26).

Talking Mats provide a highly accessible and inexpensive resource for advocacy-related activity. Murphy and Cameron (2002b) give a direct quote from a participant in one of their courses: 'It increased equality between the two partners as it's predominately a visual language system which makes the more verbal partner throw away the security and reliance on their verbal skills' (Murphy and Cameron, 2002b: 19).

In short, it offers an approach to advocacy that has potential applications across the range of client groups. It provides a potential medium for supporting both clinical and life-course decision-making, particularly where there may be some dispute with regard to what constitutes 'the best interests' of the individual.

Finding a place in society

Finding a place in society is about developing awareness of human and civil rights. Advocacy, and the many different approaches and activities associated with it, provides a vehicle for some individuals. The ultimate goal of advocacy, the distance to which an individual is prepared to travel and the speed of journey will vary according to the needs, ambitions and scope of the individual and significant other(s). Not everyone who participates in self-advocacy wants to 'bang a drum' at those in power. For some it is about asserting self and challenging practices in the here and now of daily life; for others it is about influencing the policy-makers.

The process of advocacy is centred on equality of wellbeing, where participation and inclusion are key accomplishments. Advocacy is not simply about the independence of the person representing his or her own views and opinions; rather it involves many different types of collaborative relationship between the individual and others: between people who have experiences in common, between service provider and user, between marital partners, and between parent and child. Each relationship is concerned with self-expression and mutual regard such that the human worth of individuals who have disabilities is upheld.

Chapter 10
Integrated intervention

Any one cycle of intervention experienced by a person(s) is made up of numerous facets that represent critical points on a journey from one position to another. The type of journey experienced by an individual will be affected by person-centred factors, including personality and individual characteristics; state of health and wellbeing; age and relevant life-course stage; life-course characteristics and experiences; and type and severity of communication difficulty (Basso and Marangolo, 2000; Byng, 1995). External factors of influence are to be found at the various levels of partnership, environment and society.

A complicated journey!

To view intervention as a fixed route between two stations would be to oversimplify what is essentially a multi-faceted process. Horton and Byng's (2000) use of the descriptor 'organic' (referred to in Chapter 1) promotes the view of an ever-changing, mutating intervention cycle. Taking the analogy of a train journey, it is a voyage that negotiates multiple junction points and where sideways detours may be an essential part of reaching the final destination. Clinical decisions are made at each junction point: the journey thus far is reviewed with the options for moving ahead. Together the therapist and client navigate the intervention journey by weighing up all the relevant factors. It probably has a great deal in common with an expedition to the North Pole!

Journey characteristics

Each account, regardless of the centre of influence, the presenting needs of service users, the approach used and the specialism or service location of the SLT, features:

- An *integrated approach* to intervention: there are explicit connections between various aspects of the intervention.
- *Many turning points* in an intricate journey: clinical decisions define the way as relevant factors are considered carefully.
- *Strategic moves* along the assessment–therapy continuum: the relationship between assessment activities and therapy activities is not linear, and the former does not always precede the latter. Activities are

constructed that are variously weighted according to the presenting needs of the individual(s) and the corresponding decision-making.

- *Continuous negotiation* between therapist and service user(s): the construction and progression of the intervention cycle is the outcome of the contributions of all participants.

Intervention journeys

Some detailed accounts of intervention journeys with people from a variety of client groups are presented here. The stories have been told by different SLTs. Some therapists elected to write up their account; others told the story through conversation with the author. Each story has been drawn from the therapist's perspective and therefore it must be acknowledged that only one side of the story is represented. Nevertheless, each account demonstrates the uniqueness of the intervention journey, whilst also recognizing the common frameworks that are used to make clinical decisions.

Intervention journey 1: Peter, a man with acquired language impairment

Peter, a 25-year-old man, married with one young child, was referred to the rehabilitation centre after a cerebrovascular accident which occurred during neurosurgery after an open head injury, resulting in an acquired language disability. Up to the time of the referral Peter was living with his wife and child in a rural setting. Since the time he had left school at 16 Peter had been employed as a farm worker.

Background
Peter had suffered an open-head injury as a result of an accident at work. He had originally been referred to an inpatient rehabilitation facility, where he had had intensive therapies for movement and communication disabilities. He made a good recovery over the months, regaining his ability to walk, and becoming a fluent communicator, albeit with some residual word-finding and fluency difficulties.

After he was discharged home he went for further neurosurgery. During surgery he had a cerebrovascular accident, after which his communication became severely impaired. He was briefly re-admitted to the inpatient rehabilitation facility, but became very distressed at being kept in hospital. He was able to go home to the care of his wife after a few days. He was able to walk, but needed help in some self-care. He had developed either a visual field or visual perceptual impairment, and was severely aphasic.

Outpatient therapy
Peter agreed to come for outpatient therapy. It was soon clear that he did not need or would not be able to benefit from any physical or cognitive

therapies, i.e. physiotherapy or occupational therapy. He attended speech and language therapy.

It was agreed between Peter, his wife and the two therapists (Mark and Erica) at the outpatient rehabilitation facility that Peter would see one of the therapists, Erica, for direct language/communication-related therapy, and the other, Mark, for non-directive counselling.

Language/communication therapy

Erica and Mark worked in close conjunction with each other, although Erica carried out most of the language-related therapy in the initial stages. Peter came for language therapy once a week.

Conventional (formal) assessments yielded some initial information about Peter's language and communication abilities. The type of assessments used (Event Perception Test; Sentence Comprehension Test; PALPA) sought to reveal something about his ability to understand speech and language and to express himself verbally, as well as to reveal underlying semantic and event-processing abilities/disabilities. However, his visual perceptual difficulties made it difficult to use formal assessment materials very successfully. Peter was unable to read or use written language, and found it hard to make sense of pictures initially. He also seemed to have difficulties with motor–speech co-ordination, and was, apart from some occasional formulaic expressions (such as 'OK', 'right', 'bye'), generally non-verbal.

The conclusions Erica drew from informal assessment activities (e.g. picture category sorting; odd-one-out) were that Peter had underlying semantic, and very likely sentence processing, difficulties. They began work on improving word-finding (production) through various semantic judgement activities, the rationale being that improvements in Peter's lexical semantic ability would enable more precise access to the phonological word-form, and thus improve word production. They also worked specifically on verb semantics in an effort to target his limited ability to express thematic relationships.

Non-directive counselling

Mark and Peter also met once a week. Peter and his family felt that it would be better to keep work on language separate from the opportunity to 'talk about' his circumstances. Peter's mood shifted between anger and being very low. The purpose of Peter and Mark working together was to try and enable Peter to express his feelings in any way possible: non-verbally through gesture or use of visual analogues, or verbally with support from Mark – for example, using the occasional word or fragment of a word that Peter was able to express, in conjunction with what Mark knew about Peter and his family life. Peter was still angry about the cause of and the circumstances surrounding his original head injury, but the main focus of his anger was the hospital where his neurosurgery had been carried out. His anger continued for many months and eventually found expression in the commencement of legal proceedings against the hospital. This ultimately came to nothing.

Peter's low mood was strongly associated with his loss of language – not being able to 'chat', as he put it – but also about his loss of role, as a worker, and especially in the family. His wife had now taken on all the tasks he had previously had – from the family finances to all the driving and some of the farm work. She was offered support through the local speech and language therapy relatives group, but was not really able to attend given her extensive family commitments.

Peter and Mark continued to meet, and as Peter started to be able to express himself more precisely and extensively (although still in a very limited way, verbally) he could expand more on how he felt. Peter and his wife would occasionally meet Mark together.

Changes to the intervention

When Erica left to go to a new job, Mark continued to see Peter. Peter was apparently less keen to talk about how he felt, or to continue work on language and communication. He said he wanted a break from coming up to the hospital. Mark and he agreed to a break in therapy, and that Peter should make contact when he felt he wanted to return.

About four months later Peter's wife got in touch and said that Peter wanted to come back for more therapy. Mark met them and they discussed what the purpose of more therapy might be. Peter was clear that he wanted to be able to 'say more', i.e. work on language and communication. It was agreed that, having set clear goals and taken some baseline assessments, they would work on language and communication. Mark also proposed that they make a non-language-related assessment of how Peter felt about his communication and the impact of his communication disability, and, on the same parameters, how his wife felt too.

Mark and Peter devised a series of semantic differentials rated on a visual analogue scale; these covered areas such as: communication, 'how others see me', and 'how I feel about myself'. Peter was asked to place a cross on the line where he felt he 'stood' in relation to, for example, 'I find it easy to chat to strangers' (at one end) and 'I find it very hard to chat to strangers' (at the other). Mark and Peter used this as a baseline against which to measure the impact of therapy.

Moving on

One feature of therapy which Peter asked to change, and which was pivotal in his 'moving on', was that he no longer wanted to come to hospital/clinic. He associated hospital with all the bad things that had happened to him. He and Mark agreed to have once-weekly therapy at Peter's home.

Therapy essentially concentrated on language/communication, working on expanding Peter's ability to express himself in phrases and sentences, with an emphasis on him applying his ability to understand

and produce words in conversational contexts. Thus the work in each session had two main stages: (1) formal sentence-processing work; (2) 'conversational' exchanges using some themes from the first part of the session. These were not conversations in the true sense, but rather practice conversations used to expand the context of the language work.

Broadening horizons

It became apparent to Mark while working with Peter that Peter was still very isolated. He felt safe and well supported within his family but had had little exposure communicating in everyday life outside the family. Mark and Peter discussed the possibility of working in a group with other people with aphasia, not on language impairment, but on communicative use and living-with-aphasia issues. Peter agreed to this approach, although it meant him having to go to a group, which took place at the hospital.

Peter worked once a week with one and then two other people who had non-fluent aphasia, in a group with Kate, another SLT. In the group they addressed issues of using communication and communication strategies, as well as issues around the impact of aphasia on their lives. The one-to-one therapy also continued once-weekly on a domiciliary basis.

Outcomes

Peter did show some improvements on formal assessments of language and language processing, but the most striking changes showed up on the informal assessment of impact, especially in the areas of how Peter felt about himself and how others perceived him. His self-esteem had clearly improved, as had his ability to engage in communication with others, even though his ability to 'chat' had only shown slight improvements. He was now a ready contributor to the group, and continued to attend for a little while even when he moved out of the area.

The intervention story

It is difficult as a therapist not to be moved by what are often disastrous events in other people's lives. In these circumstances, it is sometimes difficult to maintain objectivity, and keep realistic objectives for yourself and your client. It was very important for Peter to feel that he was making progress, but the criteria he was using in the first instance related entirely to 'saying more words'. Using a means of measuring the impact of therapy on parameters that Peter himself had established was an important way of maintaining an objective stance in relation to whether the therapy was effective or not, and thus whether it continued to be viable.

Another important feature of intervention with Peter was being able to be flexible in the approach. Flexibility allowed for different approaches to carry on concurrently (i.e. two different types of individual intervention – individual and group therapy), as well as allowing domiciliary and hospital-based work.

Intervention journey 2: Ahmet, a pre-school child with recently diagnosed hearing impairment

Ahmet was a little boy of 20 months at the time of his referral to speech and language therapy. He had very recently been diagnosed with a profound sensorineural hearing impairment. There was a peripatetic teacher of the deaf (ToD) already involved with Ahmet and his family, and it was she who brought the case to the attention of the specialist speech and language therapy service.

Background
Ahmet was born to a Turkish family who had lived in England for the past five years. There was an older sister of six. The father ran his own business and the mother was full-time in the home, looking after the children. Both the mother and father spoke good English although Turkish was the language used at home. At the time of the referral, there had been no experience of deafness in the family or within the extended family. Other agencies involved in Ahmet's care were the teacher of the deaf and the audiological services at the local hospital. Ahmet had been prescribed with two post-aural hearing aids.

First impressions
The first contact between Ahmet's family and the speech and language therapy service came very early after the initial diagnosis of hearing impairment. The parents presented as highly anxious and distressed about the situation they faced with their youngest child. They were unsure how, as a family, they would cope with Ahmet's disability. At the same time, the parents expressed a desire for help and guidance in supporting their son.

The first session was spent gathering case history information from the parents. The parents described Ahmet as a healthy child who was developing quite normally in all other areas apart from communication. There seemed to be no obvious cause for the hearing impairment and diagnostic investigations were continuing with an early appointment for a CT scan. They had also been offered genetic counselling as a routine service by the local hospital. After their initial anxiety, the parents came across as extremely keen to get started on ways to help Ahmet. One of their first questions was: Do you think signing will help our son? It was quite unusual for parents of a child so early on in the intervention process to be considering alternatives to conventional speech.

During the first session it was noted that Ahmet was very clingy to his mother, preferring to sit on her lap rather than engage with the toys that were present in the room. The parents stated that they were not convinced that the hearing aids actually made any difference to Ahmet's hearing but agreed that it was early days as yet and therefore too soon to reject something that might be potentially useful.

Collaboration between professionals

Discussions between the ToD and speech and language therapist (SLT) were ongoing. Based on the views expressed by the parents and the presenting needs of Ahmet and his family, it was decided that the ToD would continue with weekly visits to the family, supporting Ahmet and his family on issues to do with hearing aid-management. Family counselling was continuous throughout this period, providing the parents with the opportunity to express their concerns and to give vent to their uncertainty. The SLT would provide weekly contact until the time when it was feasible for Ahmet to start specialist educational provision for deaf and hearing-impaired children. The focus would be on the communication/interaction partnerships with Ahmet in the home setting: namely the parental and sibling interactions with Ahmet. Sessions were carried out in the home and also the clinic setting, and usually involved the mother and sister with Ahmet.

Interaction in the home

The main goal of SLT was derived from the early discussions that took place with the parents. It was to establish accessible communicative input for Ahmet in his home environment through the communication partnerships that were most significant to him. The parents had also requested some input on signing and had been helped to access a training course on British Sign Language (BSL).

Essentially, assessment and therapy activities were combined to yield information about the needs of the familiar communication partnerships in Ahmet's life at the same time as facilitating their development. Intervention activities usually involved the mother, sister, Ahmet and the SLT. A principal aim was to help Ahmet to realize that communication was taking place. The therapist modelled communication styles that were heavily annotated with visual cues. Strategies included:

- waiting for Ahmet to look at the person's face before starting a communication act;
- holding an object or toy near the face in order to direct his attention to facial expression and other visual cues that might form part of the interaction;
- use of heavily intonated speech to support use of any residual hearing and to emphasize non-verbal aspects of the communication.

Video recordings were made of interactions during the session, which the mother and therapist appraised together. Initially the mother appeared reluctant to experiment with ways of interacting with her child, preferring to observe the therapist. Gradually, after a few sessions, as her confidence in the techniques grew, she became more participative. Early on, she expressed positive feelings about the way the intervention was progressing and, once she had got over her initial reserve at being videotaped, she was able to be more active. Positive aspects of the interaction were identified so that the mother could build on them.

Interactions between Ahmet and his elder sister were promoted through their mutual love of videos. A commercially available video of signing for beginners was provided for the family. The format was derived from a popular children's television show. The content of the video was designed to be participative, providing signed renditions of some familiar nursery rhymes set in meaningful contexts, e.g. 'Old MacDonald's Farm' sung/signed by an actor in farmer's costume on location. The video provided both siblings with a focus for their conversations and for developing their relationship.

Addressing culture and language

Although Turkish was the language usually spoken at home, therapy sessions were conducted in English. This was not ideal; however, time was given to asserting that the sessions were designed to highlight the *principles* of positive interaction to be used in *Turkish*. The importance of maintaining the native language of the home was stressed repeatedly. Use of the home context in the initial stages meant that the intervention activities were developed from *within* the family culture, making them highly relevant.

Broadening the social network

As the intervention progressed, the location of the sessions was shifted to the clinic setting. This was so that Ahmet and his family would have the chance to meet others who shared similar experiences. Initially, individual appointments were arranged with the idea that contacts would occur at the changeover points between the scheduled appointments of the day. Later on the parents were invited to share an appointment time with another family to work on specific aspects of communication, such as attention and listening skills. This was an important step for Ahmet and his family as it opened out the world of people with hearing impairments and provided them with the opportunity to share their concerns, triumphs and hopes for the future.

Outcomes

Ahmet was very responsive to the visual strategies recommended in the intervention. He quickly learned to look at the person in order to initiate an interaction. His visual searching for cues was clearly evident. Looking at the proffered object was always followed by establishing eye contact with the person. The mother was clearly delighted with her son's progress and felt more confident in her own expertise as a hearing mother of a deaf child, although she admitted some frustration at her limited signing skills which she felt held her back.

Challenges of therapy

The main challenges were in having to conduct therapy sessions in English. This meant that it was difficult to ensure the translation of therapy principles into the Turkish language and culture, although activities were devised as a result of constant negotiation between therapist and family. The situation was helped by the very good use of spoken English amongst the family members.

The mother's initial reluctance to participate actively in the sessions needed to be overcome. There was a tendency to view the therapist as the 'expert' and to not believe in her own natural expertise as a parent, although this changed over time. It appeared that the mother needed to know enough in order to have a go herself, and as her confidence grew she became an active participant and skilled communicator with her son.

The intervention story

Speech and language therapy was withdrawn when Ahmet started at a school for deaf children that importantly had a bilingual signing policy. One year after the initial referral, Ahmet was offered a cochlear implant as it had been established that he was deriving almost no benefit from his hearing aids. The parents talked to others who had been through the same process, and deliberated long and hard before making their decision. Unusually, the parents decided against such a course of action. They felt that it would be too difficult to explain such an invasive operation to their very young son. Ahmet was progressing well as a child *with* a hearing impairment: he was acquiring signing skills at an age-appropriate rate, and as a family they had accommodated his different communication needs. The identity of their young son was emerging and changing along with that of the family unit. Visual communication was now an established part of the home communication environment.

Intervention journey 3: Valerie, a woman with moderate aphasia

Valerie was a 43-year-old woman who was referred to a community-based SLT service that offered group therapy for people with aphasia. Valerie had had a stroke approximately nine months before. At the time of her stroke Valerie was living alone, as she had done for much of her adult life.

Background

Prior to her stroke, Valerie worked in the public sector in a job that carried a high level of responsibility and long working hours. She had recently completed an MA and up to the time of her stroke was debating whether to pursue a PhD. Valerie described herself as someone who liked to work hard and also to invest time and energy in socializing with her network of colleagues and friends. Valerie had been unable to work since her stroke and was supported by state benefits.

Post-onset of stroke, Valerie received good acute hospital care, after which she was referred on to a residential rehabilitation unit for the purposes of intensive therapy. She spent six months in the unit before returning to live in her own home. The SLT in the rehabilitation unit referred her for group therapy. At the time of the referral, Valerie was described as having moderate aphasia, characterized by specific word-finding difficulties and problems in reading and writing. Valerie was portrayed as having an immense drive to work on and improve her speech and language, to the exclusion of all other aspects of her life. It was clear to those who worked with her that Valerie's main passion was for pursuing the 'normalization' of her speech and language. The danger of her becoming a speech and language therapy 'junkie' was recognized, and the SLT felt that Valerie would benefit from a broader approach to therapy that focused on *learning to live with disability*.

Initial impressions

On her first day at the community clinic, Valerie presented as a fully mobile woman who was able to travel independently. Communicating with Valerie, it emerged that independence, in all aspects of life, was of tremendous value to her. The stick she used for support in walking symbolized that she had been 'robbed' of something she held dear to herself. Before the stroke, Valerie had been a keen hill walker; now she experienced the loss of a pastime that asserted her independent and mobile self. Valerie articulated a strong desire to work on her communication impairment. The restitution narrative was alive and kicking in the individual goals she defined for herself; however, it was the SLT's impression that Valerie's sense of progress and achievement in regaining her pre-stroke language skills was gradually tailing off.

Individual expectations

The individual sessions offered to Valerie ran as a series of in-depth interviews so that Valerie's personal issues could be highlighted and her own 'therapy' agenda externalized. The first individual session with Valerie gave her the opportunity to identify the issues that were pertinent to her experience of aphasia and her own life course. In conversation with one of the therapists, she identified her problems with word-finding and reading as priorities for therapy. She requested work sheets and exercises so that she could continue to work on aspects of her speech and language. The issues raised by Valerie were listened to and followed up by the therapist. Valerie stated that aphasia made her feel stupid and made others, friends and former colleagues, treat her as a 'charity case'.

Valerie was also invited to participate in one of the established therapy groups, which had eight members in total. At first, Valerie expressed her reluctance to join the group, although at the same time recognizing that 'here was a good place to come'. She described herself as 'not really a group person'. During the orientation phase, Valerie was exposed to the voiced concerns and experiences of her fellow group members. The agenda of *learning to live with disability* was annoying and frustrating to her at times. Following group discussions was challenging for Valerie and this made her angry at her so-called 'stupidity'. The contrast in her life before and after her stroke was a constant source of sadness and anger for Valerie. During group sessions she would invariably 'switch off' and appear alternatively irritated or bored by the contributions of others. To her, the *living with* agenda felt like 'abandoning ship' and giving up all that she held dear.

The SLT felt that Valerie could benefit from counselling. This was suggested to Valerie, who responded by saying that she was not ready yet because she felt too sad. In accordance with Valerie's wishes, counselling was placed as an option for consideration at a later date.

'Tracks' of the journey

The first major point in Valerie's intervention journey was exploring the role of conversation partners. This formed the major topic of group sessions during a ten-week period. Together with the group facilitator and her fellow participants, Valerie started to consider the possibility of placing her experience of communication difficulties outside herself. This was a new idea to Valerie and gradually her vocabulary extended to terms such as 'barrier' to describe her experiences of communicating with others. The dominant position occupied by what she saw as *her impairment* was starting to give way to the problems that were located in others and society. 'People ignoring you' was defined as a barrier rather than a by-product of impairment. A 'lack of competence' was used to refer to the significant others who were uninformed about aphasia and lacked the ability to adjust communication to presenting needs.

The second period of ten weeks focused on the development of an aphasia-friendly leaflet. It followed on from the discussions of the previous term's theme in that it started to address some of the barriers already identified. The question of how to explain what aphasia means to the uninformed was central to the group's activity. Valerie became an energetic and enthusiastic contributor to the group's project. Her need for impairment-focused support was still apparent in her individual sessions, and work was carried out consecutively on semantic therapy, sentence processing and reading comprehension, and understanding and summarizing articles. Throughout this period, it was recognized that Valerie's impairment-drive, though still strong, was at last connecting to wider disability issues.

Defining moment

It was during one particular session, where the group was being encouraged to look at some leaflets that had been produced on the subject of aphasia, that Valerie had a truly seminal moment in her intervention journey. The therapist offered the aphasia-friendly leaflet from the Toronto Aphasia Centre (Kagan, Winckel and Schumway, 1996) for scrutiny by the group members. The meaning behind one particular phrase struck Valerie above everything: 'When you have aphasia you are still a competent person'. The realization for Valerie was that aphasia had not affected her intelligence in the way she feared. This was a defining moment in her intervention journey, which she followed up by writing to the voluntary group formerly known as Action for Dysphasic Adults (ADA), recently renamed 'Speakability'. She requested 20 copies of their information leaflet 'What is aphasia?' and sent them out to selected friends. Around this time, Valerie also completed a series of group sessions that looked at assertiveness and aphasia.

Rediscovering the arts

The next theme that the group concentrated on came directly from the expressed interests of the group members. In common with her colleagues in the group, Valerie had been interested in many forms of artistic expression before her stroke. She declared her love of reading, and described the large store of books that filled the shelves of her home and which she had not touched since her stroke. It emerged that she was not the only one in this position.

The group started to address the question of whether it was still possible to enjoy poetry when you have a language impairment. Various dramatic renditions of ancient ballads by invited readers opened up the many ways of understanding and appreciating poetry, e.g. through touch and texture, through movement and rhythm, through sound and cadence, etc. At the last session of the term, Valerie brought along a funny and witty poem by Wendy Cope. She read aloud a well-rehearsed and prepared rendition of the poem that was appreciated by one and all. Her concluding comment, 'I never thought that I would read my poetry books again,' was indicative of a reconnection between her pre- and post-stroke lives.

Reconnecting

It was about this time that Valerie was offered counselling once more, and she decided to take up the option. Personal energy and time was devoted to exploring issues related to life-course change. Valerie decided to return to work and secured a part-time job. She recognized that her capacity for work had altered but also felt that she wanted to give it a go. From flourishing on the hustle and bustle of work prior to her stroke, she expressed a need for less contact with work colleagues and all that entailed. One of the challenges facing Valerie at work was the outcome of the technological explosion that had occurred in her absence from the workplace over the previous couple of years. Individual therapy responded to the new set of issues at this turning point in Valerie's life and focused on e-mail therapy as one of the key forms of communication that Valerie would be using at work.

Despite the enormous changes and turning points in Valerie's intervention journey, she remained reluctant to talk about her stroke. The last group that Valerie participated in was a personal portfolio group. Members chose words that described their perceptions of one another.

The words 'intelligent' and 'hard worker' were assigned to Valerie. Individuals were encouraged and supported to construct a portfolio that reflected their life course, personal turning points and self-image. Valerie put in many hours of work on developing her personal portfolio at home. During the last session of the term, each member agreed to present a section to the others. Valerie brought along a beautifully crafted portfolio in the form of a photographic album. It displayed photographs of her early life and also more recent ones. The aspect she chose to present was her stroke because, as she told the group, she hated it and had never wanted to think about it. She went on to talk about her experience in the acute and rehabilitation centres in the first six months post-stroke. These were important times, and she had strong memories of the therapy staff and their approaches, and whether she had liked or disliked them. A photograph of her walking stick propped up against a wall was accompanied by a commentary expressing 'onwards and upwards'. This was her last day in the group, as Valerie had decided to leave. She was keen to move on and was about to start her new job. The SLT recognized her ongoing fragility and she was offered a contact point with the clinic as 'someone to touch base with' on a monthly or less-than-monthly basis as required.

Moving on

A year later, Valerie has moved away from the 'hustle and bustle' of city life to a gentler pace in a small town on the edge of the countryside. She shares her home with two cats and finds new value in her changed lifestyle. She joined a women's group being run for and by people with aphasia, keen to maintain some ongoing contact with others living with similar issues. Her life is reconnected and she has indeed 'moved on'.

Intervention journey 4: Maria, a child with specific language impairment in mainstream education

Maria was a young girl of six and a half. She attended an inclusive resource base located in mainstream provision that had been established by the local education authority (LEA). The aim was that she should spend time in age-related classes as a default option with the flexibility for extra support from the established resource. There were six children at Key Stage 1 who attended the resource base. They were dispersed through the reception class and Year 1.

Background

Maria lived at home with her mother, father and younger brother (three years old). They lived in a two-bedroom council flat in an inner city area. Her parents were originally from the Philippines although they had lived in England for the past six years. Both parents were fully conversant in English. The language of the home tended to be a mixture of Spanish and

English. The father worked as a domestic orderly in a local hospital and the mother managed the home. The mother reported that Maria was more fluent in English than in Spanish.

Circumstances of referral

When Maria was two years old, she and her mother participated in a series of pre-school workshops that focused on parent–child interaction. The service was offered on an ongoing basis by the pre-school SLT service and was supplemented by some one-to-one sessions. In the initial stages, Maria was described as non-verbal with underdeveloped play, characterized by repetitive actions and ordering of play items. Her play was reported as being non-imaginative with a preference for construction toys.

Maria was subsequently referred on to the mainstream SLT service. The referral came in the form of the statutory assessment report for Maria's Statement of Special Educational Needs. She was described as having some limited language skills at the point of transfer, with single-word comprehension evident when contextual cues were present. She was below the baseline on the many standardized assessments that had been attempted with her, e.g. the British Picture Vocabulary Scales (BPVS), sub-tests of the CELF-R UK, amongst others. Maria's expressive skills were extremely limited. She used extensive chunks of apparently 'learned' phrases, many acquired from television programmes, e.g. she would announce in a broadcaster-type voice – 'Today is Tuesday!' She exhibited both immediate and delayed echolalia, which showed age-appropriate phonology although relevance to context was somewhat hit and miss. She was also capable of supplying her own needs in terms of goods and services by using single words. The educational psychologist's report stated that Maria's non-verbal problem-solving ability was appropriate for her age.

Initial impressions

Maria was initially seen by the SLT in the resource base. It was noted that Maria communicated in what could only be described as a 'strange way'. She evidently was motivated to engage with the teaching staff as demonstrated by her tugging at a person's sleeve, or pulling on the hand to gain attention. Her use of language was linguistically 'bizarre' and placed the onus for interpretation largely on the communication partner. Both the SLT and teaching staff described the challenge of deciphering Maria's often obscure communicative attempts.

Early on, contact was made with the mother, who brought Maria to school each day. A meeting was set up that included the SLT and the specialist teacher employed in the resource base. The mother expressed her relief at the placement despite some early concerns that it was not at the local Catholic school, which would have been their preferred choice. The tension between meeting Maria's special needs and meeting her religious educational needs was apparent.

Maria presented as a child who experienced difficulties in the semantic and pragmatic aspects of language. She was evidently a highly visually oriented child, who used the many environmental reference points around her. She pointed at objects and could recognize her printed name on her peg and work tray. Listening time in the classroom posed the greatest challenge to Maria. She would frequently remain standing whilst her peers sat cross-legged on the carpet in front of the teacher. She was observed to watch whatever was going on and appeared 'wary' in her body language.

Exploratory therapy

From observations and formally reported information, the SLT hypothesized that Maria's communication difficulties stemmed from a disorder of semantics that was affecting her pragmatics. This informed the direction of the intervention journey. The therapist decided against carrying out formal assessments with Maria – if the recent referral report was anything to go by, she would be off the scale anyway, proving such an exercise meaningless. A language processing framework provided the underpinning of the diagnostic therapy approach. The aim was to investigate the source of Maria's difficulties and through this to identify strategies that would help to circumvent the problem.

Inclusion at every level

The philosophy of the resource base was to promote inclusion at every level and so intervention was duly located in the classroom. Although it was mere coincidence, it was incredibly fortunate that the school's special educational needs co-ordinator (SENco) was in fact the class teacher as well!

The SLT, specialist teacher and the SENco engaged in active collaboration from the earliest stage. They met frequently to ensure an even spread of responsibilities, and the allocation of time and resources. The class teacher expressed his concern regarding Maria's access to and engagement with the curriculum-based activities. Maria's poor ability to sit with her classmates was a problem. It was agreed to instigate a system of rewards for achievement of desirable attention/sitting behaviours for which he was responsible. In terms of supporting Maria's access to the curriculum, it was decided that the specialist teacher would support development of the language of numeracy, whilst the SLT would intervene in the area of Maria's central language processing through activities within the literacy hour, which was an area of particular concern to the class teacher. Together they surveyed the timetabled sessions week by week and allocated their extra support time for Maria to the literacy and numeracy hours.

The long-term goals for Maria were:

to establish functional access to the taught curriculum and engagement in the learning process;

- to enable Maria to draw on the positive factors in her skill set by using her visual recognition to support difficulties in auditory processing;
- to provide Maria with the tools to circumvent language processing difficulties whilst also revealing more information about the nature of her difficulties.

Locating intervention in the classroom

The SLT input to the literacy hour was helped by the class teacher, who identified a particular book for the class to work on each week. The daily sessions of one hour comprised different break-out activities, such as cutting and sticking, computer-based activities and picture story telling. The SLT worked with whichever activity Maria and her peers were engaged in. It was her job to provide facilitation so that Maria could participate in the mainstream learning. The techniques used were designed to address Maria's difficulties with semantics and attention maintenance. Her attempts at tasks were probed and extended. Modelling and recasting of responses were used to highlight the key characteristics of the target response. Differential feedback provided useful information about her progress and helped to refine target responses. Visual cues helped to support Maria shifting her attention between activities, particularly in a situation where she was likely to become fixated, e.g. on computer-based activities.

An individual SLT session was offered to Maria every day in order to recap on the activities relating to the focal book of the week. This would include picture sequencing, supported narrative, drawing and other such related activities. The purpose was to help Maria use her language skill to review her day's learning. A visit to an art gallery was followed up by constructing a narrative based on artefacts of the school trip and some pictures – Maria was helped to sequence the bus tickets, picture of a packed lunch, and postcards of paintings looked at so that she could recount the visit.

Progress

This approach to therapy was taken across two terms. During this time Maria's attention and listening skills were variable. There were days when she appeared to disengage from the activity on offer and would sometimes wander off; however on a good day, she was observed to maintain her attention for a ten-minute period.

Progress was monitored at the Individual Education Plan review meetings (IEPs) that happened every six weeks during term time. At these meetings, Maria's goals were identified in terms of what she needed to achieve in the short term, how the goals would be attained, and the key people who would facilitate the process. In this way, the active support being offered to Maria was made current and timely.

Over time, it became apparent that Maria's naming vocabulary was expanding steadily. It consisted mainly of single words. Although her accuracy in labelling items was improving, some semantic errors remained. There was one memorable occasion when the children were identifying the fruit and vegetables on a market stall – Maria referred to a 'green pepper' as a 'salt', showing a classic semantic error. Her written work was a strength and she achieved age-appropriate skills in a short time.

During the course of the intervention episode, Maria mixed well with other children in the playground. She ran around with them and some nurturing of Maria by the other girls was observed. Both teachers and therapist noticed an increase in Maria's social confidence. She initiated interactions with her peers increasingly and required less monitoring during group sessions. It seemed that she was aware of developing competencies and able to approach set tasks independently. The therapist described Maria as being on a 'positive spiral' of learning and development.

Next stage on the journey

Some formal assessments were used to evaluate Maria's language skills. She achieved a score on the BPVS of within normal limits for her age, although difficulties in sentence comprehension persisted. It was decided to look more closely at Maria's comprehension of verbs and prepositions. This revealed some confusion regarding thematic roles: her assignment of agent and goal was found to be fairly random. Subsequently, the SLT and class teacher met to discuss the next stage in therapy. It was agreed to introduce sentence frames for all the children in the class to develop their narrative skills. This tapped into Maria's difficulty in generating sentences by providing a facilitating structure where she was encouraged to identify the agent, the action and the goal.

Maria's language skills were becoming more appropriate although she still persisted in uttering parrot-like phrases lifted from popular television shows. Interestingly, this won her the engagement of the other children, who were frequently amused by her enacted television monologues. It appeared to have a great deal of 'street cred' with the other children!

Mechanism for change

Great value was placed on the careful and efficient co-ordination of Maria's intervention. The teachers and therapist worked closely together, with Maria placed very firmly at the centre of the process. This enabled her communication difficulties to be attacked at every level: the diagnostic approach to therapy meant a constant revealing of information about the nature of Maria's communication deficit, which in turn prompted the use of strategies to circumvent her difficulties. This occurred within an iterative process of daily contact between the SLT and teachers, ensuring continuity and cohesion of approach. The therapist reflected on the rewarding experience of working with Maria where resources, both teaching and therapy, were adequate to meet the needs of the child, and were matched by the commitment of all concerned.

Moving on

Eventually, Maria was able to transfer over to the local Roman Catholic junior school that was her parents' initial preference. Her written skills were very strong, and in this respect the emphasis placed on literacy in the national curriculum stood her in good stead. The therapist predicted that Maria would experience further difficulties as she progressed through later key stages of the curriculum where language becomes increasingly abstract.

Intervention journey 5: Winston, a man with severe learning disabilities and profound hearing impairment

Winston was a man of Afro-Caribbean background in his late twenties. He had severe learning disabilities and was also profoundly deaf. His hearing impairment was such that he could not derive any positive use from wearing hearing aids. Winston lived in a community house with one other resident of similar age and ethnic origin, supported by a staff team of ten. There was a minimum of two staff on duty at any one time.

Background

Winston had moved from a long-stay institution approximately five year previously. The ethnicity of the two residents was reflected in the recruitment of some members of staff who were of similar ethnic and cultural background. Winston had a long history of challenging behaviour which showed itself in aggression to others and destruction of property. His housemate was also known to have high support needs in relation to general behaviour, communication and daily activity. Previous SLT had concentrated on teaching Winston signs and introducing a core vocabulary of Makaton to the immediate staff team. After initial interest by individual members of staff, there was a lack of consistent carryover in Winston's daily life, and the intervention fell flat.

Circumstances of referral

At the time of the referral, the overall manager of the service was concerned with the high level of client need in the house and the corresponding low morale of the staff team. The general attitude of the wider service towards Winston's house was negative: it was viewed as 'difficult' house to work in and it was bad luck if you were assigned to work a shift there.

The service manager and the support staff team leader made contact with the SLT service through the local community team for people with learning disabilities. They felt that Winston's support service was at risk unless something could be done to reverse the negative spiral that existed amongst the team of support staff. The referral requested some form of staff training that was tailored specifically to the needs of Winston.

Preparation for intervention
Negotiation between the SLT service and the managers of Winston's support service resulted in an agreement to set up an intensive training course for all the staff. The purpose was to create a positive environment in Winston's home by establishing the use of total communication strategies amongst the staff. A primary aim of the intervention was to establish a home culture that was sensitive to Winston's profound hearing impairment.

The service committed the entire staff team to a whole week's intensive training, off site from the supported house. A relief staff team was established to cover the support needs of Winston and his housemate during the appointed week, thereby ensuring the attendance of every single member of staff. The aims of the course were defined as a result of the ongoing negotiation between the support service and the SLTs. The staff team was encouraged to articulate the goals that would take effect in Winston's house.

The service manager participated in the first and last sessions of the week. A training venue was secured off site in a community centre that ran a range of different activities. The SLT assistant prepared the training materials under the guidance of the SLTs and through consultation with the staff team. This involved identifying communication topics that were relevant to Winston's daily life, and compiling a set of resource books of signs, symbols and pictures of those topics.

Baseline measurements of the interactions taking place in the house were taken before the intervention, using systematic observation methods. These concentrated on the proportion of time that staff members and Winston spent using visual communication strategies, such as formal signs, objects of reference and visual attention calls as well as the range of communication functions used.

Training methods
The main aim of the intervention was to locate visual communication in real-life situations. Right from the start, it was agreed that the only communicative exchanges in the training context could be ones that drew on the principles of visual communication. It was felt important to establish Winston's communication needs at the centre of all the training activities that would occur that week.

The training employed a combination of problem-solving scenarios and direct training on communication tactics for people with a hearing impairment. Staff had generated the problem situations in the preparation phase.

They were encouraged to identify the critical issues in each situation and to select the most amenable and relevant total communication strategies to ameliorate the difficulties. Sometimes the solutions involved the manipulation of certain setting conditions, such as the source of natural light and the positioning of the interactants. In recognition of the difficulty in predicting a reliable outcome for the selected strategy, the participants were also encouraged to identify suitable contingencies should a strategy fail. The participants also identified a sign to represent their individual names.

Staff response to intervention

Staff expressed their enthusiasm at participating in the training week During the course of the week and later on during the initial implementation phase, staff attitude to their work and to Winston changed dramatically. There was a collective feeling that they were becoming an expert team in total communication and this renewed their energies to work with Winston. The image of Winston changed from one where challenging behaviour dominated, to one where deafness was the main barrier to building a positive relationship. This represented an important shift for staff: Winston's challenging behaviour was now understood in the context of his particular 'hearing' needs.

Changing communication environment

Other adaptations were introduced to the environment, such as installing a flashing-light doorbell. Repeated observational measures one year after the training course revealed a dramatic increase in the proportion of visual communication strategies used by the staff with Winston. Winston himself did not use any more signs at this stage, although he used more visual searching in his environment. He also started to use some familiar objects of reference to communicate basic meanings.

One direct result of the intervention was the establishment of a deaf culture within the house. The next member of staff to be recruited was woman who herself was prelingually deaf and who communicated primarily through British Sign Language for the deaf (BSL). This represented major development in Winston's support service and provided the assurance that the positive changes brought about by the intervention would not only be maintained but extended.

Commitment to change

This was an extremely well-resourced piece of work that demonstrated high level of commitment by all the stakeholders involved in supporting Winston. The role played by senior managers was extremely important Their organization of a relief staff team and their attendance at the start and close of the intervention week demonstrated a high level of commitment and a real desire to change practice. This was matched by the mobilization of SLT resources.

Integrated intervention

The intervention journeys recounted in this chapter serve to illustrate the unique qualities of each one. Common to each story is the fact that it is *not* just about the communication skills of the individuals concerned: many other factors come into play.

Identity and self-image

Identity is viewed as an integral part of the intervention process: as a variable of influence on every decision and action taken, and as an indicator of the effectiveness and suitability of a course of action. Inextricably linked to a person's communication skills as it is, identity or sense of self is affected by the interactions that take place with others.

More relevant relationships

The emerging identity of the 20-month-old Ahmet (Intervention journey 2) was supported by the development of more relevant communication partnerships with his parents and sister. This finds resonance in the story of Winston (Intervention journey 5), where the staff team learned to look at him as someone who was deaf, as opposed to challenging. This brought about a shift in the attitudes of staff towards Winston to the point that his challenging behaviour seemed almost reasonable in the context of a primarily auditory environment.

Power of public narratives

Journey 3, which retells the story of Valerie, demonstrates the powerful influence of the prevailing narratives in society. It also shows how an acquired impairment can tear an individual's life course in two. In the early days post-stroke, Valerie viewed herself as an impaired human being. The problem was hers, and she needed SLT to restore her to her former self. It raises the question for all individuals who live with disability: how does one square a robust identity with the popular public narratives where restitution and normalization are prevalent? On her journey, Valerie wrestled with different concepts of the person with aphasia. The defining moment in Valerie's journey was when an alternative narrative was introduced: when you have aphasia you are still competent. Her journey had reached a turning point and reconnection of the two pieces of her life was possible.

Importance of self-image

The importance of self-image is demonstrated in Peter's story – Intervention journey 1. At one point it was acknowledged that his 'low mood' was associated with his lack of ability to 'chat'. Later he was encouraged to evaluate his own communication skills so that the impact of his disability on his own self-perceptions and lifestyle could be ascertained. This was deemed important to the next phase of intervention that Peter had directed towards being able to 'say more'. In Intervention journey 2, the emergence of Ahmet's identity as a deaf child who signs was an integral part of his family unit to the point where a cochlear implant was rejected.

Interestingly, in Maria's story (Journey 4), it was her use of learned phrases from popular TV shows that helped her to engage with peers. Other children perceived this manifestation of her language impairment as a positive part of her character. Her story also reveals some tensions between an identity that stems from special needs, i.e. her language difficulties, and one that is derived from family values, i.e. committed Roman Catholics. This made for a difficult choice, between meeting Maria's educational needs and her religious needs, that was really only resolved when she 'moved on'.

Whose expertise?

Ongoing negotiation between client and therapist is a feature of all the intervention journeys. Expertise is distributed between client and therapist in their working relationship: the therapist contributing theoretical knowledge, clinical reasoning and professional experience; the client and significant others sharing expert knowledge based on the lived experience, personal history and insights into current difficulties.

Personal goals and initiatives

Ongoing negotiation between the key players is a feature of all the journeys, with the client occupying the pivotal point at the centre of the decision-making process. Valerie's drive for impairment-focused work could be seen in opposition to the referred need to *live with* disability however, Valerie was not ready to give up her quest for better speech at this time. Similarly her rejection of counselling as an option was respected. The individual and group approaches to intervention ran alongside each other initially, but in time their routes crossed over. Regular review and the opportunity to re-determine priorities, particularly at critical stages of her journey, brought both Valerie and her therapist to the negotiating table.

The story of Ahmet (Intervention journey 2) and Winston (Intervention journey 5) demonstrate how the ideas of significant others may be instrumental in shaping an intervention. It was Ahmet's family (Intervention journey 2) that proposed the early introduction of signing, and interestingly, further down the line, it was they who also declined the option of a cochlear implant for their child, underpinned by a clear rationale from the family's perspective. The intensive training of Winston's staff team (Intervention journey 5) came about because of a direct request from the service manager to which the SLT team responded.

Role of culture and ethnicity

The culture and ethnicity of the individual and significant others not only provide the backdrop for all aspects of the intervention, but also inform the way therapy proceeds. For Ahmet and his family (Intervention journey 2) the home culture provided a context for therapy. This was important, particularly in the early days, so that activities were relevant. Once established, there was a strategic move to the deaf culture, with appointments taking place in a community clinic where there was the opportunity to meet other families with similar issues. In some ways, the role of culture in Maria's intervention journey (Intervention journey 4) was made subordinate to meeting her special educational needs, because of constraints in the location of the resource base. Fulfilment of Maria's cultural needs was seen in her transfer to an RC school at a later date. Intervention journey 5 provides an interesting take on culture. Before the intervention, some members of the staff team shared Winston's ethnic and cultural background; however, his membership of the deaf culture had gone unheeded. It wasn't until after the completion of the staff training programme that a deaf member of staff was recruited.

Shifting centre of influence

Describing the intervention process as 'dynamic' and 'organic' (see Chapter 1) implies a process that is far from static. An initial focus on one centre of influence gives rise to a *ripple effect* that describes the movement of therapeutic effect from the individual to the outer centres of influence, and vice versa. The intervention journeys recounted here are plotted on Figure 10.1.

Interrelated and bi-directional

Having a particular focus on a centre of influence does not exclude others. Centres of influence are viewed as interrelated and bi-directional, i.e. intervention activities centred on the partnership may affect the individual(s) as well as the communication environment. In Journey 5, the targeting of the communication environment had implications for the partnerships in Winston's life and ultimately for him. Ahmet's intervention (Journey 2) initially focused on the familiar partnerships in the home context and on Ahmet himself; however, as the venue for therapy changed, other communication partnerships were made possible, and ultimately he moved on to a communication environment where his signing needs could be met.

Ripple effects'

Movement emanates from the chosen centre rather like the ripple effect of a pebble thrown into a pond. Valerie's story (Intervention journey 3)

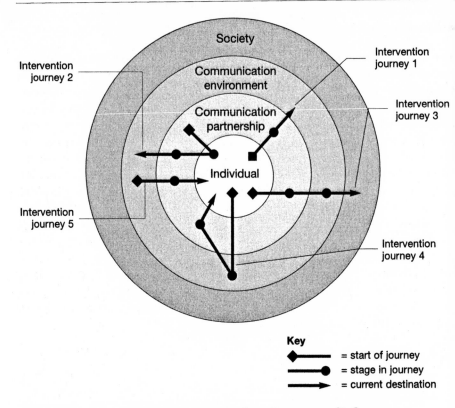

Figure 10.1 Intervention journeys mapped on the centres of influence

illustrates this effectively: how a preferred focus on individual therapy wa broadened to include the communication partnerships in a group setting which then moved outwards to the communication environment, and finally to society as self-advocacy activities supported her to 'live with disability'. Peter's progression (Intervention journey 1) follows a simila trajectory to the point where he participates in a group. The explorator nature of Maria's therapy (Intervention journey 4) demonstrates a complex interaction between a number of centres of influence: the individua communication partnerships and the broader educational environment The investigation of Maria's communicative strengths and difficulties is a the epicentre of all therapeutic activity – prefacing the strategic utilizatio of the educational context and the involvement of the main communica tion partners and, afterwards, where Maria's individual profile is reviewe so that the next stage of therapy may be planned.

It is clear that changes in one area of the person's functioning ma impact on others, e.g. conversation coaching of communication partner may give rise to collateral growth in the individual's linguistic skill restructuring person-centred planning meetings for improved access an participation may affect the quality of opportunities provided within th communication partnership.

A complex journey

The intervention stories in this chapter demonstrate the complexities of each journey. By looking across at each account, certain distinguishing features are noted, such as the aetiology of the condition, the primary disorder, the critical point in the person's life course, and associated personal and background factors. Each story is unique in its own way, although certain aspects resonate. Negotiation is a common feature. The therapist works in partnership with the client and/or significant others and other relevant professionals. This means that the expertise of the SLT is placed with the expertise of the key players in the intervention. Movement across different centres of influence corresponds to the changing needs of the individual and key factors affecting their presentation at any point in time. The culture of the individual provides a backdrop for intervention practice and features in all negotiations between therapist, client and/or significant others. Finally, the person's sense of self and how other people identify with them are critical pathways in the intervention process, because how we respond and how we communicate says something about who we are.

Appendix
Glossary of enactment processes

Category by function	Enactment processes
A. Engagement	A.1 Attention call A.2 Inclusion call
B. Modification	B.1 Adapting communication B.2 Ascribing meaning B.3 Checking interpretation B.4 Checking understanding
C. Facilitation	C.1 Encouraging contribution C.2 Modelling C.3 Production call C.4 Assisting contribution
D. Feedback	D.1 Checking contribution D.2 Differential feedback D.3 Evaluative feedback D.4 Summative feedback D.5 Acknowledging contribution
E. Personal maintenance	E.1 Emotional acknowledgement/support E.2 Physical and sensory acknowledgement/support E.3 Behavioural acknowledgement/support
F. Context maintenance	F.1 Equipment organization F.2 Setting organization
G. Transaction	G.1 Soliciting information G.2 Giving information/advice G.3 Providing instructions G.4 Framing/negotiating G.5 Explaining/rationalizing G.6 Recording

Category A: Engagement

A.1 Attention call

Definition:
There is the active seeking or maintenance of the client's attention by verbal or non-verbal means. The therapist may use a positive strategy to direct the person's attention to the specific content, location or properties of the stimulus item. A reverse strategy is when the therapist acts on an item in an unexpected or unconventional manner, such as might be used with a child, e.g. pretends to pick up a miniature object as if it was very heavy. Both have the intended purpose of attracting the person's attention.

Rationale:
Communication is about channelling ideas so that contributions are relevant and timely. The individual may experience attention difficulties due to a variety of reasons, e.g. fatigue, inflexible attention, level of distraction or developmental delay. Alternatively, comprehension difficulties or the effort of communicating may cause the individual to disengage from the main activity or conversation.

Examples:
The therapist employs technical skills for *attention call*, including:
- use of gesture linking the individual's eye gaze to materials;
- use of touch, speech, vocalization, gesture, body language to distract the client from an ongoing activity;
- particular or unusual presentation of materials to attract attention, e.g. producing an object from behind the back in dramatic fashion.

A.2 Inclusion call

Definition:
There is the positive acknowledgement of a person's presence by verbal or non-verbal signal. Typically this technique is used when the therapist's attention is divided between the client and another person or activity.

Rationale:
There are variations in the degree of engagement and participation of people due to differences in personality, confidence, communicative ability and demands of the situation. The therapist is sensitive to these individual differences and uses techniques to signal individual inclusion and to maintain the engagement of individuals, whether in a group setting or in an individual session. In individual sessions, activities such as clearing away therapy materials or responding to another stimulus, e.g. a ringing telephone, may cause the therapist's attention to be diverted from the person briefly. In group or individual sessions where a significant other is present, the therapist may use inclusion calls to the other person(s) who is not immediately engaged in the interaction.

Examples:
The therapist employs technical skills for *inclusion call*, including:
• a verbal or non-verbal gesture such as head nod or smile to a participant(s) who is not currently and actively contributing to an interaction;
• verbal or non-verbal behaviour that accompanies an introduction, change or closure to an activity so that it is imparted to all group members;
• disengaging briefly from ongoing activity to acknowledge presence of other person.

Category B: Modification

B.1 Adapting communication

Definition:
There is the introduction of different modes of communication, selecting accessible vocabulary, modifying the content and structure of utterances according to the observed needs of the individual. This is different from facilitation, which targets a specific contribution made by the client or the stimulus demands presented.

Rationale:
Asymmetry in the communication partnership is a possibility when one participant experiences communication difficulties. In order to address unevenness in communicative exchanges, the therapist makes a deliberate attempt to reflect the individual's communication skills. This is done by suspending the usual way of communicating and employing different modes, e.g. visual and graphic, and using vocabulary and structures that are consistent with the person's style of communication and what is currently know about their support needs.

Examples:
The therapist employs technical skills for *adapting communication*, including:
- use of signs, gestures, pointing and body language;
- use of writing, drawing, pictures and objects;
- use of modified language that is more accessible – simplified phrases and concrete vocabulary, slower pace of delivery.

B.2 Ascribing meaning

Definition:
There is the ascription of meaning by responding to the client's turn in such a way that the meaning is inferred, but the flow of conversation or communicative exchange is unimpeded.

Rationale:
There are times when a therapist may ascribe meaning online without checking the veracity of the communication in order to preserve the mutuality, balance and flow of exchange, as well as to provide the client with the experience of being a valued contributor. The context provides sufficient clues such that checking is not required.

Examples:
The therapist employs technical skills for *ascribing meaning*, including:
- during social routine exchanges the meaning of an unintelligible act is 'fitted' within that routine – the meaning is taken as read;
- completion of missing data because the client has provided sufficient information to make an online interpretation possible.

B.3 Checking interpretation

Definition:
An interpretation of a previous communication act is offered back to the client for scrutiny. The therapist may use a questioning intonation pattern in order to check the accuracy of an interpretation.

Rationale:
Ascription of meaning happens continuously in social communication exchanges; however, the likelihood of ambiguity is greater in exchanges with people with communication disabilities. It may be the case that the therapist has to 'second guess' the meaning and therefore needs to check whether they have got it right or not.

Examples:
The therapist employs technical skills for *checking interpretation*, including:
- suggesting an interpretation with a rising intonation and/or questioning facial expression;
- offering a written or drawn suggestion to the client for approval, rejection or modification;
- soliciting client's approval/rejection by saying 'Did you mean ...?'

B.4 Checking understanding

Definition:
The therapist checks that the client has understood a previous utterance, conversational turn or piece of information.

Rationale:
The ability to understand is important to active participation in the intervention process. Appropriate execution of activities and tasks is dependent on the client understanding what is required.

Examples:
The therapist employs technical skills for *checking understanding*, including:
- directly soliciting confirmation of client's understanding, e.g. 'Did you get that?'
- use of rhetorical utterances, e.g. 'So then you place the card on the pile, OK?'

Category C: Facilitation

C.1 Encouraging contribution

Definition:
There is the verbal or non-verbal encouragement of the client, designed to support confidence in 'having a go'.

Rationale:
Living with a communication disability may affect confidence levels because of the experience of communication struggle, effort, breakdown and failure. The therapist recognizes this and provides gentle persuasion, giving the person courage to have a go.

Examples:
The therapist employs technical skills for *encouraging contribution*, including:
- using persuasive utterances such as 'have a go';
- using verbal or non-verbal signals to indicate that the client is on the right track and should keep going, such as nodding the head, smiling, and saying 'yes' with a rising intonation;
- reminding the client of achievements so far.

C.2 Modelling

Definition:
The therapist demonstrates the target response or an example that is close to the target. The demands of the task or communication act may be simplified by providing a modelled example as an illustration of how to go about the task or activity, or how to frame an appropriate response.

Rationale:
In a similar way to *assisting contribution*, modelling or demonstrating provides support for the individual attempting a particular response type. It includes recasting and expanding the previous utterance or communication act of the individual.

Examples:
The therapist employs technical skills for *modelling*, including:

- demonstrating a target sign, gesture, word, phrase or social behaviour in view of the client;
- recasting or expanding a previous utterance;
- drawing a picture, writing a word, etc. to demonstrate use of a communication mode to the client;
- carrying out a social routine in role-play or other to provide client with target model;
- performing action(s) on objects, items or other materials as an example from the range of possible responses.

C.3 Production call

Definition:
There is a request for the client to attempt a task or the target response. Thi may be combined with a demonstration of the target by the therapist (*modelling technique*) to prompt an imitation or else simply to manipulate the current interaction thereby creating an opportunity for the client to respond or contribute.

Rationale:
Altering the functional use of communication skills involves a complex process. Directly soliciting an attempt on target or creating an opportunity for the client to respond may be a suitable follow-on stag from *modelling*.

Examples:

The therapist employs technical skills for *production call*, including:

- soliciting a production attempt to improve intelligibility of communication acts, e.g. sounds, speech, sign/symbol use, etc.;
- soliciting the use of a particular skill by use of prompt, e.g. turn taking – 'you do it now!';
- presenting a stimulus to solicit a communication act, e.g. picture, word, etc.;
- withdrawing an item, inserting a pause, non-verbally inviting the client to respond by creating the opportunity;
- starting a sentence for the client to complete.

C.4 Assisting contribution

Definition:

The therapist offers a support cue to the client so that he/she can produce or finish a contribution or communication act, or respond to a stimulus. It includes all forms of multi-modal communication.

Rationale:

Guidance or support is offered to promote the use of available skills by the person with a communication disability. The therapist observes the client's communication behaviours and constantly checks the level of verbal comprehension, expressive skills and where communication breaks down. Facilitation strategies are selected and applied so that the person is able to access a communication opportunity and to contribute to an otherwise difficult communicative exchange.

Examples:

The therapist employs technical skills for *assisting contribution*, including:

- rephrasing or simplifying a communication act to promote understanding;
- use of facial, hand and vocal gesture to cue in response;
- use of graphic skills, writing, drawing;
- use of environmental reference points, e.g. objects of reference, pointing at relevant people, photographs, symbols, line drawings;
- offering pen and paper as appropriate to client's needs;
- making suggestions for client to access self-help strategies;
- fine manipulation or adjustment of the presented materials, e.g. reducing an array of pictures or objects, covering certain aspects, gradually revealing parts of a sentence;
- providing verbal cues to client, including initial sound/syllable, semantic links, sentence completion;
- helping the client to prepare for a response attempt by reminding them of the key features.

Category D: Feedback

D.1 Checking contribution *Definition*:
The therapist reflects back the client's response for their review or else questions the contribution, i.e. 'Did you mean to say this?' This is different from checking interpretation when meaning has been ascribed, in that no interpretation is offered. The client's act is preserved, no matter how unintelligible or incomprehensible to the therapist.

Rationale:
It is sometimes difficult or even impossible for the therapist to try out an interpretation of the client's communication act because it is unintelligible or incomprehensible. Reflecting back provides the opportunity for the client to review the original intention and the resulting communication act, and to problem solve and attempt repair as appropriate.

Examples:
The therapist employs technical skills for *checking contribution*, including:
- reflecting back client's communication act (words, sound string, gesture, point, etc.) with a rising intonation/questioning facial expression;
- returning client's drawing, writing, object for approval or rejection with a rising intonation/questioning facial expression;
- soliciting client's clarification by saying 'What do you mean by ...?';
- questioning the accuracy of the client's previous turn or response.

D.2 Differential feedback

Definition:
The therapist provides the client with information about the quality of their contribution or response. This may include using written or graphic feedback with the individual.

Rationale:
Learning and change demands an improving ability to deal with errors (Dockrell and Messer, 1999). Differential feedback is designed to raise the person's awareness of the quality of their own communication acts and to help them to monitor and improve their communication skills.

Examples:
The therapist employs technical skills for providing *differential feedback*, including

- identifying the positive features of the communication act – commenting on the aspects that promoted success in the exchange;
- identifying the points of difficulty or where the quality of the communication act is not so good – commenting on the aspects that impaired the quality and may contribute to breakdown;
- identifying aspects or features that are missing in a communication act – pointing out the significant features in a drawing that are missing and which therefore constrain the interpretation.

D.3 Evaluative feedback

Definition:
The therapist makes qualitative comment on the selection/use of materials, the demands of a communication activity/opportunity, the contextual features or the use of a therapeutic technique in relation to the person's responses.

Rationale:
Evaluative feedback is used to articulate the relative value and demands of the selected aspect of therapy to the client. It provides the means for acknowledging any difficulties or lack of challenge experienced by the person.

Examples:
The therapist employs technical skills for providing evaluative feedback, including:
- making qualitative comments on the materials used – dimensions, features, layout, content;
- making qualitative comments on the demands placed on the person and their experience – 'That was difficult', 'You found that one easy'.

D.4 Summative feedback

Definition:
The therapist summarizes critical aspects of the content, process and context of therapy.

Rationale:
Summative feedback provides the opportunity for recapitulation of learning so that therapeutic principles may be taken forward.

Examples:
The therapist employs technical skills for providing *summative feedback*, including:
- providing a synopsis of the client's responses to one activity immediately, after its close and before the next activity;
- providing a synopsis of the activities carried out and the individual's, responses to them at the end of a session;
- providing a synopsis of the main points of the consultation and highlighting the critical issues to take forward.

D.5 Acknowledging contribution

Definition:
The therapist observes the client and is sensitive to any contributions made or the effort entailed in attempting a task, whether verbal or non verbal.

Rationale:
Communication is a process of mutually co-ordinated social exchange where there are at least two participants who make contributions. The therapy agenda is sufficiently flexible to accommodate initiations made by the client.

Examples:
The therapist employs technical skills for *acknowledging contribution*, including:
• switching from a verbal focus to a non-verbal one on the basis of the client's action, e.g. client offers newspaper for discussion of headline, child offers toy for interaction;
• making a relevant comment or sharing an experience that extends the theme introduced by the client;
• following the individual's initiated behaviour by responding verbally or non-verbally in a way that shows evidence of notice;
• acknowledging the client's effort by commenting, e.g. 'You've really tried hard'.

Category E: Personal maintenance

E.1 Emotional acknowledgement/ support

Definition:
The therapist gives evidence of notice with regard to the individual's emotional state and related expressive behaviours. The type of emotional acknowledgement or support varies according to the way the individual expresses his/her internal state and what is already known about him/her.

Rationale:
The internal psychological state of the participants in an interaction will affect their contributions. Emotional expression may require the therapist to divert from the current focus, in order to support the expressive act of the person before rejoining the agenda.

Examples:
The therapist employs technical skills for providing *emotional acknowledgement/ support*, including:

- acknowledging the pain or sadness of the other person by notice, e.g. 'I can see this is painful for you', 'This is a very difficult time for you';
- providing physical comfort for the person, e.g. tissues for person's tears, touch contact if appropriate;
- offering the person the opportunity to talk further about their feelings or experiences, e.g. 'Do you want to talk about it?';
- diverting from current focus of session by verbal enquiry after person's feelings or experiences, e.g. 'What is it that makes this difficult for you?';
- checking the person's general emotional wellbeing, e.g. 'How do you feel today?'

E.2 Physical and sensory acknowledgement/support

Definition:
The therapist acknowledges the individual's sensory or physical needs and provides support according to the presenting needs of the individual.

Rationale:
The physical and sensory needs of the individual will affect the interaction. The individual may exhibit signs of discomfort or difficulty. The therapist observes the individual and accommodates their needs appropriately.

Examples:
The therapist employs technical skills for providing *physical and sensory acknowledgement/support*, including:
- checking the individual's use of vision and hearing, and any aids that are normally worn/used, e.g. hearing aid, glasses;
- adjustment of physical comfort – adjust client's seated position, enquire after client's level of comfort, provide cushion for back support, offer drink;
- adjustment of sensory comfort – prompt use of glasses or other aid, adjust placement/visual display of materials, check hearing aid, adjust source of light;
- rearranging therapy materials or modifying communication style in response to visual or hearing difficulties displayed by the individual, e.g. moving closer to person's better ear, moving a stimulus into the person's visual field;
- checking the person's level of physical comfort, e.g. fit of dentures, sitting position, body heat, thirst;
- checking the person's level of arousal and general state of health and wellbeing, e.g. fatigue, tiredness, lack of energy, distractibility.

E.3 Behaviour acknowledgement/support

Definition:
The therapist observes and responds to the individual's behavioural needs as appropriate.

Rationale:
The behaviour of the individual may affect his/her ability to contribute to an interaction. In order to support or manage the behaviour of the person, the therapist may need to divert from the activity in focus, and use a behavioural support technique before rejoining the agenda.

Examples:
The therapist employs technical skills for providing *behaviour acknowledgement/support*, including:

- breaking up a particular behavioural pattern by physical intervention, e.g. adjusting the person's seated position, guiding the person's head position, removing an offending item;
- verbally checking the undesirable behaviour, e.g. 'Sit down', 'Let's leave that alone now', 'That's enough now';
- soliciting appropriate action from a significant other in relation to the undesirable behaviour, e.g. asking the mother of a highly distracted child: 'Perhaps he'll sit on your lap?'

Category F: Context maintenance

F.1 Equipment organization/ maintenance

Definition:
The therapist introduces, organizes, sets out or adjusts the materials or other relevant equipment so that they are accessible to the individual.

Rationale:
The equipment used in assessment and therapy activities is only as effective as the way it is used. The therapist focuses on the perspective of the client(s), and orders, manipulates, moves and arranges the materials and other relevant equipment so that it is accessible to them.

Examples:
The therapist employs technical skills for providing *equipment organization/ maintenance*, including:
- arranging a display of materials, e.g. placing objects or pictures in an accessible array;
- moving items into the person's visual and auditory field of operation, e.g. showing a picture around the various members of a group, placing an auditory stimulus closer to a person's better functioning ear.

F.2 Setting organization/ maintenance

Definition:
The therapist organizes the immediate environment so that it is conducive to optimal therapeutic interaction. This is usually in response to observations and knowledge of the client.

Rationale:
The physical space and furnishings may affect how the individual responds to assessment and therapy activities. If the room is too hot or airless it may affect the client's level of arousal. If the room is too dim it may affect the accuracy of the client's visual processing. The therapist focuses on the perspective of the client(s), and moves and organizes the furniture, adjusts the lighting and room temperature, and generally maintains a comfortable space.

Examples:
The therapist employs technical skills for providing *setting organization/ maintenance*, including:
- rearranging the furniture, e.g. adjusting the therapist's chair to establish a better orientation to the client;
- adjusting the lighting or room temperature, e.g. opening a window, closing a door, turning on the light, adjusting the blinds.

Category G: Transaction

G.1 Soliciting information

Definition:
The therapist solicits information that is relevant to the individual's intervention. Questions are posed and verbal probes are used in order to expand the client's information base.

Rationale:
In order to ensure the relevance and timing of intervention activities, the therapist needs to access relevant information about the client and significant others.

Examples:
The therapist employs technical skills for *soliciting information*, including:

- asking questions about lifestyle issues of significance, e.g. occupation, play preferences, care arrangements;
- probing issues to do with possible precipitating and/or maintaining factors concerning the individual's communication difficulties;
- learning about other aspects of the person's functioning (physical/sensory conditions, family background, social/educational/occupational issues, associated medical background, developmental history);
- identifying the person's current needs, the involvement of other professionals and recent or existing interventions.

G.2 Giving information/ advice

Definition:
The therapist gives information and advice that is relevant to the individual's communication difficulties. It includes summarizing the person's communication difficulties or the findings from an assessment activity. Information may be supported by text or graphic representations.

Rationale:
The giving of information and advice is designed to clarify relevant issues and to help the individual to participate in the therapy process.

Examples:
The therapist employs technical skills for *giving information/advice*, including:
- suggesting self-help strategies to the person, e.g. carrying a communication passport to help communicating with unfamiliar others;
- providing helpful advice to the parent of a child, e.g. language stimulation games to be carried out at home;
- outlining a particular technique or procedure that the person will be going through, e.g. what is entailed in the surgical procedure for a complete laryngectomy;
- profiling the individual's communication difficulties so that the person can appreciate the reasons for their difficulties and the relevant implications, e.g. drawing together information from various assessment activities into an integrated profile of the person's communication skills.

5.3 Providing instructions

Definition:
The therapist provides instructions and guidance on how to approach a given task or activity.

Rationale:
In order to meet the demands of a task or activity, the individual needs to understand what is required. The therapist does not take it for granted that the person knows what to do, and therefore provides clear directions and guidance for the individual.

Examples:
The therapist employs technical skills for *giving instructions*, including:

- setting out the rules of a turn-taking game with a child;
- outlining how a person's language skills should be used in relation to a task, e.g. in sentence construction – 'What you must do is select the person, then the verb and then the object.'

G.4 Framing/negotiating

Definition:
The therapist demarcates the scope, structure, timing and content of the session for appraisal with the client. Framing/negotiating is a process that considers the client's views and responses.

Rationale:
The provision of SLT requires an appropriate degree and manner of therapeutic control. Framing/negotiating techniques are used to establish and articulate the goals of therapy, the content of therapy and the mechanisms for change in the therapy process, with reference to individual needs and preferences.

Examples:
The therapist employs technical skills for *framing/negotiating activity*, including:

- providing/negotiating an outline of a session or therapy plan;
- deliberately closing/introducing a task so that the client is prepared;
- deliberate pausing at the change-over point between activities;
- providing general feedback on what has happened during the session, or else on a previous occasion, as a preface or link to the current agenda.

G.5 Explaining/ rationalizing

Definition:
The therapist explains the purpose of assessment or therapy activities. There is the reasoning of activities in terms of content and demands with reference to the individual's communication skills.

Rationale:
The 'why' of therapy is crucial to the engagement of the individual in the therapy process. By providing rationales for therapy activities the therapist is helping the person, as a key agent of change, to understand the basic principles of the therapeutic process.

Examples:
The therapist employs technical skills for *explaining/rationalizing therapy*, including:
- explaining the reasons underlying a particular task, activity or recommended course of action;
- explaining how therapeutic change will occur;
- explaining what has been revealed by the individual's responses to certain activities or assessment schedules;
- negotiating and articulating the demands that will be placed on the client in a new activity or in the change-over between activities.

G.6 Recording

Definition:
The therapist notes the individual's responses to an activity, or completes an entry on a form that provides a record of progress.

Rationale:

There may be times during a session that the therapist needs to record what has been said, how the person has responded and any achievements or difficulties that have been observed.

Examples:

The therapist employs technical skills for *recording* aspects of intervention practice, including:

- narrative record of session as in a diary description;
- operating technology such as an audio or video camera to produce a faithful record of the session;
- completing a checklist that defines the scope of the therapist's observations.

Bibliography

brahamsen AM, Romski MA, Sevcik RA (1989) Concomitants of success in acquiring an augmentative communication system: changes in attention, communication and sociability. American Journal on Mental Retardation 93: 475–96.

budarham S, Hurd A (eds) (2002) Management of Communication Needs in People with a Learning Disability. London: Whurr Publishers Ltd.

cheson D (1998) Independent Inquiry into Inequalities in Health. London: The Stationery Office.

hmad Waqar IU (ed) (2000) Ethnicity, Disability and Chronic Illness. Buckingham: Open University Press.

hmad WIU, Atkin K, Chamba R (2000) Causing havoc among their children: parental and professional perspectives on consanguinity and childhood disability. In WIU Ahmad (ed) Ethnicity, Disability and Chronic Illness. Buckingham: Open University Press, pp. 28–44.

hmad WIU, Darr A, Jones L (2000) 'I send my child to school and he comes back an Englishman': minority ethnic deaf people, identity politics and services. In WIU Ahmad (ed) Ethnicity, Disability and Chronic Illness. Buckingham: Open University Press, pp. 67–84.

li Z, Fazil Q, Bywaters P, Wallace L, Singh G (2001) Disability, ethnicity and childhood: a critical review of research. Disability & Society 16: 949–68.

lm N, Newell AF (1996) Being an interesting conversation partner. In S. von Tetzchner, M. Hygum Jensen (eds) Augmentative and Alternative Communication – European Perspectives. London: Whurr Publishers Ltd. pp. 171–81.

rmstrong L, Jans D, MacDonald A (2000) Parkinson's disease and aided AAC: some evidence from practice. International Journal of Language & Communication Disorders 35: 377–90.

rthur M, Butterfield N, McKinnon DH (1998) Communication intervention for students with severe disability: results of a partner training program. International Journal of Disability, Development and Education 45: 97–113.

tkinson D (1998) The Life Story Interview. London: Sage.

tkinson D (1999) Advocacy: A Review. Brighton: Pavilion with Joseph Rowntree Foundation.

tkinson D (2002) Self-advocacy and research. In B Gray, R Jackson (eds) Advocacy & Learning Disability. London: Jessica Kingsley, pp. 120–36.

tkinson D, McCarthy M, Walmsley J, Cooper M, Rolph S, Aspis S, Barette P, Coventry M, Ferris G (eds) (2000) Good Times, Bad Times: Women with Learning Difficulties Telling their Stories. Kidderminster: BILD.

Atkinson D, Jackson M, Walmsley J (1997) Forgotten Lives – Exploring the History of Learning Disability. Kidderminster: BILD.

Atkinson JM, Heritage J (eds) (1984) Structures of Social Action: Studies in Social Action. Cambridge: Cambridge University Press.

Ayer S, Alaszewski A (1984) Community Care and the Mentally Handicapped – Services for Mothers and their Mentally Handicapped Children. London: Croom Helm.

Baillie D, Strachan VM, Gordon R (2002) The legal context of the advocacy service. In B Gray, R Jackson (eds) Advocacy & Learning Disability. London: Jessica Kingsley, pp. 89–103.

Baker K, Donnelly M (2001) The social experiences of children with disability and the influence of environment: a framework for intervention. Disability & Society 16: 71–85.

Ballard K (1991) Assessment for early intervention: evaluating child development and learning in context. In D Mitchell, RI Brown (eds) Early Intervention Studies for Young Children with Special Needs. London: Chapman Hall, pp 127–59.

Barnes C (1996) Visual impairment and disability. In G Hales (ed) Beyond Disability: Towards an Enabling Society. London: Sage Publications, pp. 36–44

Barnlund DC (1976) The mystication of meaning: doctor–patient encounters Journal of Medical Education 91: 898–902.

Baron RJ (1985) An introduction to medical phenomenology: 'I can't hear you when I'm listening'. Annals of International Medicine 103: 606–11.

Barron K (2001) Autonomy in everyday life, for whom? Disability & Society 16 431–47.

Bartlett C, Bunning K (1997) The importance of communication partnerships: a study to investigate the communicative exchanges between staff and adult with learning disabilities. British Journal of Learning Disabilities 25: 148–153

Basil C, Soro-Camats E (1996) Supporting graphic acquisition by a girl with multiple impairments. In S von Tetzchner, MH Jensen (eds) Augmentative and Alternative Communication: European Perspectives. London: Whurr Publishers Ltd, pp. 270–91.

Basso A, Marangolo P (2000) Cognitive neuropsychological rehabilitation: the emperor's new clothes? Neuropsychological Rehabilitation 10: 219–29.

Bastien J, Cross-cultural communication between doctors and peasants in Bolivia Social Science & Medicine 24: 1109–18.

Baxter C, Poonia K, Ward L, Nadirshaw Z (1990) Double Discrimination: Issue and Services for People with Learning Difficulties from Black and Ethnic Minority Communities. London: Kings Fund and Commission for Racial Equality.

Beazley S, Frost R, Halden J (2001) Working with deaf children. In M Kersner, Wright (eds) Speech and Language Therapy: The Decision Making Process when Working with Children. London: David Fulton Publishers, pp. 163–76.

Becker RE, Heimberg RG, Bellack AS (1987) Social Skills Training for Treatment of Depression. New York: Pergamon.

Beckett C, Wrighton E (2000) 'What matters to me is not what you're talking about' – maintaining the social model of disability in 'public and private' negotiations. Disability & Society 15: 991–9.

Begum N (1992) Something to be Proud of: The Lives of Asian People and Carers in Waltham Forest. London Borough of Waltham Forest: Race Relations and Disability Unit.

Beukelman DR, Mirenda P (1998) Augmentative and Alternative Communication: Management of Severe Communication Disorders in Children and Adults. Baltimore: Paul H. Brookes.

Bhakta P, Katbamna S, Parker G (2000) South Asian carers' experiences of primary health care teams. In Waqar IU Ahmad (ed) Ethnicity, Disability and Chronic Illness. Buckingham: Open University Press, pp. 123–38.

Bhui K (ed) (2002) Racism & Mental Health: Prejudice and Suffering. London: Jessica Kingsley.

Bignall T, Butt J, Pagarani D (2002) Peer support groups and young black and minority ethnic disabled and deaf people. Joseph Rowntree Foundation – Findings: July (762).

Biklen D (1990) Communication unbound: autism and praxis. Harvard Education Review 60: 291.

Bishop DVM (1982) The Test for the Reception of Grammar. Manchester University Press.

Bjorck-Akesson E, Granlund M, Olsson C (1996) Collaborative problem solving in communication intervention. In S von Tetzchner, MH Jensen (eds) Augmentative and Alternative Communication: European Perspectives. London: Whurr, pp. 324–54.

Black People First (1993) Conference Report. London: People First.

Blackstone S (1999) Communication partners: email survey. Augmentative and Alternative Communication 12: 6–7.

Booth S, Swabey D (1999) Group training in communication skills for carers of adults with aphasia. International Journal of Language & Communication Disorders 34: 291–310.

Borland J, Ramcharan P (1997) Empowerment in informal settings: the themes. In P Ramcharan, G Roberts, G Grant, J Borland (eds). Empowerment in Everyday Life: Learning Disability. London: Jessica Kingsley, pp. 88–97.

Bott C, Farmer R, Rohde J (1997) Behaviour problems associated with lack of speech in people with disabilities. Journal of Intellectual Disability Research 41: 3–7.

Bourgeois MS (1992) Evaluating memory wallets in conversations with persons with dementia. Journal of Speech and Hearing Research 35: 1344–57.

Bowen C, Cupples L (1999) Parents and children together (PACT): a collaborative approach to phonological therapy. International Journal of Language & Communication Disorders 34: 35–54.

Boyle M (1999) What's in a name? Not much if it's not well defined. Aphasiology 13: 132–4.

Bradshaw J (1998) Assessing and intervening in the communication environment. British Journal of Learning Disabilities 26: 62–6.

Bradshaw J (2000) A total communication approach: towards meeting the communication needs of people with learning disabilities. Tizard Learning Disability Review 5: 27–30.

Bradshaw J (2002) The management of challenging behaviour within a communication framework. In S Aburdarham, A Hurd (eds) Management of Communication Needs in People with a Learning Disability. London: Whurr Publishers Ltd, pp. 246–75.

Bray M, Ross A, Todd C (1999) Speech and Language Clinical Process and Practice. London: Whurr Publishers Ltd.

Bricker D (1992) The changing nature of communication and language intervention. In SF Warren, J Reichle (eds) Causes and Effects in Communication and Language Intervention. Volume 1. Maryland: Paul H Brookes Publishing Co. Inc, pp. 332–61.

Bronfenbrenner U (1979) The Ecology of Human Development: Experiments by Nature and Design. Cambridge, MA: Harvard University Press.

Brown L (1998) Carer communication – making the change. Speech and Language Therapy in Practice (summer): 4–7.

Brown L (2002) Communication education. RCSLT Bulletin, September: 12–13.

Brown P, Levinson S (1978) Universals in language usage: politeness phenomena. In EN Goody (ed) Questions and Politeness: Strategies in Social Interaction. Cambridge: Cambridge University Press.

Brulle AR, Repp AC (1984) An investigation of the accuracy of momentary time sampling procedures with time series data. British Journal of Psychology 75: 481–5.

Brumfitt S (1999) The Social Psychology of Communication Impairment. London: Whurr Publishers Ltd.

Bruner J (1975) The ontogenesis of speech acts. Journal of Child Language 2: 1–19.

Bryan K, Maxim J (1996) Communication Disability and the Psychiatry of Old Age. London: Whurr Publishers Ltd.

Bryan K, Axelrod L, Maxim J, Bell L, Jordan L (2002) Working with older people with communication difficulties: an evaluation of care worker training. Aging & Mental Health 6: 248–54.

Buckley S, Emslie M, Haslegrave G, LeProvost P (1993) The Development of Language and Reading Skills in Children with Down's Syndrome. Portsmouth: University of Portsmouth.

Bunning K (1996) Development of an Individualised Sensory Environment for Adults with Learning Disabilities and an Evaluation of its Effects on the Interactive Behaviours. Unpublished thesis, City University, London.

Bunning K (1997) The role of sensory reinforcement in developing interaction. In M Fawcus (ed) Children with Learning Difficulties: A Collaborative Approach. London: Whurr Publishers Ltd, pp. 97–129.

Bunning K (2002) Communication profiling: capturing interactions between carer and client. Paper presented at the Inaugural Conference of IASSID Europe 12–15 June, Dublin: Eire.

Bunning K, Grove N (2002) Making connections: understanding and promoting communication. In S Carnaby (ed) Learning Disability Today. Brighton: Pavilion Publishing, pp. 83–94.

Button G, Casey N (1984) Generating topic: the use of topic initial elicitors. In J Atkinson, J Heritage (eds) Structures of Social Action: Studies in Social Action. Cambridge: Cambridge University Press, pp. 167–90.

Byng S (1995) What is aphasia therapy? In C Code, D Muller (eds) Treatment of Aphasia: From Theory to Practice. London: Whurr Publishers Ltd, pp. 3–17.

Byng S, Black M (1995) What makes a therapy? Some parameters of therapeutic intervention in aphasia. European Journal of Disorders of Communication 30: 303–16.

Byng S, Cairns D, Duchan J (2002) Values in practice and practising values. Journal of Communication Disorders 35: 89–106.

Byng S, Pound C, Parr S (2000) Living with aphasia: a framework for therapy interventions. In I Papathanasiou (ed) Acquired Neurogenic Communication Disorders: A Clinical Perspective. London: Whurr Publishers Ltd, pp. 49–75.

Byng S, Swinburn K, Pound C (eds) (1999) The Aphasia Therapy File. Hove: Psychology Press.

Byng S, van der Gaag A, Parr S (1998) International initiatives in outcomes measurement: a perspective from the United Kingdom. In C Frattali (ed) Measuring Outcomes in Speech–Language Pathology. New York: Thieme Medical Publishers, pp. 558–78.

Byrne EA, Cunningham CC, Sloper P (1988) Families and their Children with Down's Syndrome: One feature in common. London: Routledge.

Calculator SN, Bedrosian JL (eds) (1988) Communication Assessment and Intervention for Adults with Mental Retardation. London: Taylor Francis.

Calkins MP (2001) The physical and social environment of the person with Alzheimer's disease. Aging & Mental Health 5 (Supplement 1): S74–8.

Campbell J (2002) Valuing diversity: the disability agenda – we've only just begun. Disability & Society 17: 471–8.

Campbell J, Oliver M (1996) Disability Politics: Understanding Our Past, Changing Our Future. London: Routledge.

Casserley C The disability discrimination act: an overview in J Cooper (ed) (2000) Law, Rights & Disability. London: Jessica Kingsley, pp. 139–64.

Chamba R, Ahmad WIU (2000) Language, communication and information: the needs of parents caring for a disabled child. In Waqar IU Ahmad (ed) Ethnicity, Disability and Chronic Illness. Buckingham: Open University Press, pp. 85–102.

Chamba R, Ahmad WIU, Jones L (1998) Improving Services for Asian Deaf Children – Parents' and Professionals' Perspectives. York: Joseph Rowntree Foundation.

Chamberlain L, Chung MC, Jenner L (1993) Preliminary findings on communication and challenging behaviour in learning difficulty. British Journal of Developmental Disabilities XXXIX, Part 2, 77: 118–25.

Charmaz K (1995) The body, identity, and self: adapting to impairment. Sociological Quarterly 36: 657–80.

Charness N, Holley P (2001) Human factors and environmental support in Alzheimer's disease. Aging & Mental Health 5 (Supplement 1): 65–73.

Chiat S, Law J, Marshall J (eds) (1997) Language Disorders in Children and Adults. London: Whurr Publishers Ltd.

Clark C (ed) (2001) Adult Day Services and Social Inclusion: Better Days. London: Jessica Kingsley.

Clement T (2002) Exploring the role of values in the management of advocacy schemes. In B Gray, R Jackson (eds) Advocacy & Learning Disability. London: Jessica Kingsley, pp. 50–71.

Cockerill H, Fuller P (2001) Assessing children for augmentative and alternative communication. In H Cockerill, L Carroll-Few (eds) Communication Without Speech: Practical Augmentative & Alternative Communication. London: MacKeith Press, pp. 73–87.

Cogher L (1999) The use of non-directive play in speech and language therapy. Child Language Teaching and Therapy 15: 7–15.

Coll X, Child B (2002) Please don't let me be misunderstood: importance of acknowledging racial and cultural difference. In K Bhui (ed) Racism and Mental Health – Prejudice and Suffering. London: Jessica Kingsley, pp. 129–38.

Commission for Racial Equality (1997a) CRE Factsheet: Employment and Unemployment. London: CRE.

Commission for Racial Equality (1997b) CRE Factsheet: Criminal Justice in England and Wales. London: CRE.

Connect – the Communication Disability Network (www.connect.org).

Cooper J (ed) (2000) Law, Rights & Disability. London: Jessica Kingsley.

Corker M (1993)Integration and deaf people: the policy and power of enabling environments. In J Swain, V Finkelstein, S French, M Oliver (eds) Disabling Barriers, Enabling Environments. London: Open University Press and Sage Publications, pp. 145–54.

Corker M, French S (eds) (1999) Disability Discourse. Buckingham: Philadelphia Press.

Coupe O'Kane J, Goldbart J (1998) Communication Before Speech – Development and Assessment. London: David Fulton.

Cramp DG, Carson ER (1985) The patient/clinician relationship, computing and wider healthcare system. In ER Carson, DG Cramp (eds) Computers and Control in Clinical Medicine. New York: Plenum Press, pp. 245–55.

Crossley R (1997) Remediation of communication problems through facilitated communication training: a case study. European Journal of Disorders of Communication 32: 61–88.

Crossley R, Remington-Gurney J (1992) Getting the words out: Facilitated Communication Training. Topics in Language Disorders 12: 29.

Crutchley A (2000) Bilingual children in language units: does having 'well informed' parents make a difference? International Journal of Language & Communication Disorders 35: 65–82.

Cuckle P, Wilson J (2002) Social relationships and friendships among young people with Down's syndrome in secondary schools. British Journal of Special Education 29: 66–71.

Cullen C (1988) A review of staff training: the emperor's old clothes. Irish Journal of Psychology 9: 309–23.

Cummins K, Hulme S (2001) Managing pre-school children in community clinics. In M Kersner, J Wright (eds) Speech and Language Therapy: The Decision Making Process when Working with Children. London: David Fulton Publishers, pp. 53–62.

Cunningham CC, Davis H (1985) Working with Parents: Frameworks for Collaboration. London: Open University Press.

Cunningham CC Glenn SM (1985) Parent involvement and intervention. In I Lane, B Stratford (eds) Current Approaches to Down's Syndrome. Eastbourne: Holt, Rinehart and Winston.

Cunningham CC, Morgan PA, McGucken RB (1984) Down's syndrome: is dissatisfaction with disclosure of diagnosis inevitable? Developmental Medicine and Child Neurology 26: 33–9.

Daker-White G, Beattie AM, Gilliard J, Means R (2002) Minority ethnic groups in dementia care: a review of service needs, service provision and models of good practice. Aging & Mental Health 6: 101–8.

Dalrymple J, Burke B (1995) Anti-Oppressive Practice: Social Care and The Law. Buckingham: The Open University Press.

Daniels H, Sandow S (1987) Backlash: will circular 6186 frustrate the 1981 Act. British Journal of Special Education 14: 10.

Datlow-Smith M, Haas P, Belcher R (1994) Facilitated communication: the effect of facilitator knowledge and level of assistance on output. Journal of Autism and Developmental Disabilities 24: 357–67.

Davies P, van der Gaag A (1992) The professional competence of speech therapists. III: skills and skill mix possibilities. Clinical Rehabilitation 6: 311–23.

Davis JM, Watson N (2001) Where are the children's experiences? Analysing social and cultural exclusion in 'special' and 'mainstream' schools. Disability & Society 16: 671–87.

Department for Education and Employment (DfEE) (1994) Code of Practice on the Identification and Assessment of Special Needs. London: HMSO.

Department for Education and Employment (DfEE) (1997) Excellence for all children. London: Stationery Office.

Department for Education and Employment (DfEE) (1998) Human Rights Act. London: HMSO.

Department for Education and Employment (DfEE) (2000) Provision of SALT Services to Children with Special Needs (England) Report of the Working Group. London: Stationery Office.

Department for Education, Employment and Skills (DfES) (2001) Special Educational Needs and Disability Rights Act. London: Stationery Office.

Department for Education and Skills (DfES) (1995) Disability Discrimination Act. London: Stationery Office.

Department of Health (DoH) (1989) Caring for People. Community Care in the Next Decade and Beyond. London: HMSO.

Department of Health (DoH) (1999) Reform of the Mental Health Act 1983. Proposals for consultation. London: Department of Health Publications.

Department of Health (DoH) (2000) A Quality Strategy for Social Care. London: Stationery Office.

Department of Health (2001a) The National Service Framework for Older People. London: Stationery Office.

Department of Health (2001b) Valuing People: A New Strategy for Learning Disability in the 21st Century. London: Department of Health Publications.

Department of Health (2001c) Involving Patients and the Public in Healthcare: A Discussion Document. September, London: HMSO.

Department of Health (2001d) The NHS Plan – creating a 21st century health service. London: Department of Health Publications.

Department of Health and Social Security (DHSS) (1980) Mental Handicap: Progress, Problems and Priorities. A review of mental handicap services in England since the 1971 White Paper 'Better services for the mentally handicapped'. London: HMSO.

Department of Health, Social Services Inspectorate (1998) Disabled Children: Directions for their Future Care. London: HMSO.

Desrochers MN, Hile MG, Williams-Moseley TL (1997) Survey of functional analysis procedures used with individuals who display mental retardation and severe problem behaviors. American Journal on Mental Retardation 101: 535–46.

Deutsch T, Carson E, Ludwig E (1994) Dealing with Medical Knowledge – Computers in Clinical Decision Making. London: Plenum Press.

DiLillo A, Neimeyer RA, Manning WH (2002) A personal construct psychology view of relapse: indications for a narrative therapy component to stuttering treatment. Journal of Fluency Disorders 27: 19–42.

Disability Rights Task Force (1999) From Exclusion to Inclusion: Final Report. December: 1–40.

Dobson S (2001) When effectiveness is hard to prove. Speech & Language Therapy in Practice, Winter: 4–6.

Dobson S (2002) Using an interdisciplinary approach to training to develop the quality of communication with adults with profound learning disabilities by care staff. International Journal of Language & Communication Disorders 37: 41–58.

Dockrell J, Messer D (1999) Children's Language and Communication Difficulties: Understanding, Identification and Intervention. London: Continuum.

Dodd B (1995) Differential Diagnosis and Treatment of Children with Speech Disorders. London: Whurr Publishers Ltd.

Dodd B, Bradford A (2000) A comparison of three therapy methods for children with different types of phonological disorder. International Journal of Language & Communication Disorders 35: 189–210.

Dowling M, Dolan L (2001). Families with children with disabilities – inequalities and the social model. Disability & Society 16: 21–35.

Dowson S (1997) Empowerment within services – a comfortable delusion. In P Ramcharan, G Roberts, G Grant, J Borland (eds) Empowerment in Everyday Life – Learning Disability. London: Jessica Kingsley, pp. 101–20.

Duchan J (2000) Impairment and social views of speech–language pathology clinical practice re-examined. Advances in Speech–Language Pathology 3: 37–45.

Dundas R, Morgan M, Redfern J, Lemic-Stojcevic N, Wolfe C (2001) Ethnic differences in behavioural risk factors for stroke: implications for health promotion. Ethnicity & Health 6: 95–103.

Dunn LM, Whetton C, Pintillie O (1982) The British Picture Vocabulary Scales. Windsor: NFER-Nelson.

Dunnet CP, MacKenzie K, Robinson K, Sellars GC, Wilson JA (1997) Voice therapy for dysphonia – still more art than science? European Journal of Disorders of Communication 32: 333–44.

Edmundson A, McIntosh J (1995) Cognitive and neuropsychological approaches. In C Code, D Muller (eds) Treatment of Aphasia: From Theory to Practice. London: Whurr Publishers Ltd, pp. 137–63.

Emerson E (1995) Challenging Behaviour: Analysis and Intervention in People with Learning Difficulties. Cambridge: Cambridge University Press.

Emerson E, McGill P, Mansell J (1994) Severe Learning Disabilities and Challenging Behaviours: Designing High Quality Services. London: Chapman & Hall.

Enderby P (1992) Outcomes measures in speech therapy: impairment, disability, handicap and distress. Health Trends 24: 61–64.

Enderby P, Emerson J (1995) Does Speech and Language Therapy Work? London: Whurr Publishers Ltd.

Enderby P, John A (1997) Therapy Outcomes Measures for Speech and Language Therapists. San Diego: Singular Press.

Enderby PM, John A (1999) Therapy outcome measures in speech and language therapy: comparing performance between providers. International Journal of Language & Communication Disorders 34: 417–30.

Fazil Q, Bywaters P, Ali Z, Wallace L, Singh G (2002) Disadvantage and discrimination compounded: the experience of Pakistani and Bangladeshi parents of disabled children in the UK. Disability & Society 17(3): 237–53.

Felce D (1993) Ordinary housing: a necessary context for meeting service philosophy and providing an effective therapeutic environment. In RSP Jones, C

Eayrs (eds) Challenging Behaviour and Intellectual Disability: A Psychological Perspective. Kidderminster: BILD, pp. 121–147.

Ferguson A (1999) Clinical forum: Learning in aphasia therapy: it's not so much what you do as how you do it! Aphasiology 13(2): 125–50.

Ferns P (1992) Promoting race equality through normalisation. In H Brown, H Smith (eds) Normalisation: a Reader for the Nineties. London: Routledge.

Fey ME, Proctor-Williams K (2001) Recasting, elicited imitation and modelling in grammar intervention for children with specific language impairments. In DVM Bishop, LB Leonard (eds) Speech and Language Impairments in Children: Causes, Characteristics, Intervention and Outcome. Hove: Psychology Press Ltd, pp. 177–94.

Finkelstein V, French S (1993) Towards a psychology of disability. In J Swain, V Finkelstein, S French, M Oliver (eds) Disabling Barriers, Enabling Environments. Open University Press and Sage Publications, pp. 26–33.

Fishman S, Timler G, Yoder D (1985) Strategies, prevention and repair of communication breakdown in conversations with communication board users. Augmentative and Alternative Communication 1: 38–51.

Fogel A (1993) Two principles of communication: co-regulation and framing. In J Nadel, L Camaioni (eds) New Perspectives in Communication Development. London: Routledge, pp. 9–22.

Frattali C (1998a) Outcomes measurement: definitions, dimensions, and perspectives. In C Frattali (ed) Measuring Outcomes in Speech–Language Pathology. New York, NY: Thieme Medical Publishers, pp. 1–27.

Frattali C (1998b) Measuring modality-specific behaviours, functional abilities, and quality of life. In C Frattali (ed) Measuring Outcomes in Speech–Language Pathology. New York, NY: Thieme Medical Publishers, pp. 55–88.

Frazier-Norbury C, Chiat S (2000) Semantic intervention to support word recognition: a single case study. Child Language Teaching and Therapy 16: 141–63.

French S (1994) On Equal Terms: Working with Disabled People. Oxford: Butterworth: Heinemann.

French S (1996) The attitudes of health professionals towards disabled people. In G Hales (ed) Beyond Disability – Towards an Enabling Society. London: Sage Publications.

French Gilson S, Depoy E (2000) Multiculturalism and disability: a critical perspective. Disability & Society 15(2): 207–18.

Garner P, Sandow S (eds) (1995) Advocacy, Self-Advocacy and Special Needs, London: David Fulton.

Gascoigne M (2001) Managing children with communication problems in mainstream schools and units. In M Kersner, JA Wright (eds) Speech and Language Therapy: The Decision Making Process when Working with Children. London: David Fulton, pp. 63–78.

Gerard KA, Carson ER (1990) The decision-making process in child language assessment. British Journal of Disorders of Communication 25: 61–75.

Gersch IS, Gersch B (1995) Supporting advocacy and self-advocacy: the role of the allied professions. In P Garner, S Sandow (eds) Advocacy, Self-Advocacy and Special Needs. London: David Fulton, pp. 126–52.

Gibbs Levitz B, Schwartz AA (1995) Linking parents with parents: the family connection casebook of best practices. In L Nadel, D Rosenthal (eds) Down Syndrome – Living and Learning in the Community. Chichester: John Wiley, pp. 84–90.

Goble C (2002) Professional consciousness and conflict in advocacy. In B Gray, R Jackson (eds) Advocacy and Learning Disability. London: Jessica Kingsley, pp 72–88.

Goffman E (1955) On face work. Psychiatry 18: 213–31.

Goldbart J (1996) Reading the communication of people who are non-verbal issues of interpretation. Paper presented at a seminar on Interpreting the Communication of People who are Non-Verbal: Issues of Validation. London University Institute of Education, 17 May.

Golding E (1989) Middlesex Elderly Assessment of Mental State. Bury St Edmunds: Thames Valley Test Company.

Gompertz J (1997) Developing communication: early intervention and augmentative signing from birth to five years. In M Fawcus (ed) Children with Learning Difficulties: A Collaborative Approach to their Education. London: Whurr Publishers Ltd, pp. 64–96.

Goodley D (1996) Tales of hidden lives: a critical examination of life history research with people who have learning disabilities. Disability & Society 11(3): 333–48.

Goodley D (2000) Self-advocacy in the Lives of People with Learning Difficulties. Buckingham: Open University Press.

Goodley D, Rapley M (2001) How do you understand learning difficulties Towards a social theory of impairment. American Journal on Mental Retardation 39: 229–32.

Goodwin C (1981) Conversational Organisation: Interaction Between Speaker and Hearers. New York: Academic Press.

Gordon JK (1999) Can learning theory teach us about aphasia therapy Aphasiology 13: 134–9.

Granlund M, Bjorck-Akesson E, Olsson C, Rydeman B (2001) Working with families to introduce augmentative and alternative communication systems. In J Cockerill, L Carroll-Few (eds) Communication Without Speech: Practical Augmentative and Alternative Communication. London: MacKeith Press, pp. 88–102.

Gray B, Jackson R (eds) (2002) Advocacy and Learning Disability. London: Jessica Kingsley.

Gray B, Ridden G (1999) Lifemaps of People with Learning Disabilities. London: Jessica Kingsley.

Greenbaum C, Auerbach J (1998) The environment of the child with mental retardation: risk, vulnerability and resilience. In J Burack, R Hodapp, E Zigler (eds) Handbook of mental retardation and development, pp. 583–605.

Griffiths M (1994) Transition to Adulthood: The Role of Education for Young People with Severe Learning Difficulties. London: David Fulton.

Grove N (1998) Literature For All. London: David Fulton.

Grove N, Peacey N (1999) Teaching subjects to pupils with profound and multiple learning difficulties – considerations for the new framework. British Journal of Special Education 26: 83–6.

Grove N, Bunning K, Porter J (2001) Interpreting the meaning of behavior by people with intellectual disabilities: theoretical and methodological issues. In Columbus (ed) Advances in Psychology Research, Volume 7. New York: Nova Sciences Publishers, Inc, pp. 87–126.

Grove N, Bunning K, Porter J, Olsson C (1999) See what I mean: Interpreting the meaning of communication by people with severe and profound intellectual disabilities. Journal of Applied Research in Intellectual Disabilities 12: 190–203.

Grove N, Bunning K, Porter J, Morgan M (2000) See What I Mean: Guidelines to Aid Understanding of Communication by People with Severe and Profound Learning Disabilities. Kidderminster: BILD & Mencap.

Hales G (ed) (1996) Beyond Disability: Towards an Enabling Society. London: Sage Publications.

Halliday S, Leslie JC (1986) A longitudinal semi-cross-sectional study of the development of mother–child interaction. British Journal of Developmental Psychology 4: 211–22.

Hamilton BL, Snell ME (1993) Using the milieu approach to increase spontaneous communication book use across environments by an adolescent with autism. Augmentative and Alternative Communication 9: 259–72.

Hanley-Maxwell C, Whitney-Thomas J, Mayfield Pogoloff S (1995) The second shock: a qualitative study of parents' perspectives and needs during their child's transition from school to adult life. Journal of the Association of Persons with Severe Handicaps 20: 3–15.

Harding A, Cheasman C, Logan J (2002) On being your own person. Winter/Spring Issue, Speaking Out (www.stammering.org)

Hargie O (ed) (1997) The Handbook of Communication Skills (2nd edn). London: Routledge.

Hargie O, Saunders C, Dickson D (1994) Social Skills in Interpersonal Communication (2nd edn). London: Routledge.

Harris M (1992) Language Experience and Early Language Development – From Input to Uptake. Hove: Lawrence Erlbaum.

Harris SJ (2001) Self-advocacy for people who stammer. RCSLT Bulletin, Issue 596: 12–14.

Harris-Cooksley R, Catt R (1995) Classroom strategies for teacher and pupil support. In P Garner, S Sandow (eds) Advocacy, Self-Advocacy and Special Needs. London: David Fulton Publishers, pp. 43–65.

Harter S (1999) The Construction of Self: A Developmental Perspective. London: The Guildford Press.

Hastings RP, Remington B (1994) Staff behaviour and its implication for people with learning disabilities and challenging behaviours. British Journal of Clinical Psychology 33: 423–38.

Hayes A (1998) Families and disabilities: another facet of inclusion. In A Ashman, J Elkins (eds) Educating Children with Special Needs (3rd edn). Sydney: Prentice Hall, pp. 611–20.

Health of the Nation (1991) A consultative document for health in England. London: HMSO.

Heath C (1984) Talk and recipiency: sequential organization in speech and body movement. In JM Atkinson and J Heritage (eds) Structures of Social Action: Studies in Social Action. Cambridge: Cambridge University Press, pp. 247–65.

Herbert M (1998) Clinical Child Psychology: Social Learning, Development and Behaviour (2nd edn). Chichester: John Wiley.

Hickman J (2002) Issues of service delivery and auditing. In S Aburdarham, A Hurd (eds) Management of Communication Needs in People with a Learning Disability. London: Whurr Publishers Ltd, pp. 1–32.

Higgs J (1992) Developing clinical reasoning competencies. Physiotherapy 78: 575–81.

Hill M (1994) Getting things right. Community Care Inside, 31 March.

Hitchings A, Spence R (1991) The Personal Communication Plan for People with a Learning Disability. Windsor: NFER-Nelson.

Hogan A (1999) Carving out a space to act: acquired impairment and contested identity. In M Corker, S French (eds) Disability Discourse. Buckingham Philadelphia Press, pp. 79–91.

Holland A (1991) Pragmatic aspects of intervention in aphasia. Journal of Neurolinguistics 6: 197–211.

Holland A (1998) Why can't clinicians talk to aphasic adults? Comments on supported conversation for adults with aphasia: methods and resources for training conversational partners. Aphasiology 12: 844–7.

Holland A, Thompson CK (1998) Outcomes measurement in aphasia. In C Frattali (ed) Measuring Outcomes in Speech–Language Pathology. New York, NY Thieme Medical Publishers, pp. 245–66.

Holloway S (2001) The experience of higher education from the perspective of disabled students. Disability & Society 16: 597–615.

Holman A with Bewley C (1999) Funding Freedom 2000: People with Learning Difficulties Using Direct Payments. London: Values into Action.

Honey P, Mumford A (1992) The Manual of Learning Styles. Peter Honey.

Hopper T, Holland A, Rewega M (2002) Conversational coaching: treatment outcomes and future directions. Aphasiology 16: 745–61.

Hornby G (1991) Parent involvement, in D Mitchell and RI Brown (eds) (1991) Early Intervention Studies for Young Children with Special Needs. London Chapman and Hall, pp. 206–24.

Horowitz F, Haritos C (1998) The organism and the environment: implications for understanding mental retardation. In J Burack, R Hodapp, E Zigler (eds) Handbook of Mental Retardation and Development, pp. 20–40.

Horton S, Byng S (2000) Examining interaction in language therapy. International Journal of Language & Communication Disorders 35: 355–75.

Howard D (1999) Clinical forum: Learning theory is not enough. Aphasiology 13: 140–43.

Howard D, Hatfield FM (1987) Aphasia Therapy: Historical and Contemporary Issues. Hove: Lawrence Erlbaum.

Howard D, Patterson K, Franklin S, Orchard-Lisle V, Morton J (1985) The facilitation of picture naming in aphasia. Cognitive Neuropsychology 2: 49–80.

Hulme S, Rahman-Jennings Z, Thomas D (2001) Alternative methods. RCSLT Bulletin, August: 10–12.

Hunt J (1999) Drawing on the semantic system: the use of drawing as a therapy medium. In S Byng, K Swinburn and C Pound (eds) The Aphasia Therapy File Hove: Psychology Press, pp. 41–60.

Hunter S, Tyne A (2001) Advocacy in a cold climate: a review of some citizen advocacy schemes in the context of long-stay hospital closures. Disability & Society 16: 549–61.

Hurd A (1995) The influence of signing on adult/child interaction in a teaching context. Child Language, Teaching and Therapy 11: 319–30.

Hussain Y, Atkin K, Ahmad W (2002) South Asian Young Disabled People and their Families. Joseph Rowntree Foundation Findings, July: (742).

Hutchby I, Wooffitt R (1998) Conversation Analysis: Principles, Practices and Applications. Cambridge: Polity Press.

Jackson RN (1988) Perils of 'pseudo-normalisation'. Mental Handicap 16: 148–50.

Johansson I (1994) Language Development in Children with Special Needs – Performative Communication. Translated by E Thomas. London: Jessica Kingsley.

Johnson JA, Pring T (1990) Speech therapy and Parkinson's disease: a review and further data. British Journal of Disorders of Communication 25: 183–94.

Jones EV, Byng S (1989) The practice of aphasia therapy: an opinion. CSLT Bulletin 449: 2–4.

Jones J (2000) The total communication approach: towards meeting the communication needs of people with learning disabilities. Tizard Learning Disability Review 5: 20–26.

Jones J (2001) The communication gap – a paper exploring the fundamental nature of communication in achieving the 'New Vision' of the White Paper 'Valuing People' (www.learningdisabilities.org.uk)

Jones J, Turner J, Heard A (1992) Making communication a priority. CSLT Bulletin 478: 6–7.

Jones L, Atkin K, Ahmad WIU (2001) Supporting Asian deaf young people and their families: the role of professionals and services. Disability & Society 16: 51–70.

Jones S (1990) Intecom. Windsor: NFER-Nelson.

Jordan L, Kaiser W (1996) Aphasia – A social Approach. London: Chapman & Hall.

Kagan A (1995) Revealing the competence of aphasic adults through conversation: a challenge to health professionals. Topics in Stroke Rehabilitation 2: 15–28.

Kagan A (1998) Supported conversation for adults with aphasia: methods and resources for training conversation partners. Aphasiology 12: 817–30.

Kagan A, Gailey GF (1993) Functional is not enough: training conversation partners for aphasic adults. In AL Holland, MF Forbes (eds) Aphasia Treatment World Perspectives. California: Singular Publishing Group, pp. 199–226.

Kagan A, LeBlanc K (2002) Motivating for infrastructure change: toward a communicatively accessible, participation-based stroke care system for all those affected by aphasia. Journal of Communication Disorders 35: 153–69.

Kagan A, Winckel J, Schumway E (1996) Pictographic Resources Manual. Toronto: North York Aphasia Centre.

Katbamna S, Bhakta P, Parker G (2000) Perceptions of disability and care-giving relationships. In WIU Ahmad (ed) Ethnicity, Disability and Chronic Illness. Buckingham: Open University Press, pp. 12–27.

Katz RC, Hallowell B, Code C, Armstrong E, Roberts P, Pound C, Katz L (2000) A multinational comparison of aphasia management practices. International Journal of Language and Communication Disorders 35: 303–14.

Kay J, Lesser R, Coltheart M (1992) Psycholinguistic Assessments of Language Processing in Aphasia. London: Lawrence Erlbaum.

Kelly A (1996) Talkabout: A Social Communication Skills Package. Oxford: Winslow Press Ltd.

Kelly A (2000) Working with Adults with a Learning Disability. Oxon: Speechmark Publishing Ltd.

Kelly G (1963) A Theory of Personality: The Psychology of Personal Constructs. New York: Norton.

Kendrick M (2002) Integrity and advocacy. In B Gray, R Jackson (eds) Advocacy and Learning Disability. London: Jessica Kingsley, pp. 189–205.

Kenworthy J, Whittaker J (2000) Anything to declare? The struggle for inclusive education and children's rights. Disability & Society 15: 219–31.

Kersner M (2001) The decision-making process in speech and language therapy. In M Kersner, J Wright (eds) Speech and Language Therapy: The Decision Making Process when Working with Children. London: David Fulton Publishers, pp. 3–11.

Kersner M, Wright J (eds) (2001) Speech and Language Therapy: The Decision Making Process when Working with Children. London: David Fulton Publishers

Kolb D (1984) Experiential Learning: Experience as the Source of Learning and Development. Englewood Cliffs NJ: Prentice Hall.

Kraat AW (1987) Communication Interaction Between Aided and Natural Speakers: A State of the Art Report. Toronto: Canadian Rehabilitation Council for the Disabled.

Lantsbury M (2001) Crossing the culture barriers. RCSLT Bulletin, September: 7

Launonen K (1996) Enhancing communication skills of children with Down syndrome: early use of manual signs. In S von Tetzchner, MH Jensen (eds) Augmentative and Alternative Communication: European Perspectives London: Whurr Publishers Ltd, pp. 213–31.

Lasker JP, Bedrosian JL (2000) Acceptance of AAC by adults with acquired disorders. In D Beukelman, K Yorkston, J Reichle (eds) Augmentative Communication for Adults with Neurogenic and Neuromuscular Disabilities Baltimore: Paul H Brookes, pp. 107–36.

Lasker JP, Bedrosian JL (2001) Promoting acceptance of augmentative and alternative communication by adults with acquired communication disorder Augmentative and Alternative Communication 17: 141–53.

Law J (1997) Evaluating intervention for language impaired children: a review of the literature. European Journal of Disorders of Communication 32: 1–14.

Law J (2000) Developmental language disorders: the preschool years. In Rinaldi (ed) Language Difficulties in an Educational Context. London: Whurr Publishers Ltd, pp. 22–40.

Law J, Lindsay G, Peacey N, Gascoigne M, Soloff N, Radford J, Band S, Fitzgerald L (2000) Provision for Children with Speech and Language Needs in England and Wales: Facilitating Communication between Education and Health Services. Nottingham: DfEE Publications.

Law J, Lindsay G, Peacey N, Gascoigne M, Soloff N, Radford J, Band S (2002) Consultation as a model for providing speech and language therapy in school: a panacea or one step too far? Child Language Teaching and Therapy 18: 145–6

Law J, Byng S, Bunning K, Farrelly S, Heyman B, Bryars R (2003) Making sense primary care. Project report to NHS Executive, London.

Lawson R, Fawcus M (1999) Increasing effective communication using a total communication approach. In S Byng, K Swinburn, C Pound, (eds) The Aphasia Therapy File. Hove: Psychology Press, pp. 61–71.

Le Provost P (1993) The use of signing to encourage first words. In S Buckley, Emslie, G Haslegrave, P Le Provost (eds) The Development of Language and Reading Skills in Children with Down's Syndrome. Portsmouth: University Portsmouth, pp. 29–37.

ees J (2002) Crossing the cultural divide. RCSLT Bulletin, October: 11–12.

eonard L (1981) Facilitating linguistic skills in children with specific language impairment. Applied Psycholinguistics 2: 89–148.

esser R, Perkins L (1999) Cognitive Neuropsychology and Conversation Analysis: An Introductory Casebook. London: Whurr Publishers Ltd.

etts C (2001) Multicultural issues in assessment and management. In M Kersner, JA Wright (eds) Speech and Language Therapy: The Decision Making Process when Working with Children. London: David Fulton, pp. 177–87.

eudar I (1989) Communicative environments for mentally handicapped people. In M Beveridge, G Conti-Ramsden, I Leudar (eds) Language and Communication with People with Learning Disabilities. London: Routledge.

évesque L, Gendron C, Vézina J, Hébert R, Ducharme F, Lavoie JP, Gendrom M, Voyer L, Préville M (2002) The process of a group intervention for caregivers of demented persons living at home: conceptual framework, components and characteristics. Ageing & Mental Health 6: 239–47.

ight J (1989) Towards a definition of communicative competence for individuals using augmentative and alternative communication systems. Augmentative and Alternative Communication 5: 137–44.

ight J, Collier B, Parnes P (1985) Communication interaction between young non-speaking physically disabled children and their primary caregivers: Part 1 – Discourse patterns. Augmentative and Alternative Communication 1: 125–34.

indsay G, Dockrell J (2002) Meeting the needs of children with speech language and communication needs: a critical perspective on inclusion and collaboration. Child Language Teaching and Therapy 3: 91–101.

indsay G, Dockrell J, Letchford B, Mackie C (2002) Self-esteem of children with specific speech and language difficulties. Child Language Teaching and Therapy 18: 125–43.

ingard T (2001) Does the Code of Practice help secondary school SENCos to improve learning? British Journal of Special Education 28: 187–90.

ivneh H (1991) A unified approach to existing models of adaptation to disability: a model of adaptation. In RP Martinelli and AE Dell Orto (eds) Psychological and Social Impact of Disability. New York: Springer.

ord S (2002) Recipe for conversation. RCSLT Bulletin 602: 10–11.

ourenco L, Faias J, Afonsoo R, Moreira A, Ferreira JM (1996) Improving communication and language skills of children with developmental disorders: family involvement in graphic language intervention. In S von Tetzchner, MH Jensen (eds) Augmentative and Alternative Communication: European Perspectives. London: Whurr Publishers Ltd, pp. 309–23.

ucas PJ, Lucas AM (1980) Down's syndrome: Telling the parents. British Journal of Mental Subnormality 26: 21–31.

udlow BL, Herr SS (1988) Advocacy and rights to habituation. In Ludlow BL, Turnbull AP, Luckasson R (eds) Transition to Adult Life for People with Mental Retardation: Principles and Practices. Baltimore: Paul H Brookes.

und NJ, Duchan JF (1988) Assessing Children's Language in Naturalistic Contexts (2nd edn). Englewood Cliffs: Prentice Hall.

yon JG (1995) Drawing: its value as a communication aid for adults with aphasia. Aphasiology 9: 33–50, 84–94.

Lyon JG, Cariski D, Keisler L, Rosenbek J, Levine R, Kumpula J, Ryff C, Coyne S, Levine J, (1997) Communication partners: enhancing participation in life and communication for adults with aphasia in natural settings. Aphasiology 11: 693–708.

MacMillan L, Bunning K, Pring T (2000) The development and evaluation of a deaf awareness training course for support staff. Journal of Applied Research in Intellectual Disabilities 13: 283–91.

Maneta A, Marshall J, Lindsay J (2001) Direct and indirect therapy for word sound deafness. International Journal of Language & Communication Disorders 36: 91–106.

Manolson A (1983) It Takes Two to Talk. Toronto: Hanen Early Language Resource Centre.

Marks D (1999) Disability: Controversial Debates and Psychosocial Perspectives. London: Routledge.

Marshall J, Chiat S, Pring T (1997) An impairment in processing verbs' thematic roles: a therapy study. Aphasiology 11: 855–76.

Martin P, Bateson P (1986) Measuring Behaviour – An Introductory Guide. Cambridge: Cambridge University Press.

Martinsen H, von Tetzchner S (1996) Situating augmentative and alternative communication. In S von Tetzchner, MH Jensen (eds) Augmentative Communication: European Perspectives. London: Whurr Publishers Ltd, pp 65–87.

McCall F, Moodie E (1998) Training staff to support AAC users in Scotland: current status and needs. Augmentative and Alternative Communication 14: 228–38.

McCartney E (ed) (1999) Speech/Language Therapists and Teachers Working Together. London: Whurr Publishers Ltd.

McCartney E, van der Gaag A (1996) How shall we be judged? Speech and language therapists in educational settings. Child Language Teaching and Therapy 12: 314–27.

McConkey R, Purcell M, Morris I (1999) Staff perceptions of communication with a partner who is intellectually disabled. Journal of Applied Research in Intellectual Disabilities 12: 204–10.

McCool S (1999) Collaboration with parents. In E McCartney (ed) Speech Language Therapists and Teachers Working Together. London: Whurr Publishers Ltd, pp. 150–61.

McCormick L, Schiefelbusch R (1990) Early Language Intervention: An Introduction (2nd edn). Columbus, OH: Merill/Macmillan.

McIntosh P (2002) An archi-texture of learning disability services: the use of Michel Foucault. Disability & Society 17: 65–79.

McLean J, Snyder-McLean L (1978) A Transactional Approach to Early Language Training. Columbus, OH: Merill/MacMillan.

McLeod H, Houston M, Seyfort B (1995) Communicative interactive skills training for caregivers of nonspeaking adults with severe disabilities. International Journal of Practical Approaches to Disability 9: 5–11.

Meichenbaum D (1977) Cognitive Behavior Modification: An Integrative Approach. New York: Plenum Press.

Mencap Report, March (1997) Left in the Dark: A Mencap Report on the Challenges Facing the UK's 400,000 Families of Children with Learning Disabilities. Executive Summary. London: Mencap.

Mental Health Foundation (2000) Myths in Madness. (www.mentalhealth.org.uk)

Menzies Lyth I (1990) Social systems as a defence against anxiety: an empirical study of the nursing service of a general hospital. In E Trist, H Murray (eds) The Social Engagement of Social Science, Vol. 1, The Social–Psychological Perspective. London: Free Association Books.

Mey J (1993) Pragmatics: An Introduction. Oxford: Basil Blackwell.

Miles M (2000) Disability on a different model: glimpses of an Asian heritage. Disability & Society 15(4): 603–18.

Millar S (2001) Supporting children using augmentative and alternative communication in school. In H Cockerill, L Carroll-Few (eds) Communicating Without Speech: Practical Augmentative and Alternative Communication. London: MacKeith Press, pp. 103–24.

Millar S, Caldwell M (1997) Personal communication passports. Paper first presented at the SENSE Conference, Westpark Centre, University of Dundee, 13 September. (www.callcentrescotland.org.uk)

Miller AB, Keys CB (1996) Awareness, action, and collaboration: how the self-advocacy movement is empowering for persons with developmental disabilities. Mental Retardation 34: 312–19.

Miller C (1999) Teachers and speech and language therapists: a shared framework. British Journal of Special Education 26: 141–6.

Mittler P (1984) Evaluation of services and staff training. In J Dobbing (ed) Scientific Studies in Mental Retardation. London: MacMillan.

Molkhia M, Oakeshott P (2000) A pilot study of cardiovascular risk assessment in Afro-Caribbean patients attending an inner city general practice. Family Practice 17: 60–62.

Money D (2002) Management models. In S Abudarham, A Hurd (eds) Management of Communication Needs in People with a Learning Disability. London: Whurr Publishers Ltd, pp. 82–102.

Morton-Cooper A, Bamford M (1997) Excellence in Health Care Management. Oxford: Blackwell Science.

Mosely J (1994) You Choose. Cambridge: LDA.

Muller E, Soto G (2002) Conversation patterns of three adults using aided speech: variation across partners. Augmentative and Alternative Communication 18: 77–90.

Murphy J (1998) Talking mats. Speech and Language Therapy in Practice, Autumn: 11–14.

Murphy J (1999) Enabling people with motor neurone disease to discuss their quality of life. Communication Matters 13: 2–6.

Murphy J (2000) Enabling people with aphasia to discuss quality of life. British Journal of Therapy and Rehabilitation 7: 454–7.

Murphy J, Cameron L (2002a) Let your mats do the talking. Speech & Language Therapy in Practice, Spring: 18–20.

Murphy J, Cameron L (2002b) Talking Mats and Learning Disability: a Low-Tech Resource to Help People to Express their Views and Feelings. Scotland: University of Stirling.

Murray S, O'Neill J (2000) Four assistants and an NVQ. RCSLT Bulletin 573: 11–21.

Nadirshaw Z (2000) Learning disabilities in multi-cultural Britain. In D Bhugra, R Cochrane (eds) Multi-cultural Psychiatry in Britain. London: Gaskell Publications.

Naugle RI (1991) Denial in rehabilitation: its genesis, consequences and clinical management. In RP Martinelli, AE Dell Orto (eds) Psychological and Social Impact of Disability. New York: Springer.

Neill KG (2000) In the shadow of the temple: cross-cultural sensitivity in international health program development. Ethnicity & Health 5: 161–71.

Nickels L (1997) Evaluating lexical semantic therapy: BOXes, arrows and how to mend them. Aphasiology 11: 1083–9.

Nickels L, Best W (1996) Therapy for naming disorders (Part II): specifics, surprises and suggestions. Aphasiology 10: 109–36.

Nicoll A (2001) Imprints of the mind. Speech and Language Therapy in Practice Winter: 14–18.

Nind M, Hewett D (1994) Access to Communication. London: David Fulton.

Nind M, Hewett D (1998) Interaction in Action: Reflections on the Use of Intensive Interaction. London: David Fulton.

Nind M (1996) Efficacy of intensive interaction: Developing sociability and communication in people with severe and complex learning difficulties using an approach based on care giver infant interaction. European Journal of Special Needs Education 11(1): 48–66.

Nind M, Hewett D (2001) A Practical Guide to Intensive Interaction. Kidderminster: British Institute of Learning Disabilities.

Nofsinger RE (1991) Everyday Conversation. London: Sage Publications.

Norwich B (1996) Special needs education or education for all: connective specialisation or ideological impurity. British Journal of Special Education 23 100–109.

O'Brien J (1987) A guide to lifestyle planning: using the activities catalogue to integrate services and natural support systems. In B Wilcox, GT Bellamy (eds) A Comprehensive Guide to the Activities Catalogue for Youth and Adults with Severe Disabilities. Baltimore: Paul H Brookes, pp. 175–89.

Office for National Statistics (ONS) (1996) Social Focus on Ethnic Minorities. London: HMSO.

Oliver M (1990) The Politics of Disablement. London: Macmillan.

Oliver M (1996a) Defining impairment and disability: issues at stake. In C Barnes G Mercer (eds) Exploring the Divide: Illness and Disability. Leeds: The Disability Press.

Oliver M (1996b) Understanding Disability: From Theory to Practice. London: Macmillan.

Oliver M, Barnes C (1998) Disabled People and Social Policy: From Exclusion to Inclusion. London and New York: Longman.

Olney MF, Kim A (2001) Beyond adjustment: integration of cognitive disability into identity. Disability & Society 16: 563–83.

Onslow M, O'Brian S, Harrison E (1997) The Lidcombe Programme of early stuttering intervention: methods and issues. European Journal of Disorders of Communication 32: 231–66.

Orange JB, Ryan JB, Meredith SD, McLean MJ (1995) Application of the communication enhancement model for long-term care residents with Alzheimer disease. Topics in Language Disorders 15: 20–35.

Osgood CE (1957) Motivational dynamics of language behavior. In NM Jones (ed) Nebraska Symposium on Motivation. Lincoln, NB: University of Nebraska Press.

Panagos JM (1996) Speech therapy discourse – the input to learning. In MD Smith, JS Damico (eds) Childhood Language Disorders. New York: Thieme Medical Publishers, pp. 41–63.

Parr S, Byng S (2002) Breaking new ground in familiar territory: a comment on 'Supported conversation for adults with aphasia' by Aura Kagan. Aphasiology 12: 847–50.

Parr S, Byng S, Gilpin S, with Ireland C (1997) Talking About Aphasia. Buckingham: Open University Press.

Partners in advocacy, www.partnersinadvocacy.co.uk

Patterson A (2001) Training and educating colleagues. In M Kersner, JA Wright (eds) Speech and Language Therapy: The Decision Making Process when Working with Children. London: David Fulton, pp. 112–21.

Pearson V, Wong YC, Perini J (2002) The structure and content of social inclusion: voices of young adults with learning difficulties in Guangzhou. Disability & Society 17: 365–82.

Penn C (1998) Clinician–researcher dilemmas: comment on 'Supported conversation for adults with aphasia'. Aphasiology 12: 839–44.

Pennington L, McConachie H (1999) Mother–child interaction revisited: communication with non-speaking physically disabled children. International Journal of Language & Communication Disorders 34: 391–416.

Perkins L (1995) Applying conversational analysis to aphasia: clinical implications and analytic issues. European Journal of Disorders of Communication 30: 372–83.

Peters S (1996) The politics of disability identity. In L Barton (ed) Disability & Society: Emerging Issues and Insights. Essex: Addison Wesley Longman Ltd, pp. 215–34.

Pomerantz A (1984) Pursuing a response. In JM Atkinson, J Heritage (eds) Structures of Social Action. Studies in Conversation Analysis. Cambridge: Cambridge University Press, pp. 57–101.

Porter J, Ouvry C, Morgan M, Downs C (2001) Interpreting the communication of people with profound and multiple learning difficulties. British Journal of Learning Disabilities 29: 12–16.

Porter L, McKenzie S (2000) Professional Collaboration with Parents of Children with Disabilities. London: Whurr Publishers Ltd.

Pound C, Parr S, Duchan J (2001) Using partners' autobiographical reports to develop, deliver, and evaluate services in aphasia. Aphasiology 15: 477–93.

Pound C, Parr S, Lindsay J, Woolf C (2000) Beyond Aphasia: Therapies for Living with Communication Disability. Buckinghamshire: Winslow Press.

Powell G (2001) Children with severe learning disabilities. In M Kersner, JA Wright (eds) Speech and Language Therapy: The Decision Making Process when Working with Children. London: David Fulton, pp. 244–55.

Priestley M (1999) Discourse and identity: disabled children in mainstream high schools. In M Corker, S French (eds) Disability Discourse. Buckingham: Open University Press, pp. 92–102.

Prior R, Cummins M (1992) Questions about facilitated communication and autism. Journal of Autism and Developmental Disorders 22: 331.

Purcell M, McConkey R, Morris I (2000) Staff communication with people with intellectual disabilities: the impact of a work-based training programme. International Journal of Language and Communication Disorders 35: 147–58.

Quine L, Rutter DR (1994) First diagnosis of severe mental and physical disability: a study of doctor–parent communication. Journal of Child Psychology and Psychiatry 35: 1273–87.

Radford J, Tarplee C (1995) The management of conversational topic by a ten year old: implications of social knowledge. In M Kersner, S Peppe (eds) Work in Progress Vol. 5 Department of Human Communication Science, UCL, London.

Rai-Atkins A (2002) Mental health advocacy for black and minority ethnic users and carers. Joseph Rowntree Foundation Findings, March: (352).

Rahman-Jennings Z, Hulme S (2001) Involve and deliver. RCSLT Bulletin, June: 12–14.

Ramcharan P, McGrath M, Grant G (1997) Voices and choices – mapping entitlements to friendships and community contacts. In P Ramcharan, G Roberts, G Grant, J Borland (eds) Empowerment in Everyday Life – Learning Disability. London: Jessica Kingsley,pp. 48–69.

Ramcharan P, Roberts G, Grant G, Borland J (1997a) Empowerment in Everyday Life – Learning Disability. London: Jessica Kingsley.

Ramcharan P, Roberts G, Grant G, Borland, J (1997b) Citizenship, empowerment and everyday life – deal and illusion in the new millennium. In P Ramcharan, G Roberts, G Grant, J Borland (eds) Empowerment in Everyday Life – Learning Disability. London: Jessica Kingsley, pp. 241–58.

Rao S (2001) 'A little inconvenience': perspectives of Bengali families of children with disabilities on labelling and inclusion. Disability & Society 16(4): 531–48.

Rinaldi W (1992) The Social Use of Language Programme. Windsor: NFER Nelson.

Rosen A, Proctor E (1981) Distinctions between treatment outcome and their implications for treatment evaluation. Journal of Consulting and Clinical Psychology 49: 418–25.

Royal College of Speech and Language Therapists (RCSLT) (1993) Audit: A Manual for Speech and Language Therapists. London: RCSLT.

Royal College of Speech and Language Therapists (1996) Communicating Quality 2. London: RCSLT.

Read J (2000) Disability, the Family and Society – Listening to Mothers Buckingham: Open University Press.

Rees S (1991) Achieving Power: Practice and Policy in Social Welfare. London: Allen and Unwin.

Rendall D (1997) Fatherhood and learning disabilities: A personal account of reaction and resolution. Journal of Learning Disabilities for Nursing, Health and Social Care 1: 77–83.

Richardson K, Klecan-Aker JS (2000) Teaching pragmatics to language-learning disabled children: a treatment outcome study. Child Language, Teaching & Therapy 16: 23–42.

Rinaldi W (2000) Language Difficulties in an Educational Context. London: Whurr Publishers Ltd.

Robson, C (1993) Real World Research. Oxford: Blackwell.

Robson J, Pring T, Marshall J, Morrison S, Chiat S (1998a) Written communication in undifferentiated jargon aphasia: a therapy study. International Journal of Language & Communication Disorders 33(3): 305–28.

Robson J, Marshall J, Pring T, Chiat S (1998b) Phonological naming therapy in jargon aphasia: positive but paradoxical effects. The Journal of the International Neuropsychological Society 4: 675–86.

ogers CR (1951) Client-Centred Therapy. London: Constable.

ondal J, Edwards S (1997) Language in Mental Retardation. London: Whurr Publishers Ltd.

oulstone S (2001) The role of speech and language therapists working in community clinics, child development centres, and hospitals. In M Kersner, J Wright (eds) Speech and Language Therapy: The Decision Making Process when Working with Children. London: David Fulton Publishers.

oux J (1996) Working collaboratively with teachers: supporting the newly qualified speech and language therapist in a mainstream school. Child Language Teaching and Therapy 12: 48–59.

ustin L, Kuhr A (1989) Social Skills and the Speech Impaired. London: Whurr Publishers Ltd.

yan S (1995) The study and application of clinical reasoning research. British Journal of Therapy and Rehabilitation 2: 265–71.

absay S, Kernan KT (1983) Communicative design in the speech of mildly retarded adults. In KT Kernan, M Begab and R Edgerton (eds) Environments and Behavior: The Adaptation of Mentally Retarded Persons. Baltimore: University Park Press, pp. 283–94.

acchett C, Byng S, Marshall J, Pound C (1999) Drawing together: evaluation of a therapy programme for severe aphasia. International Journal of Language & Communication Disorders 34: 265–89.

acks H, Schegloff EA, Jefferson G (1978) A simplest systematics for the organization of turn-taking for conversation. In J Schenkein (ed) Studies in the Organization of Conversational Interaction. New York: Academic Press, pp. 7–55.

arno MT (1993) Aphasia rehabilitation: psychosocial and ethical considerations. Aphasiology 7: 321–34.

arno MT (1997) Quality of life in aphasia in the first post-stroke year. Aphasiology 11: 665–79.

aunders C, Caves R (1986) An empirical approach to the identification of communication skills with reference to speech therapy. Journal of Further and Higher Education 10: 29–44.

avignon SJ(1983) Communicative Competence: Theory & Classroom Practice. Reading, MA: Addison Wesley.

chegloff EA, Jefferson G, Sacks H (1977) The preference for self-correction in the organisation of repair in conversation. Language 53: 361–82.

chell BA, Cervero RM (1993) Clinical reasoning in occupational therapy: an integrative review. American Journal of Occupational Therapy 47: 605–9.

cherer MJ (1993) What we know about women's technology use, avoidance and abandonment. Women and Therapy 14: 117–32.

chiffrin D (1988) Conversation analysis. In J Frederick (ed) Linguistics: The Cambridge Survey. Cambridge: Cambridge University Press, pp. 251–76.

chubert GW, Miner AL, Till JA (1973) The Analysis of Behavior of Clinicians (ABC) System. Grand Forks: University of North Dakota.

chwartz B, Robbins SJ (1995) Psychology of Learning and Behavior (4th edn). New York: WW Norton & Co.

chwartz MF, Saffran E, Fink RB, Myers JL, Martin N (1994) Mapping therapy: a treatment programme for agrammaticism. Aphasiology 8: 19–54.

cott J, Larcher J (2002) Advocacy with people with communication difficulties. In B Gray, R Jackson (eds) Advocacy & Learning Disability. London: Jessica Kingsley, pp. 170–88.

Searle J (1983) Intentionality. Cambridge: Cambridge University Press.

Seltzer MM, Greenberg JS, Floyd FJ, Pettee Y, Hong J (2001) Life course impacts of parenting a child with a disability. American Journal on Mental Retardation 106: 265–86.

Shakespeare T, Gillespie-Sells K, Davies D (1996) The Sexual Politics of Disability London: Cassell.

Shelton, JR (1997) Comments on 'Lexical semantic therapy: BOX': a considera tion of the development and implementation of the treatment. Aphasiology 11: 1100–106.

Shevlin M, O'Moore AM (2000) Creating opportunities for contact between main stream pupils and their counterparts with learning difficulties. British Journal of Special Education 27: 29–34.

Simmons-Mackie N (1998) In support of supported conversation for adults with aphasia. Aphasiology 12: 831–8.

Simmons-Mackie N, Damico J (1995) Communicative evidence in aphasia: evi dence from compensatory strategies. In M Lemme (ed) Clinical Aphasiology Vol. 23. Austin, TX: Pr–ed, pp. 95–105.

Simmons-Mackie N, Damico JS (1998) Social role negotiation in aphasia therapy competence, incompetence and conflict. In D Kovarsky, J Duchan, Maxwell, M (Eds) Constructing (In)Competence: Disabling Evaluations in Clinical and Social Interaction. The Social Construction of Incompetence. Mahwah, NJ Lawrence Erlbaum Press, pp 313–42.

Simmons-Mackie N, Kagan A (1999) Communication strategies used by 'good' ver sus 'poor' speaking partners of individuals with aphasia. Aphasiology 13: 807–20

Simmons-Mackie N, Damico JS, Damico HI (1999) A Qualitative Study of Feed back in Aphasia Treatment. American Journal of Speech–Language Pathology 8 218–30.

Sinclair J, Coulthard RM (1975) Towards an Analysis of Discourse. The English Used by Teachers and Pupils. London: Oxford University Press.

Smith H (1994) A damaging experience: black disabled children and educationa and social services provision. In N Beegum, M Hill, A Stevens (eds) Reflections Views of Black People on their Lives and Community Care. CCETSW, Pape 32.3. Cambridge: Black Bear Press.

Smith M (2002) Self-Help Groups. http://www.stammering.org

Somers M (1994) The narrative construction of identity: a relational and networ approach. Theory and Society 23: 606–49.

Sperber D, Wilson D (2nd edn) (1995) Relevance, Communication an Cognition. Oxford: Blackwell.

Sproston KA, Pitson LB, Walker E (2001) The use of primary care services by th Chinese population living in England: examining inequalities. Ethnicity Health 6: 189–96.

Stackhouse J, Wells B (1997) Children's Speech and Literacy Difficulties: Psycholinguistic Framework. London: Whurr Publishers Ltd.

Stackhouse J, Wells B (eds) (2001) Children's Speech and Literacy Difficultie Book 2. London: Whurr Publishers Ltd.

Stalker K (2002) Inclusive daytime opportunities for people with learning di abilities. In C Clark (ed) Adult Day Services and Social Inclusion – Better Day London: Jessica Kingsley, pp 46–66.

Stamp GH, Knapp ML (1990) The construct of intent in interpersonal commur cation. Quarterly Journal of Speech 76: 282–99.

Stengelhofen J (1993) Teaching Students in Clinical Settings. London: Chapman Hall.

Stewart JA, Dundas R, Howard RS, Rudd AG, Wolfe CDA (1999) Ethnic differences in incidence of stroke: prospective study with stroke register. British Medical Journal 318: 967–71.

Strydom A, Forster M, Wilkie BM, Edwards C, Hall IS (2001) Patient information leaflets for people with learning disabilities who take psychiatric medication. British Journal of Learning Disabilities 29: 72–6.

Stuart O (1992) Race and disability: what type of double disadvantage? Disability, Handicap & Society 7: 177–88.

Sutcliffe J, Simons K (1993) Self-Advocacy and Adults with Learning Difficulties: Contexts Debates. Leicester: National Institute of Adult Continuing Education in Association with the Open University Press.

Swain J, Cameron C (1999) Unless otherwise stated: discourses of labelling and identity in coming out. In M Corker, S French (eds) Disability Discourse. Buckingham: Open University Press. pp 68–78.

Swain J, French S, Cameron C (2003) Controversial issues in a disabling society. Buckingham: Open University Press.

Swain J, Finkelstein V, French S, Oliver M (eds) (1993) Disabling Barriers – Enabling Environments. London: Sage.

Sweeney T (1995) Curriculum matters: using drama to extend the involvement of children with special educational needs. In P Garner, S Sandow (eds) Advocacy, Self-Advocacy and Special Needs. London: David Fulton Publishers. pp. 66–88.

Tajfel H (1981) Human Groups and Social Categories. Cambridge: Cambridge University Press.

Tarplee C (1993) Working on talk: collaborative shaping of linguistic skills within parent–child interaction. Unpublished DPhil thesis. Department of Language and Linguistic Science, University of York.

Tarplee C (1996) Working on child's utterances: prosodic aspects of repetition during picture labelling. In E Couper-Kuhlen, M Selting (eds) Prosody in Conversation: International Studies. Cambridge: Cambridge University Press.

Thomas C (1999) Narrative identity and the disabled self. In M Corker, S French (eds) Disability Discourse. Buckingham: Open University Press, pp 68–78.

Thomas E (1990) Early intervention in Down's syndrome. Speech Therapy in Practice, May: 4–5.

Thompson L, Lobb C, Elling R, Herman S, Jurkiewicz T, Hulleza C (1997) Pathways to family empowerment: Effects of family-centred delivery of early intervention services. Exceptional Children 64: 99–113.

Threats TT (2000) The world health organization's revised classification: what does it mean for speech–language pathology? Journal of Medical Speech–Language Pathology 8: xiii–xviii.

Traustadottir R, Johnson K (eds) (2000) Women with Intellectual Disabilities – Finding a Place in the World. London: Jessica Kingsley.

Tregaskis C (2000) Interviewing non-disabled people about their disability-related attitudes: seeking methodologies. Disability & Society 15: 343–53.

Trevarthen C (1993) The functions of emotions in early infant communication and development. In J Nadel, L Camaioni (eds) New Perspectives in Early Communication Development. London: Routledge.

Twine F (1994) Citizenship and Social Rights: The Interdependence of Self and Society. London: Sage.

Tyne A (1981) The Principle of Normalisation. London: Values into Action.

van der Gaag A (1988) The Communication Assessment of Speech Profile London: Speech Profiles Ltd.

van der Gaag A (1989) Joint assessment of communication skills: formalising the role of carer. British Journal of Mental Subnormality, XXXV Part 1, 68: 22–28.

van der Gaag A, Davies P (1994) Following the dolphins: an ethnographic study of speech and language therapy with people with learning difficulties European Journal of Disorders of Communication 29: 203–23.

van der Gaag A, Dormandy K (1993) Communication and Adults with Learning Difficulties. London: Whurr Publishers Ltd.

van Riper C (1973) The Treatment of Stuttering. Englewood Cliffs, NJ: Prentice Hall.

Vernon A (1995) Understanding simultaneous oppression, in a conference report: Disability Rights: A Symposium of the European regions. October Southampton.

Vernon A (1999) The dialectics of multiple identities and the disabled people' movement. Disability & Society 14: 385–98.

Vernon A (2002) Users' views of community care for Asian disabled people Joseph Rowntree Foundation Findings, July: (752).

Visch-Brink EG, Bajema IM, van de Sandt-Koenderman ME (1997) Lexical seman tic therapy: BOX. Aphasiology 11: 1057–78.

von Tetzchner S (1997) Historical issues in intervention research: hidden know ledge and facilitating techniques in Denmark. European Journal of Disorder of Communication 32: 1–18.

von Tetzchner S, Jensen MH (1996) Augmentative and Alternativ Communication: European Perspectives. London: Whurr Publishers Ltd.

von Tetzchner S, Martinsen H (2000) Introduction to augmentative and alterna tive communication (2nd edn). London: Whurr Publishers Ltd.

Von Tetzchner S, Grove N, Loncke F, Barnett S, Woll B, Clibbens J (1996) Prelim inaries to a comprehensive model of augmentative and alternative com munication. In S von Tetzchner, MH Jensen (eds) Augmentative an Alternative Communication: European Perspectives. London: Whur Publishers Ltd, pp. 19–36.

Vygotsky L (1978) Mind in Society: The Development of Higher Psychologica Processes. Cambridge, MA: Harvard University Press.

Vygotsky L (1981) The genesis of higher mental functions. In JV Wertsch (ed trans) The Concept of Activity in Soviet Psychology. Armonk, NY: ME Sharp Inc. (original work published in 1960), pp. 144–188

Vygotsky L (1986) Thought and language. Cambridge, MA: MIT Press (origin work published in 1934).

Waddington L (2000) Changing attitudes to the rights of people with disabiliti Europe. In J Cooper (ed) Law, Rights & Disability. London: Jessica Kingsley, p 33–58.

Walker M (1995) Surviving Secrets. Philadelphia, PA: Open University Press.

Walmsley J (1996) Doing what mum wants me to do: looking at family relatio ships from the point of view of people with intellectual disabilities. Journal Applied Research in Intellectual Disabilities 9: 324–41.

Walmsley J (2002) Principles and types of advocacy. In B Gray, R Jackson (eds) Advocacy & Learning Disability. London: Jessica Kingsley, pp. 24–37.

Walmsley J, Downer J (1997) Shouting the loudest: self-advocacy, power and diversity. In P Ramcharan, G Roberts, G Grant, J Borland (eds) Empowerment in Everyday Life: Learning Disabilities. London: Jessica Kingsley, pp. 35–47.

Ware J (1996) Creating a Responsive Environment for People with Profound and Multiple Learning Difficulties. London: David Fulton.

Ware J, Healey I (1994) Conceptualising progress in children with profound and multiple learning difficulties. In J Ware (ed) Educating Children with Profound and Multiple Learning Difficulties. London: David Fulton, pp. 1–14.

Warner R (1999) The views of Bangladeshi parents on the special school attended by their young children with severe learning difficulties. British Journal of Special Education 26: 218–23.

Watson CM, Cenery HJ, Carter MS (1999) An analysis of trouble and repair in the natural conversations of people with dementia of the Alzheimer's type. Aphasiology 13(3): 195–218.

Weismer SE (2000) Intervention for children with developmental language delay. In DVM Bishop, LB Leonard (eds) Speech and Language Impairments in Children: Causes, Characteristics, Intervention and Outcome. Hove: Psychology Press Ltd, pp. 157–76.

Weniger D (1995) Drawing the message across: a successful approach to the improvement of communicative interactions in aphasia? Aphasiology 9: 63–8.

Wheeler DL, Jacobson JW, Paglieri RA, Schwartz AA (1993) An experimental assessment of facilitated communication. Mental Retardation 31: 49–60.

White A, Deary IJ, Wilson JA (1997) Psychiatric disturbance and personality traits in dysphonic patients. European Journal of Disorders of Communication 32: 307–14.

Wilkinson R, Bryan K, Lock S, Bayley K, Maxim J, Bruce C, Edmundson A, Moir D (1998) Therapy using conversation analysis: helping couples to adapt to aphasia in conversation. International Journal of Language & Communication Disorders 33 supplement: 144–9.

Wilkinson R (1999) Introduction. Aphasiology 13(4–5): 251–8.

Williamson K (2001) Competencies Project: Support Practitioner Framework. London: RCSLT.

Wilson D (1980) Communication and the family physician. Canadian Family Physician 26: 1701–16.

Winchurst C, Stenfert Kroese B, Adams J (1992) Assertiveness training for people with a mental handicap: a group approach. Mental Handicap 20: 97–101.

Winter K (1999) Speech and language therapy provision for bilingual children: aspects of the current service. International Journal of Language & Communication Disorders 34: 85–98.

World Health Organization (1980) International Classification of Impairments, Disabilities and Handicaps (ICIDH). Geneva: WHO.

World Health Organization (1997) International Classification of Impairments, Disabilities and Handicaps – 2nd edition (ICIDH-2). Geneva: WHO.

World Health Organization (2001) International Classification of Functioning, Disability and Health. (ICF) Geneva: WHO.

Wolfensberger W (1992) A Brief Introduction to Social Role Valorisation as a High-order Concept for Structuring Human Services. USA: Syracuse University.

Worrall L, Yiu E (2000) Effectiveness of functional communication therapy by volunteers for people with aphasia following stroke. Aphasiology 14: 911–24.

Wren Y, Roulstone S, Parkhouse J, Hall B (2001) A model for a mainstream school based speech and language therapy service. Child Language, Teaching and Therapy 17: 107–25.

Wright J, Kersner M (1998) Supporting Children with Communication Problems: Sharing the Workload. London: David Fulton.

Wright J, Wood J, Stackhouse J (2000) Language and Literacy: Joining Together. London: British Dyslexia Association.

Wright L, Sherrard C (1994a) Stuttering therapy with British-Asian children. I. A survey of service delivery in the United Kingdom. European Journal of Disorders of Communication 29: 307–25.

Wright L, Sherrard C (1994b) Stuttering therapy with British-Asian children. II. Speech and language therapists' perception of their effectiveness. European Journal of Disorders of Communication 29: 325–38.

Yampolsky S, Waters G (2002) Treatment of single word oral reading in an individual with deep dyslexia. Aphasiology 16: 455–71.

Yeates S (1989) Hearing in people with mental handicaps: a review of 100 adults. Mental Handicap 17: 33–7.

Yeates S (1991) Hearing loss in adults with learning disabilities. British Medical Journal 303: 427–8.

Yeates S (1992). Have they got a hearing loss? A follow-up study of hearing in people with mental handicaps. Mental Handicap 20: 126–33.

Yeates S (1995) The incidence and importance of hearing loss in people with severe learning disability: the evolution of a service. British Journal of Learning Disability 23: 79–84.

Yoder DE (2001) Having my say. Augmentative and Alternative Communication 17: 2–10.

Young DA, Quibell R (2000) Why rights are never enough: rights, intellectual disability and understanding. Disability & Society 15: 747–64.

Index

Printed in the United Kingdom
by Lightning Source UK Ltd.
113807UKS00002B/163-243

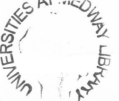

UNIVERSITIES AT MEDWAY LIBRARY

9 781861 564009